AF880726

Cephalometry in Orthodontics: 2D and 3D

Dedication

I dedicate this book to two important people in my life: my father, James A. Miller, Sr, who taught me the importance of hard work and the strength to persevere, and my husband, Theodore J. Kula, Jr, who taught me to question and to solve problems using the scientific method.

–KK

I dedicate this book to my late father and mother for the encouragement they blessed me with my entire life. I also dedicate it to my lovely wife and daughters for their continuous love and support. Lastly, a special thanks to many of my students whom I have had the pleasure of teaching and supervising.

–AG

Library of Congress Cataloging-in-Publication Data

Names: Kula, Katherine, editor. | Ghoneima, Ahmed, editor.
Title: Cephalometry in orthodontics : 2D and 3D / edited by Katherine Kula and Ahmed Ghoneima.
Description: Batavia, IL : Quintessence Publishing Co,Inc, [2018] | Includes bibliographical rewferences and index.
Identifiers: LCCN 2018021619 | ISBN 9780867157628 (hardcover)
Subjects: | MESH: Cephalometry--methods | Orthodontics--methods | Cephalometry--instrumentation | Cone-Beam Computed Tomography
Classification: LCC RK310.C44 | NLM WU 141.5.C3 | DDC 617.6/4307572--dc23
LC record available at https://lccn.loc.gov/2018021619

QUINTESSENCE PUBLISHING
USA

© 2018 Quintessence Publishing Co, Inc

Quintessence Publishing Co, Inc
411 North Raddant Road
Batavia, IL 60510
www.quintpub.com

5 4 3 2 1

All rights reserved. This book or any part thereof may not be reproduced, stored in a retrieval system, or transmitted in any form or by any means, electronic, mechanical, photocopying, or otherwise, without prior written permission of the publisher.

Editor: Leah Huffman
Design: Erica Neumann
Production: Kaye Clemens

Printed in China

CEPHALOMETRY IN ORTHODONTICS: 2D AND 3D

Edited by
Katherine Kula, MS, DMD, MS
Professor Emeritus
Department of Orthodontics and Oral Facial Genetics
Indiana University School of Dentistry
Indianapolis, Indiana

Ahmed Ghoneima, BDS, PhD, MSD
Chair and Associate Professor, Orthodontics
Hamdan Bin Mohammed College of Dental Medicine
Dubai, United Arab Emirates

Adjunct Faculty
Department of Orthodontics and Oral Facial Genetics
Indiana University School of Dentistry
Indianapolis, Indiana

QUINTESSENCE PUBLISHING

Berlin, Barcelona, Chicago, Istanbul, London, Milan, Moscow, New Delhi, Paris, Prague, São Paulo, Seoul, Singapore, Tokyo, Warsaw

PREFACE

Successful orthodontic treatment of a patient depends on accurate diagnosis and treatment planning. The purpose of this book is to provide an updated use of clinical cephalometrics, an important part of diagnosis and treatment planning. An effort was made to minimize esoteric parameters that are not frequently used in clinical orthodontics and to introduce and broaden the aspects of the role of cephalometrics in diagnosis and treatment planning.

Currently, clinical orthodontics is transitioning from the two-dimensional (2D) world to the three-dimensional (3D) world. The use of cone beam computed tomography (CBCT) has changed from a rather myopic view that the use of 3D CBCTs could be unethical to a far broader acceptance. This has happened not only because of radiation and cost reduction but also as a result of research showing the benefits of 3D CBCTs. The unknown became the known. As equipment starts to break down, the clinician also evaluates the cost and benefit of new equipment and what his or her technologically savvy market expects. However, 2D cephalometrics is still the standard for clinical orthodontics, although many practices and orthodontic programs currently take 3D CBCTs. In reality, many practices and orthodontic programs globally are using 2D cephalometric measures with the 3D CBCTs. Thus, 2D cephalometrics is still very pertinent to patient treatment.

In order to teach cephalometrics, some history of cephalometrics is necessary but not to the degree that clinicians become lost in it. Cephalometric software programs make a plethora of analyses available for use because many clinicians do not restrict their analysis to those of individual treatment camps. Indeed, many of the cephalometric analyses are based on research or writings of multiple authors. In order to teach cephalometrics, both 2D and 3D cephalometry with their advantages and limitations need to be discussed, not as a philosophy but related to the craniofacial structures and their relationships. As research and product development increase, use of 3D measures might negate the use of 2D measures.

The addition of 3D CBCTs to cephalometry presents another dimension to the identification of skeletal and soft tissue landmarks. The transverse dimension is inherently integrated with the lateral dimension and is available for almost instant review without the viewer having to stitch separate images together. The internal structures of the face, skull, and airways can be reviewed for structural abnormalities and pathologies. The internal potentially driving structures of facial morphology can be viewed and measured more precisely in 3D. The authors integrate these possibilities with cephalometry and present currently evolving concepts and processes within cephalometry that the clinician needs to be aware of. Cephalometry, a measure of straight lines and angles of the hard and soft tissue of the face and cranium, is evolving into measures of areas and volumes that will need to be interpreted for clinical decisions and evaluation of outcomes. However, clinicians need to understand 2D cephalometry to be able to apply it better in 3D cephalometry.

Acknowledgments

Our sincere appreciation to our administrative assistant, Shannon Wilkerson, for providing assistance with typing and copying as well as allowing us to focus on our writing by running interference; to the clinical supervisor and dental assistants, Gayle Massa, Brenda McClarnon, Darlene Arnold, Shelley Pennington, and all the others, who helped us with patient records; and to the business office supervisor and other personnel, Monica Eller, Karen Vibbert, and others, for helping with patient contacts.

Note on Terminology

The hyphenation standards for cephalometric terms and landmarks used in the literature are not consistent, and many publications rely on jargon that is not universally accepted. For the sake of consistency and understanding in this book, hyphens are only used when referring to angles or landmarks that require the hyphen for clarity. Every effort has been made to remove unnecessary jargon and use clinically relevant terms and landmarks.

CONTENTS

CONTRIBUTORS

Eman Allam, BDS, PhD, MPH
Postdoctoral Fellow
Department of Orthodontics and Oral Facial Genetics
Indiana University School of Dentistry
Indianapolis, Indiana

Mohamed Bazina, BDS, MSD
Assistant Clinical Professor
Department of Orthodontics
University of Kentucky

Adjunct Assistant Professor
Department of Orthodontics
School of Dental Medicine
Case Western Reserve University
Cleveland, Ohio

Eric Dellinger, DDS, MSD
Private Practice Limited to Orthodontics
Angola, Indiana

Paul C. Edwards, DDS, MSc
Professor
Department of Oral Pathology, Medicine & Radiology
Indiana University School of Dentistry
Indianapolis, Indiana

Tarek Elshebiny, BDS, MSD
Clinical Assistant Professor
Department of Orthodontics
School of Dental Medicine
Case Western Reserve University
Cleveland, Ohio

James Geist, DDS, MS
Professor
Department of Biomedical and Diagnostic Sciences
Director, Oral and Maxillofacial Imaging Center
University of Detroit Mercy
Detroit, Michigan

Ahmed Ghoneima, BDS, PhD, MSD
Chair and Associate Professor, Orthodontics
Hamdan Bin Mohammed College of Dental Medicine
Dubai, United Arab Emirates

Adjunct Faculty
Department of Orthodontics and Oral Facial Genetics
Indiana University School of Dentistry
Indianapolis, Indiana

Katherine Kula, MS, DMD, MS
Professor Emeritus
Department of Orthodontics and Oral Facial Genetics
Indiana University School of Dentistry
Indianapolis, Indiana

Manuel Lagravère, DDS, MSc, PhD
Associate Professor
Division of Orthodontics
Faculty of Medicine and Dentistry
University of Alberta
Edmonton, Alberta

Connie P. Ling, DDS, MSc
Private Practice Limited to Orthodontics
Toronto, Ontario

Juan Martin Palomo, DDS, MSD
Professor and Residency Director
Department of Orthodontics
Director of the Craniofacial Imaging Center
School of Dental Medicine
Case Western Reserve University
Cleveland, Ohio

Leena Palomo, DDS, MSD
Associate Professor
Department of Periodontology
School of Dental Medicine
Case Western Reserve University
Cleveland, Ohio

Edwin T. Parks, DMD, MS
Professor
Department of Oral Pathology, Medicine & Radiology
Indiana University School of Dentistry
Indianapolis, Indiana

Ali Z. Syed, BDS, MHA, MS
Assistant Professor
Director of Radiology
School of Dental Medicine
Case Western Reserve University
Cleveland, Ohio

Achint Utreja, BDS, MS, PhD
Assistant Professor and Director, Pre-Doctoral Orthodontics
Director, Mineralized Tissue and Histology Research Laboratory
Department of Orthodontics and Oral Facial Genetics
Indiana University School of Dentistry
Indianapolis, Indiana

Introduction to the Use of Cephalometrics

Katherine Kula, MS, DMD, MS
Ahmed Ghoneima, BDS, PhD, MSD

Cephalometrics refers to the quantitative evaluation of cephalograms, or the measuring and comparison of hard and soft tissue structures on craniofacial radiographs. It is an evolving science and art that has been woven into orthodontics and the treatment of patients. Cephalograms are an integral part of orthodontic records and are typically used for almost all orthodontic patients. The cephalometric analysis or evaluation helps to confirm or clarify the clinical evaluation of the patient and provide additional information for decisions concerning treatment.

The American Association of Orthodontists (AAO) developed the current Clinical Practice Guidelines for Orthodontics and Dentofacial Orthopedics,[1] which recommend that initial orthodontic records include examination notes, intraoral and extraoral images, diagnostic casts (stone or digital), and radiographic images. These radiographic images include appropriate intraoral radiographs and/or a panoramic radiograph as well as cephalometric radiographs. A three-dimensional cone beam computed tomograph (3D CBCT) can be substituted for a cephalometric radiograph; however, the routine use of a CBCT is not generally required in orthodontics, so cephalometric radiographs are the current standard.

The AAO Clinical Practice Guidelines[1] also recommend evaluating the patient's treatment outcome and determining the efficacy of treatment modalities by comparing posttreatment records with pretreatment records. Posttreatment records may include dental casts; extraoral and intraoral images (either conventional or digital, still or video); and intraoral, panoramic, and/or cephalometric radiographs depending on the type of treatment and other factors. Many orthodontists also take progress cephalograms to determine if treatment is progressing as expected. In addition, board certification with the American Board of Orthodontics requires cephalograms and an understanding of cephalometry to explain the decisions for diagnosis, treatment, and the effects of growth and orthodontic treatment. Therefore, it is paramount that orthodontists understand how to use cephalometrics in their practice.

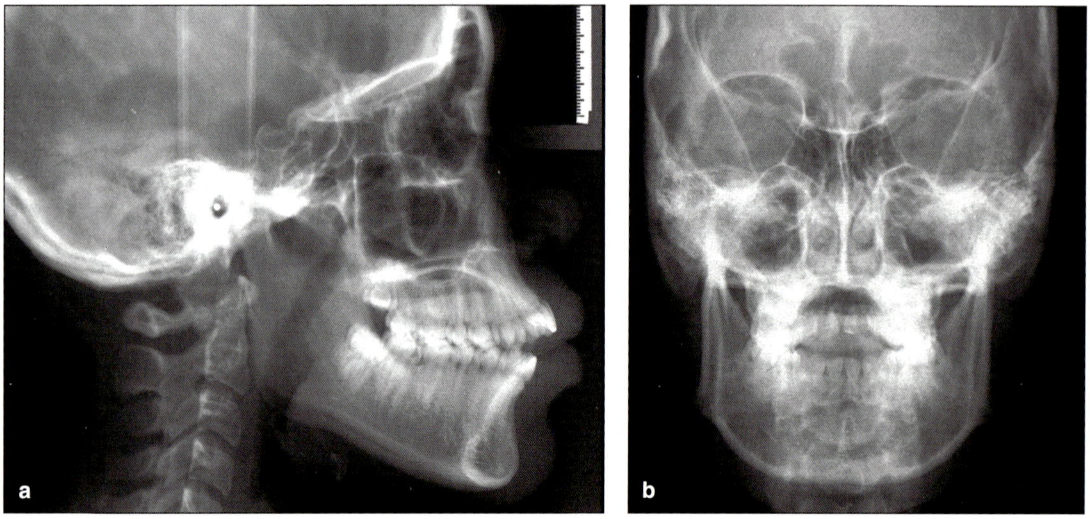

Fig 1-1 *(a and b)* Lateral and frontal cephalograms.

Basics of Cephalometrics

Cephalometrics is used to assist in *(1)* classifying the malocclusion (skeletal and/or dental); *(2)* communicating the severity of the problem; *(3)* evaluating craniofacial structures for potential and actual treatment using orthodontics, implants, and/or surgery; and *(4)* evaluating growth and treatment changes of individual patients or groups of patients. In general, a lateral cephalogram shows a two-dimensional (2D) view of the anteroposterior position of teeth, the inclination of the incisors, the position and size of the bony structures holding the teeth, and the cranial base (Fig 1-1a). A cephalogram can also provide a different view of the temporomandibular joint than a panoramic radiograph and a view of the upper respiratory tract.

In addition, cephalograms aid in the identification and diagnosis of other problems associated with malocclusion such as dental agenesis, supernumerary teeth, ankylosed teeth, malformed teeth, malformed condyles, and clefts, among others. They have also been used to identify pathology and can give some indication of bone height and thickness around some teeth. However, they are not very useful in identifying dental caries, particularly initial caries, and periodontal disease, so bitewing radiographs and periapical radiographs are needed for patients who are caries susceptible or show signs of periodontal disease. While some asymmetry can be diagnosed using a lateral cephalogram, an additional frontal cephalogram (Fig 1-1b) is needed to better identify which hard tissue structures are involved in the asymmetry.

Of course all of these conventional radiographs are 2D images. A 3D CBCT can replace multiple 2D radiographs and can allow the entire craniofacial structure to be viewed from multiple aspects (x, y, z format) with one radiograph (Fig 1-2). Intracranial and midline facial structures can be viewed without overlying confounding structures, and bilateral structures can be viewed independently. While the worldwide transition from 2D to 3D imaging is occurring quickly, it is still important for clinicians to understand what has been used for decades (2D), what additional 3D information is needed, and the limitations and potential of 3D imaging.

The general purpose of this book is to introduce the orthodontic clinician to the use and interpretation of cephalometrics, both 2D and 3D, and to show the potential benefits of using 3D CBCTs. The purpose of this chapter is to provide the background for the current and future use of cephalometrics.

History of Cephalometrics

Prior to the use of radiographs, growth and development of the craniofacial complex was essentially a study of skull measurements (craniometry) (Fig 1-3) or soft tissue. Craniometry[2] dates back to Hippocrates in the 4th century BC and is still used today in physical anthropology, forensics, medicine, and art. It is used to determine the size of cranial bones and teeth, their relationship to each other, potential differences among groups of people, and evolutionary changes in the cranium and face. Some of the current cephalometric landmarks, planes, and angles have their origin in craniometry. For example, the Frankfort plane was established in 1882 during a meeting of the German Anthropological Society as a standardized method of orienting the skull horizontally for measurements.[2] The anthropologists agreed to define the Frankfort plane as a plane from the upper borders of the auditory meati (external auditory canals) to the inferior margins of each orbit. Later, this plane was modified for cephalometry to indicate that the right and left porion and left orbitale would be used to define the horizontal plane to minimize problems that asymmetry caused.

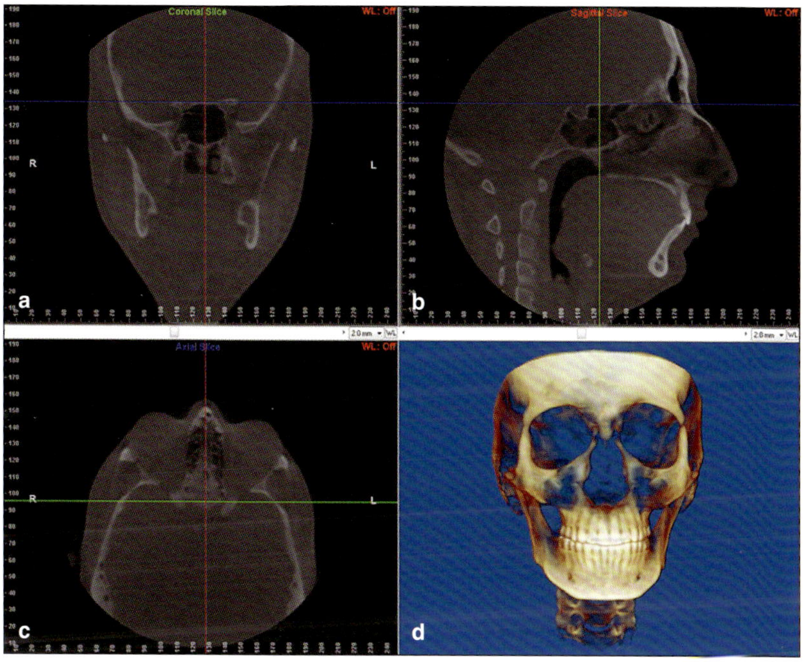

Fig 1-2 Software screen showing *(a)* coronal slice (*green line* in *b* and *c*), *(b)* sagittal slice (*red line* in *a* and *c*), *(c)* axial slice (*blue line* in *a* and *b*), and *(d)* 3D CBCT reconstruction of the same study.

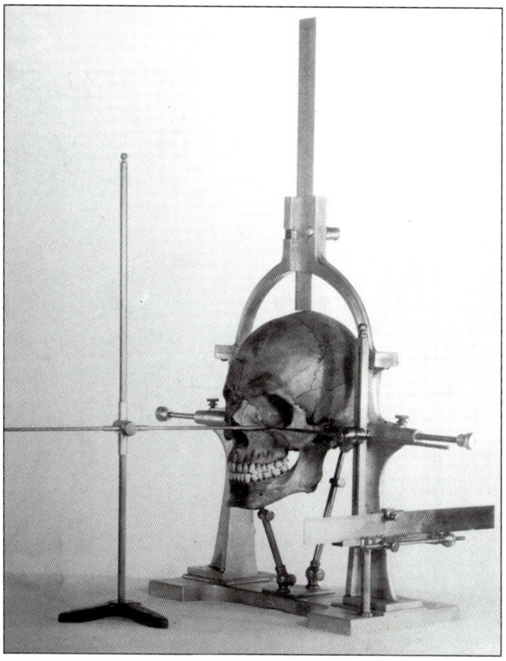

Fig 1-3 An original Broadbent craniostat used to standardize skull position and measurement. (Courtesy of Dr Juan Martin Palomo, Case Western Reserve University.)

Craniometry, however, had limitations. Each skull represented a one-time peek or snapshot at the development of one individual—in other words, a cross-sectional data point. There was little hope of a longitudinal study. Frequently, the reason for the death of the individual was unknown, resulting in an unknown effect on the growth and development of the skull. Thus, craniofacial development was interpreted based on the skulls of children who died because of trauma, disease, starvation, abuse, or genetics. Todd,[3] the chairman of the Department of Anatomy at Case Western Reserve University School of Medicine, considered the measuring of these children's skulls as studying defective growth and development; the longitudinal effect of orthodontic treatment on growth and development could not be assessed. Animal studies using dyes were obviously limited in providing interpretation of the effect of various factors on human growth and development. Soft tissue studies, particularly longitudinal, were also limited by the lack of reproducible data. Radiographs, however, provided the opportunity to study and compare multiple patients over decades.

The use and standardization of cephalograms continually evolved from their early beginnings in the late 1800s. Similarly, during that time, orthodontics had its inception as a dental specialty. Edward Hartley Angle classified malocclusion in 1899 and was recognized by the American Dental Association for making orthodontics a dental specialty.[4] Angle established the first school of orthodontics (Angle School of Orthodontia in St Louis) in 1900, the first orthodontic society (American Society of Orthodontia) in 1901, and the first dental specialty journal (*American Orthodontist*) in 1907.

Shortly after the discovery of x-rays by Wilhelm Conrad Roentgen in 1895,[5] the use of the first facial and cranial radiographs was reported as early as 1896 by Rowland[6] and later by Ketcham and Ellis.[7] By 1921, B. H. Broadbent was using lateral cephalograms in his private practice.[7] In 1922, Spencer Atkinson reported to the Angle College of Orthodontia that he used lateral facial radiographs to identify the position of the first molar below the maxilla's key ridge.[7] Because the radiographs also showed soft tissue, Atkinson suggested that these lateral radiographs had the potential of relating the mandible and the maxilla to the face and to the cranial base.

Initially, the comparison of cephalometric radiographs to show the effects of growth and treatment was difficult because head position and distance from the cephalometric film were not standardized. In an attempt to standardize head position, in 1921 Percy Brown designed a head holder for taking radiographic images of the face.[7] In 1922, A. J. Pacini reported standardizing head position for lateral radiographs by using a gauze bandage to hold the film to the head.[8] Ralph Waldron followed in 1927 by constructing a cephalometer to measure the gonial angle on a roentgenogram taken 90 degrees from the profile.[9] Martin Dewey and Sidney Riesner held the patient's head in a clamp and took a profile view with the film cassette placed against the head.[10] However, for several decades there was no universal standardization of cephalometric technique, meaning that identical radiographs of the same patient could not be reproduced.

It was obvious to Broadbent[11] that accurate and reliable longitudinal measurements of the head and face in three dimen-

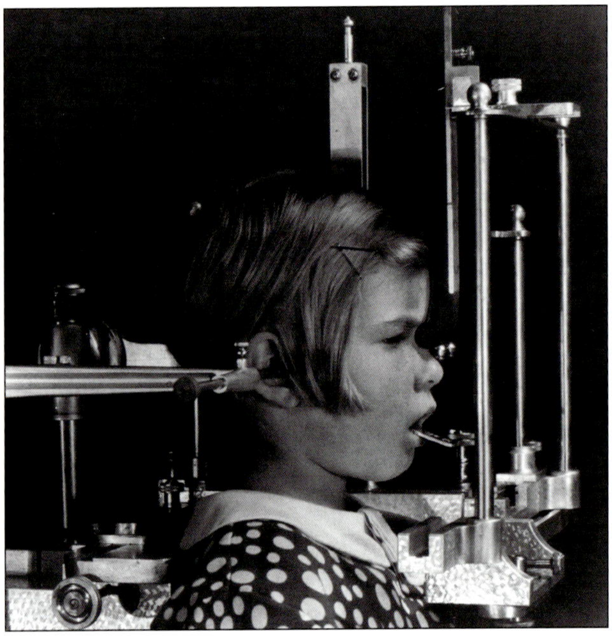

Fig 1-4 An original Broadbent cephalometric craniostat consisting of a head-holding device, two ear rods, and a nasion rest to stabilize the head of a living person relative to the radiographic film and the x-ray source. (Courtesy of Dr Juan Martin Palomo, Case Western Reserve University.)

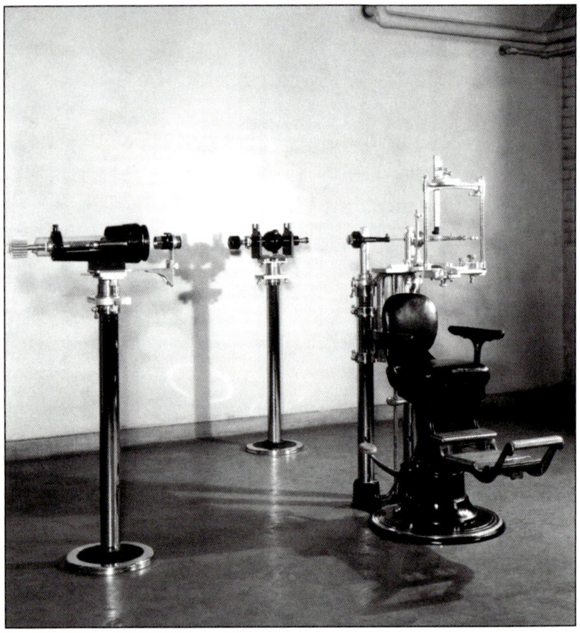

Fig 1-5 An original Bolton cephalostat modified to standardize head position for a frontal roentgenogram. (Courtesy of Dr Juan Martin Palomo, Case Western Reserve University.)

sions would be necessary to study growth and development of the teeth and the jaws as well as the effect of orthodontic treatment. Drawing on his previous experience of modifying Todd's craniostat into a craniometer to standardize skull position and measurement (see Fig 1-3), Broadbent developed a craniostat that consisted of a head-holding device, two ear rods, and a nasion rest to stabilize the head of a living person relative to the radiographic film and the x-ray source (Fig 1-4). Broadbent even took impressions of the teeth while the patient was positioned in the craniostat and related them to the maxilla and mandible. He announced in 1930 that he had used a radiographic craniostat to study the longitudinal growth of the living face[12] and published a description of the invention in 1931.[11] Bolton's cephalostat was modified later to include the standardization of head position for a roentgenogram from the frontal view (Fig 1-5). During the same year, a German orthodontist, H. Hofrath, also reported the development of a craniostat to standardize head position while taking lateral radiographs.[13]

The standardization of cephalograms allowed comparison of the same head over time. Treatment effects and comparison with other individuals could also be studied. This so impressed Congresswoman Frances Bolton that she established a long-term research study at Case Western Reserve University to examine the growth and development of the teeth and the jaws in healthy children.

Early studies by Broadbent[14] and other investigators of cranial and facial development emphasized the need to identify stable landmarks in order to superimpose the radiographs. Broadbent thought that at least in early childhood, certain cranial areas were more stable than the rapidly growing face. This led to the development of the Bolton-nasion plane of orientation and a registration point (R) in the sphenoidal area as the most fixed point in the head or face[14] (Fig 1-6). The Bolton-nasion plane was a line drawn from nasion, the most forward position of the frontonasal suture, at the midline to the highest point (Bolton point) on the profile of the right and left condyles of the occipital bone posterior to the foramen magnum. Bolton point was chosen rather than the superior tip of the auditory meatus because the cephalostat's ear rods masked the auditory canals. The bilateral occipital condyles were considered to produce a single image because they were essentially close enough to each other to be on the midplane of the skull. The center ray of the radiographic machine was considered to cause little magnification shadow. A point midway on a line drawn from the center of sella turcica on a perpendicular to the Bolton-nasion plane was called *registration point* (R) and was used to register superimpositions of the same individual or different individuals.

To measure facial changes after registering the Bolton-nasion plane on R, the Frankfort horizontal plane was added to the initial record of each child, and the perpendicular orbital plane (the plane perpendicular to Frankfort horizontal through orbitale) was passed through the dentition. Measurements of changes were taken from these two planes, not directly from the Bolton-nasion plane.

During the next few decades, multiple centers evaluating growth and development using cephalograms were started, and numerous orthodontists provided their data in various formats to best describe their analysis of the craniofacial complex. Some parameters were used primarily for research, while others were specifically used for clinical analysis. Many analyses or groups of parameters assumed the names of the orthodontist best known for promoting them but included measures previously used in craniometry or by other orthodontists. In some cases (eg, mandibular plane, length of mandible, and cranial base) various orthodontists published somewhat different methods of defining the structures. Wilton Krogman and Viken Sassouni attempted to validate the clinical usefulness of approximately 70 existing cephalometric analyses in 1957.[15] In some cases, these differences remain today because of strongly held opinions of the different schools of orthodontics. Unfortunately, this has also led to confusion for novices in this area and to intense discussion about which cephalometric values lend more to correct diagnosis and treatment analysis. In addition, comparison of various studies is complicated when different landmarks and planes are used.

Many cephalometric values were reported as simple descriptive statistics. Descriptive statistics, which are used to indicate the center or most typical value of a data set, are called *measures of central tendency* and include means and medians. The *mean* is the average of all the numbers for that data set, and the *median* is the data value in the middle of all the data arranged in ascending or descending order. Means or averages are provided more commonly than medians to clinically compare cephalometric values of groups. Research studies might report one or both values depending on the purpose and the sample in the study. However, data sets with the same mean can have considerable variation in the incorporated values. The descriptive statistics used to quantitatively describe these differences are called *measures of dispersion* (how widely the values are dispersed). The two measures of dispersion commonly used in cephalometrics are range and standard deviation. The *range* of a data set is the difference between the largest and the smallest value in that data set. The larger the difference, the greater is the dispersion of the data. The *standard deviation* tells how much deviation there is from the mean. The larger the standard deviation, the larger is the variation of the data. Usually, all data within a data set fall within three standard deviations (±3 SD) of the mean. Clinically, some orthodontists suggest that it is more difficult to treat patients whose cephalometric values are more than one standard deviation outside the mean; however, this also depends on the particular cephalometric value.

For the most part, it is assumed that the skeletal and dental cephalometric traits have values that, if plotted, would fall within a bell-shaped curve, a normal curve. That is, if the mean was determined and designated as zero, then when standard deviations are determined and marked on each side of the mean, the normal curve would be symmetric, and most of the data would fall within three standard deviations on each side. Depending on the range and the width of the standard deviations, the curve could be taller than wide or vice versa. However, normality should always be checked because not all data sets fit a bell-shaped curve. Unfortunately, many of the classic cephalometric studies did not report adequate statistics. Therefore, a careful reading of the literature is required for knowledgeable use of cephalometrics.

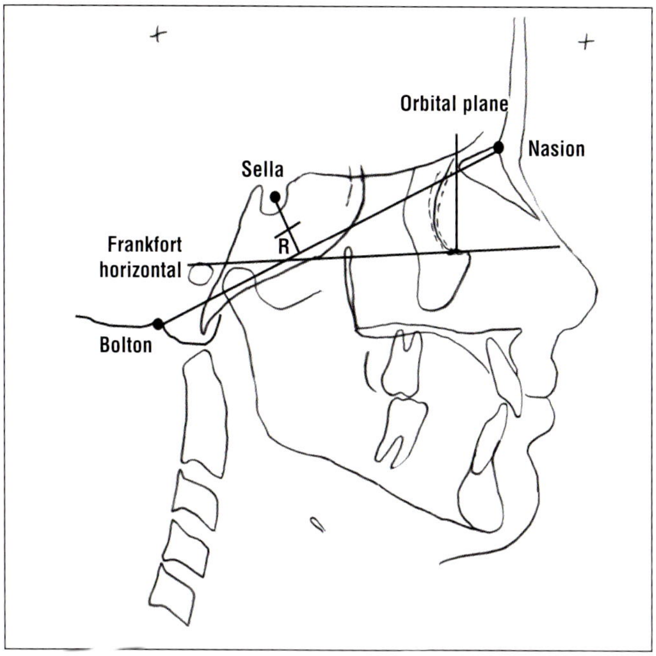

Fig 1-6 Bolton-nasion plane of orientation and registration point (R) in the sphenoidal area. The Frankfort horizontal and the perpendicular orbital plane were used for superimpositions.

Many published cephalometric studies reported descriptive statistics to quantify the results of the cephalometric parameters for samples of the population they studied. In most cases, the study included a limited number of cases (sample) compared with the entire population. Samples were used because it was too difficult or expensive to study the entire population. Obviously, the more alike the individuals in a population, the more representative the selection of the sample would be for that population. However, the criteria for the samples used in some of the early cephalometric analyses were very limiting and probably did not truly represent the population. In other cases, the samples were so small and heterogenous that the results reported appear to have little value. Some criteria for subject selection included that the subjects must have acceptable, attractive,[16] or award-winning faces.[17]

In one study[18] of 79 adults with ideal occlusions, the cephalometric measures showed a large range of values from Class II to Class III maxillomandibular relationships, high-angle to low-angle mandibles, and incisor retrusion to protrusion. Although the means measured in the study were similar to those reported in other published studies, the ranges were considerably larger. A retrospective review of the faces indicated no extremely poor or unacceptable faces, showing that good occlusion was achievable even naturally without surgery. Thus, cephalometrics alone is never used for treatment decisions.

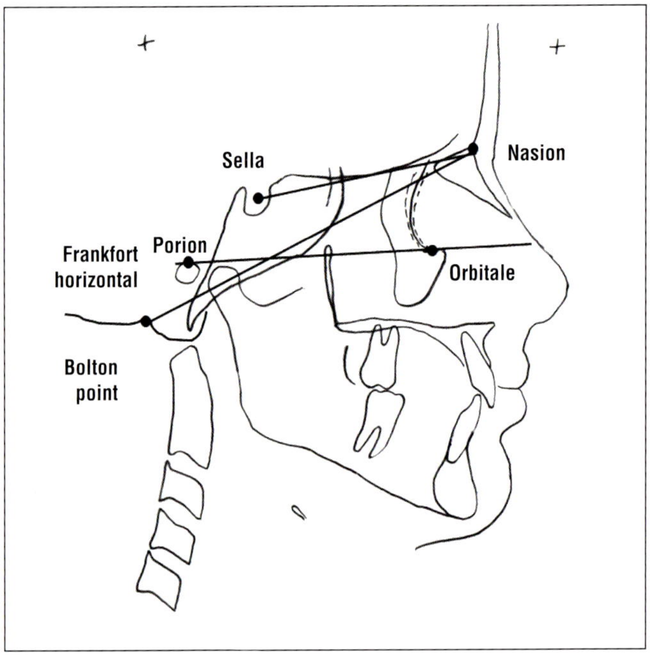

Fig 1-7 Sella-nasion, Frankfort horizontal, and Bolton-nasion reference planes.

Various factors influence cephalometric values. For example, the measurement of 2D cephalometric parameters is influenced by the diverging rays of the cephalostat striking a multidimensional object that is at a distance from the recording film, causing magnification error. Prior to standardization of the distances of the object and the film from the x-ray source, the differential was unknown unless a standardizing object was included in the film. Magnification error also varies with different machines. Some early studies did not report or correct the magnification error when they were published. (Formerly, the American Board of Orthodontics required that cases submitted for board certification show a calibration device in the cephalogram to allow for correction of magnification error.) Despite these problems, the early studies were helpful in developing a better understanding of craniofacial growth and development and provided the basis for additional investigation. However, these original publications should be analyzed carefully before they are cited or used as a basis for clinical treatment.

One of the issues in determining craniofacial changes with early cephalometrics was the selection of cephalometric reference parameters called *planes* to compare skeletal and dental changes. For example, early in the development of cephalometry, William B. Downs[19] realized that numerous measures were being used to describe the face. He sought to determine the range and the correlations of cephalometric values for individuals with excellent occlusions by comparing various cephalometric values from a group of 10 male and 10 female potentially growing adolescents (12 to 17 years old). Downs eventually came to the conclusion that he should evaluate the face by dividing the facial skeleton from the teeth and the alveolar processes. He would classify the skeletal pattern (maxilla versus mandible) alone and then determine the relationship of the teeth and alveoli to the facial skeleton. He suggested that the variability in values comparing the facial plane to sella-nasion (SN), the Frankfort horizontal, and the Bolton plane was so small that he was not sure why one was used instead of another to evaluate the face (Fig 1-7). Downs used the Frankfort horizontal because he felt that the SN and Bolton-nasion planes separated the cranium from the face, whereas the Frankfort horizontal allowed comparison of relationships involving only the face, the structures that orthodontic treatment (with or without surgery) could control. Using four faces, he demonstrated how the facial angle (facial plane to Frankfort horizontal) described the facial type better than the facial plane to SN or the facial plane to the Bolton plane when the position of the mandible was assessed (see Fig 1-7). Contrary to many cephalometric analyses that reported the mean measure, his comparisons for angle of convexity, AB plane, and mandibular plane angle were the numerical differences from the mean of the control group. For example, if the mean angle of convexity of the control group was reported as 180 degrees, a measurement of 185 degrees in a test patient would be reported as +5.0 degrees (a negative difference indicating concave profile and a positive difference indicating convex profile), not 185 degrees. Similarly, deviations from the means of the AB plane or mandibular plane angle were read as the difference from that mean without considering the variation within the control group. Downs thought that these differences would show the difficulty of treating the case. While Downs's study was small, did not look at sex differences, and used growing individuals for whom some cephalometric values could change with age, his cephalometric parameters and values are still used today. Numerous parameters have been introduced following his study.[15]

During the next few decades, numerous studies emphasized the importance of reliable and standardized landmarks, parameters, and references points to determine *(1)* the outcome of treatment for a single patient, *(2)* comparison of outcomes from multiple patients undergoing similar treatment, or *(3)* growth prediction with or without treatment. Unfortunately, some of these landmarks have changed slightly in definition or emphasis through the century of 2D cephalometry and will change for 3D cephalometry because of the addition of the third dimension. For example, in light of 3D investigation, it is currently in question whether A-point can be considered the most forward position of the maxilla.[20]

3D CBCTs

3D CBCTs were first reported in 1994 and originally introduced commercially in Europe in 1996. However, it was not until 2001 that the first 3D CBCT was introduced commercially to the United States. Prior to 2007, few articles linked 3D CBCTs to orthodontics.[21] Initial concerns about the high radiation dosage and its cost probably limited its use in orthodontics for a while but drove reengineering of the technology, which significantly reduced the radiation exposure and cost. Since 2007, hundreds of articles relating the use of 3D CBCTs to orthodontics have been published. The applicability of 3D CBCTs for associated orthognathic surgery and dental implants as well as need-specific orthodontics (eg, impacted teeth, craniofacial anomalies, bone thickness) has increased their usage in orthodontics and general dentistry. However, significant issues remain, including whether the landmarks and measures used in 2D cephalometry can be used in 3D cephalometry as well as the clinical relevance and use of 3D cephalometry for all orthodontic patients.

The evolution of 3D cephalometry has occurred more quickly than 2D cephalometry, probably due to worldwide digital communications. More than 50 years after the inception of lateral radiographs in orthodontics, Steiner[22] indicated that cephalometrics was still not being used for clinical applications but was primarily a tool for academic studies of growth and development. On the other hand, it is predicted that in just 5 years, the global CBCT market will increase from $494.4 million in 2016 to $801.2 million in 2021, although the growth will probably not be limited to orthodontics.[23]

Conclusion

Patient care is performed best by educated and discerning clinicians, so it is essential that clinicians not only understand the basics of 2D cephalometry and how it relates to 3D cephalometry but also keep up to date with the evolution of cephalometry and its associated technology, software, and applications.

References

1. American Association of Orthodontists. Clinical Practice Guidelines for Orthodontics and Dentofacial Orthopedics [amended 2014]. https://www.aaoinfo.org/system/files/media/documents/2014%20Cllinical%20Practice%20Guidelines.pdf. Accessed 25 August 2017.
2. Finlay LM. Craniometry and cephalometry: A history prior to the advent of radiography. Angle Orthod 1980;50:312–321.
3. Todd TW. The orthodontic value of research and observation in developmental growth of the face. Angle Orthod 1931;1:67.
4. American Dental Association. History of Dentistry Timeline. http://www.ada.org/en/about-the-ada/ada-history-and-presidents-of-the-ada/ada-history-of-dentistry-timeline. Accessed 25 August 2017.
5. NDT Resource Center. https://www.nde-ed.org/index_flash.htm. Accessed 25 August 2017.
6. Rowland S. Archives of Clinical Skiagraphy. London: Rebman, 1896.
7. Broadbent BH Sr, Broadbent BH Jr, Golden WH. Bolton Standards of Dentofacial Developmental Growth. St Louis: C.V. Mosby, 1975:166.
8. Pacini AJ. Roentgen ray anthropometry of the skull. J Radiol 1922;42:230–238,322–331,418–426.
9. Basyouni AA, Nanda SR. An Atlas of the Transverse Dimensions of the Face, vol. 37 [Craniofacial Growth Series]. Ann Arbor: University of Michigan Center for Human Growth and Development, 2000:235.
10. Dewey MN, Riesner S. A radiographic study of facial deformity. Int J Orthod 1948;14:261–267.
11. Broadbent BH. A new x-ray technique and its application to orthodontia. Angle Orthod 1931;1:45.
12. Broadbent BH. The orthodontic value of studies in facial growth. In: Physical and Mental Adolescent Growth [The Proceedings of the Conference on Adolescence, 17–18 October 1930, Cleveland, OH].
13. Hofrath H. Die Bedeutung der Rontgenfern und Abstandsaufname für die Diagnostic der Kieferanomalien. Fortschr Orthod 1931;1:232–258.
14. Broadbent BH. Investigations of the orbital plane. Dental Cosmos 1927;69:797–805.
15. Krogman WM, Sassouni V. Syllabus in Roentgenographic Cephalometry. Philadelphia: College Offset, 1957:363.
16. Tweed CH. The Frankfort mandibular incisor angle (FMIA) in orthodontic diagnosis, treatment planning, and prognosis. Angle Orthod 1954;24:121–169.
17. Riedal R. An analysis of dentofacial relationships. Am J Orthod 1957;43:103–119.
18. Casko JS, Shepherd WB. Dental and skeletal variation within the range of normal. Angle Orthod 1984;54:5–17.
19. Downs WB. Variations in facial relationships: Their significance in treatment prognosis. Am J Orthod 1948;34:812–840.
20. Kula TJ III, Ghoneima A, Eckert G, Parks E, Utreja A, Kula K. A 2D vs 3D comparison of alveolar bone over maxillary incisors using A point as a reference. Am J Orthod Dentofacial Orthopedics (in press).
21. Gribel BF, Gribel MN, Frazão DC, McNamara Jr JA, Manzi FR. Accuracy and reliability of craniometric measurements on lateral cephalometry and 3D measurements on CBCT scans. Angle Orthod 2011;81:26–35.
22. Steiner CC. Cephalometrics for you and me. Am J Orthod 1953;39:729–754.
23. Markets and Markets. CBCT/Cone Beam Imaging Market by Application. http://www.marketsandmarkets.com/Market-Reports/cone-beam-imaging-market-226049013.html?gclid=EAIaIQobChMI4_b899b31AIVyEwNCh1xXQseEAAYASAAEgJa0_D_BwE. Accessed 25 August 2017.

2

2D and 3D Radiography

Edwin T. Parks, DMD, MS

Two-dimensional (2D) cephalometry has been an integral component of orthodontic patient assessment since Broadbent described the technique in 1931.[1] For years the only image receptor for cephalometry was radiographic film, which limited the clinician to a 2D patient assessment. Today there are multiple receptor options such as photostimulable phosphor (PSP), charge-coupled device (CCD), and derived 2D data from cone beam computed tomography (CBCT). While CBCT allows for clinicians to evaluate the patient in three dimensions, most patient assessment is still performed on 2D data. This chapter discusses the various techniques for generating traditional 2D cephalograms, cephalograms derived from three-dimensional (3D) data, radiation exposures, and advantages/disadvantages of the various techniques and image receptors.

Patient Positioning

Regardless of image receptor, proper patient positioning is essential to producing an acceptable cephalometric image.

Lateral cephalogram

The patient's head is positioned with the left side of the face next to the image receptor, with the midsagittal plane parallel to the image receptor and the Frankfort plane parallel to the floor[2] (Fig 2-1). The patient's head should be stabilized in a cephalostat. The *cephalostat* is a device with two ear rods that are placed in the external auditory meatuses and a nasion guide. Head stabilization serves two purposes: *(1)* It diminishes patient movement, and *(2)* it ensures reproducibility to allow for sequential evaluation over time.

The radiation source is positioned so that the distance between the source and the midsagittal plane is 60 inches. The receptor (or film) should be placed 15 cm (approximately 6 inches) from the midsagittal plane. The x-ray beam should be collimated to the size of the receptor, and the center of the beam should be directed through the external auditory meatus (Fig 2-2). Because of the projection geometry, structures away from the receptor will be magnified more than the structures close to the receptor.

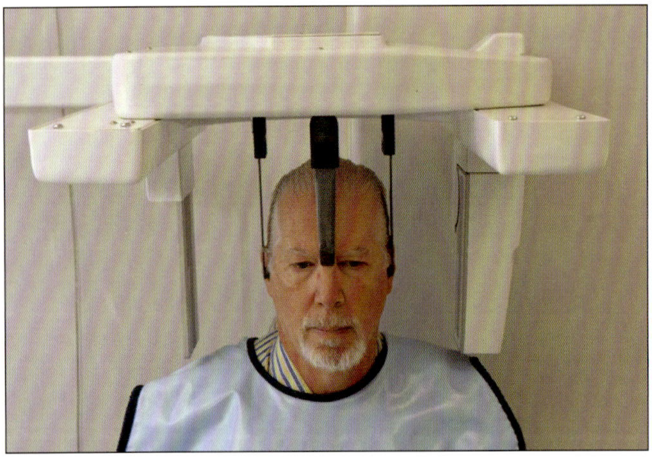

Fig 2-1 Proper patient positioning for a lateral cephalogram showing the cephalostat around the patient's head.

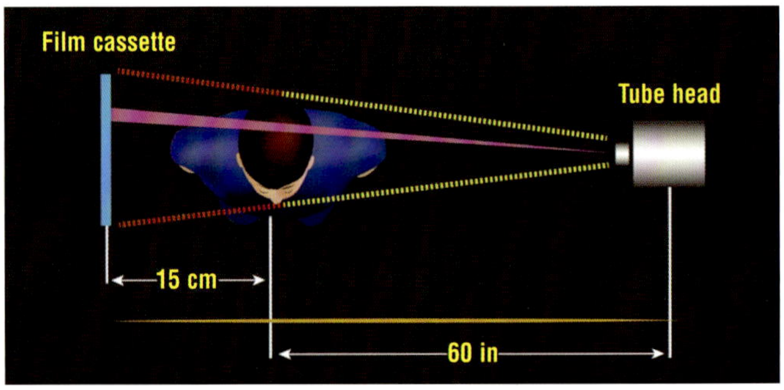

Fig 2-2 Graphic representation of patient positioning for a lateral cephalogram *(viewed from above)*.

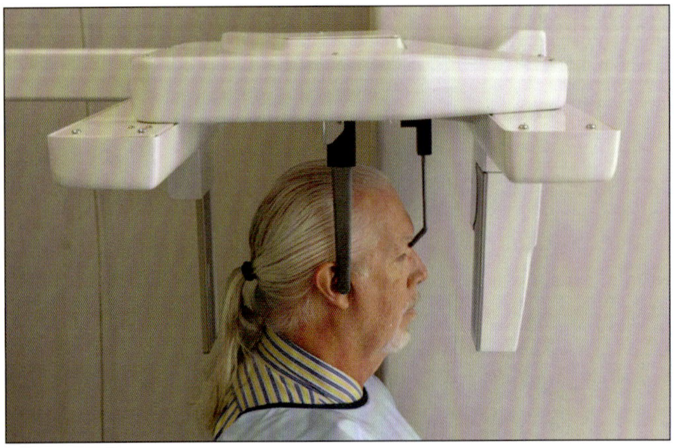

Fig 2-3 Proper patient positioning for a PA cephalogram.

Posteroanterior cephalogram

Patient positioning for the posteroanterior (PA) cephalogram uses the same armamentarium as the lateral cephalogram. The patient is positioned with the midsagittal plane perpendicular to the receptor (nose toward the receptor) and the Frankfort plane parallel to the floor (Fig 2-3). The source should be 60 inches from the ear rods, and the receptor should be positioned 15 cm from the ear rods.[2]

Patient Protection

There has been a great deal of discussion regarding the need for shielding of the patient from the primary beam. The American Dental Association,[3] National Council on Radiation Protection and Measurements,[4] and US Food and Drug Administration[3] have created fairly specific recommendations for patient shielding for intraoral imaging but not for extraoral imaging. Nevertheless, many of the factors involved in the recommendations are applicable to extraoral imaging. Use of fast image receptors and collimation of the primary beam to the size of the receptor significantly reduce the dose to the patient. However, these factors do not reduce the dose to zero. Consequently, there is slight potential for risk to the patient.

The effects of high doses of x-radiation are well documented, but the effects of low doses of radiation have only been inferred or derived from a model. The accepted model for determining risk from x-radiation is the linear, nonthreshold model. This model suggests that risk is directly related to radiation dose. The concept of threshold is that there is a level of exposure below which there is no risk. The nonthreshold model indicates that there is no safe dose of radiation to the patient. Ludlow et al calculated effective doses for commonly used dental radiographic examinations and reported effective doses of 5.6 microsieverts (µSv) for a lateral cephalogram (using PSP) and 5.1 µSv for the PA cephalogram (using PSP).[5] For comparison, they reported an effective dose for panoramic imaging (CCD) ranging from 14.2 to 24.3 µSv and 170.7 µSv for a full-mouth series using F-speed film and round collimation.[5] In a different study, Ludlow et al evaluated the effective dose from several CBCT systems and reported effective doses ranging from 58.9 to 557.6 µSv.[6] For a comparison, the paper also reported an effective dose for conventional CT of 2,100 µSv for a maxillomandibular scan.[6]

There is a huge range of effective doses for these imaging modalities for many reasons. First, all of these systems use different exposure factors (eg, kilovoltage peak [kVp], milliamperage [mA], exposure time) and cover many different critical organs. The critical organs most commonly included in dose calculation for the maxillofacial complex are the thyroid gland, salivary glands, and bone marrow. This gets complicated pretty quickly. Now imagine what it must be like for the patient and parent when you start to describe effective dose. A better way to talk to the patient and parent is the concept of benefit versus risk. Explain to the patient and/or parent the reason you need the radiographic image (eg, asymmetry, impacted teeth) and that the risk to the patient is minimal. There is even some research that indicates that the lap apron provides no added protection from scatter radiation.[7] This study, while not directly applicable, looks at the imaging modality that most closely approximates the field of view for orthodontic evaluation (panoramic). Still, it is important to realize that patients and parents are concerned about any radiation exposure. It probably takes less time to shield the patient with a lap apron than to explain why you do not need it. The thyroid collar should not be used for either 2D cephalometry or 3D CBCT.

Exposure Factors

All radiographic imaging is predicated by differential absorption of the x-ray beam by the region of interest. Multiple exposure factors need to be adjusted depending on the patient's size and bone density. These exposure factors— kVp, mA, and exposure time—are discussed below.

Kilovoltage peak (kVp)

Kilovoltage refers to the energy or penetrating power of the x-ray beam. *Peak* simply refers to the highest energy in a polyenergetic beam. The mean beam energy is generally considered to be one-third of the peak. As kilovoltage increases, the beam energy and penetrating power also increase. Conversely, lower kilovoltage produces lower beam energy and generates photons that are more likely to be absorbed by the region of interest. Kilovoltage should be increased for patients with large or dense facial bones and decreased for patients with small or less dense facial bones. Most cephalometric units function in a range of 70 to 90 kVp. CBCT units function between 90 and 120 kVp.

Milliamperage (mA) and exposure time

Milliamperage is the determinant of the tube current and controls the number of photons of x-radiation that are produced in the tube head. It is often adjusted because of the density of the soft tissues of the head and neck, and it is often reported together with exposure time (seconds). Both mA and exposure time have a direct relationship with output. It is important to remember that mAs = mAs. This simply means that as long as the product of mA and exposure time remains constant, the output of the machine will also remain constant. For example, if mA is 5 and the exposure time is 0.5 seconds, the mAs is 2.5. If the milliamperage is 10, the exposure time would need to be decreased to 0.25 seconds to maintain output.

Collimation/Soft Tissue Filtration

The shape and size of the primary beam of x-radiation is controlled by collimation of the beam. The radiation beam should be collimated to the size of the image receptor. Collimating the beam to the size of the receptor decreases the exposure and dose received by the patient. The cephalometric unit should have a mechanism to filter the soft tissues of the nose and lips. Generally, the x-ray beam is generated to penetrate bony structures and will burn out soft tissue structures. The soft tissue filter attenuates the beam prior to it contacting the patient, providing some radiation protection to the patient and decreasing the energy of the beam so that the soft tissues will be enhanced in the cephalogram.

Image Distortion/Magnification

A 2D cephalogram will contain some image distortion in the form of differential magnification because a 3D object is being imaged using diverging radiation rays. Structures away from the image receptor will be magnified much more than objects that are positioned close to the image receptor. Magnification is calculated by dividing the distance from the source of radiation to the image receptor (SID) by the distance from the source to the object of interest (SOD). Based on this calculation, it is easy to see that the right and left sides of the skull will be different sizes in a lateral cephalogram. Because there is a potential for distortion just from projection geometry, it is essential to either record the distance from the center of the cephalostat to the image receptor or to establish a standard distance when evaluating sequential cephalograms.

Image Receptors

Film-based systems

Film-based cephalometry employs indirect-exposure radiographic film positioned between two intensifying screens. Intensifying screens convert x-radiation into light. Indirect-exposure film is more sensitive to light than it is to x-radiation. As a consequence, the use of intensifying screens and indirect-exposure radiographic film allows for very low exposure times. Different types of intensifying screens emit different wavelengths of light. Care must be taken to match the spectral sensitivity of the film to the light emitted from the intensifying screens. Rare-earth intensifying screens emit either green or blue light. Traditional or par screens emit purple light. If intensifying screens emit a green light, you must use green-sensitive film to produce an acceptable image. Figure 2-4 shows examples of film-based lateral and PA cephalograms.

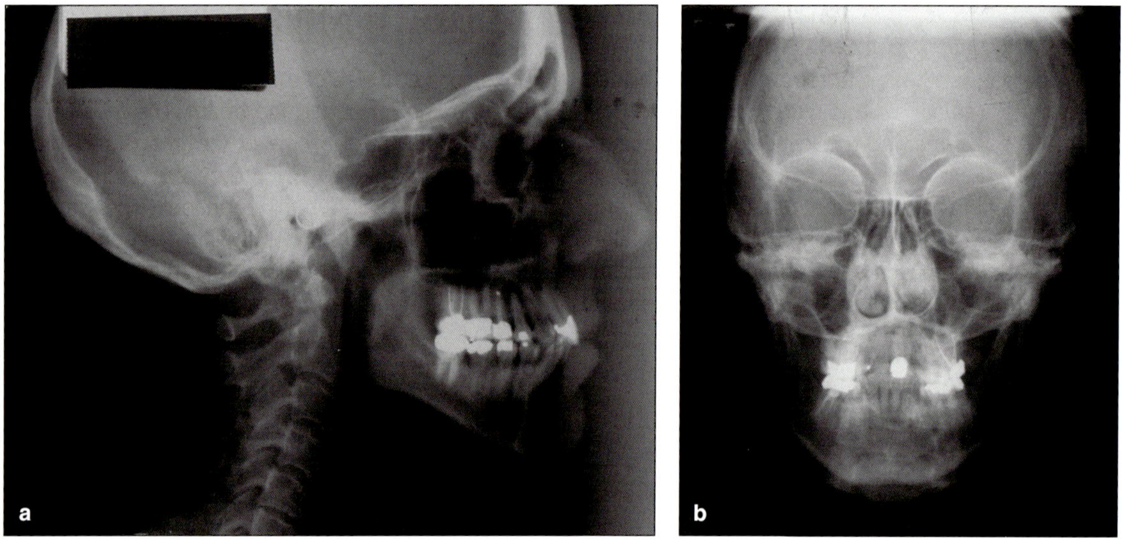

Fig 2-4 Examples of film-based lateral *(a)* and PA *(b)* cephalograms.

Box 2-1 **Advantages and disadvantages of digital cephalometric imaging**

Advantages
- Exposure reduction
- Image enhancement
- Digital image storage
- Automated analysis
- Image transmission
- Increased staff efficiency

Disadvantages
- High initial cost
- Differences in projection geometry

Darkroom procedures

As with any film-based imaging, chemical processing must be performed to convert the latent or chemical image into a visible image. All film processors go through the same steps: development, fixation rinse, and drying. The function of the developer is to convert the silver ions on the film into metallic silver. The process of fixation stops the development process and renders an archival image. The quality of correctly processed film images will not change over time; unfortunately, however, most images are not correctly processed. Quality assurance in the darkroom is essential for quality film-based imaging. Quality assurance pertains to many components of the darkroom—lighting as well as the activity of the processing chemistry. Processing chemistry must be replenished every day. Developer and fixer activity diminish due to workload rather than time, so it is essential to have an ongoing program of assessing the activity of the chemistry. Finally, because direct- and indirect-exposure films require different safelight filters, make sure that the safelight in the darkroom does not fog the film prior to processing.

Digital systems

Digital receptors are divided into two groups: indirect digital and direct digital systems. PSP plates are considered to be indirect digital sensors, whereas CCD and complementary metal oxide semiconductors (CMOS) are considered to be direct digital sensors. There are many advantages to the use of digital receptors (Box 2-1). In addition to reduced exposure, a huge advantage is the ability to enhance images once they are captured. Electronic image storage and image transmission are also advantages of digital receptors compared with film-based systems. While automated analysis can be performed on a film-based image that is converted into a digital image through a process called *analog to digital conversion*, data is lost in the process, whereas with digital images automated analysis can be performed without any lost data. Staff efficiency is also increased with the use of digital receptors: There is no downtime spent waiting for the image to be processed.

There are two potential disadvantages to the use of digital receptors: *(1)* cost and *(2)* differences in projection geometry (see Box 2-1). There is no doubt that the initial cost of a digital cephalometric unit is higher than the cost of a film-based sys-

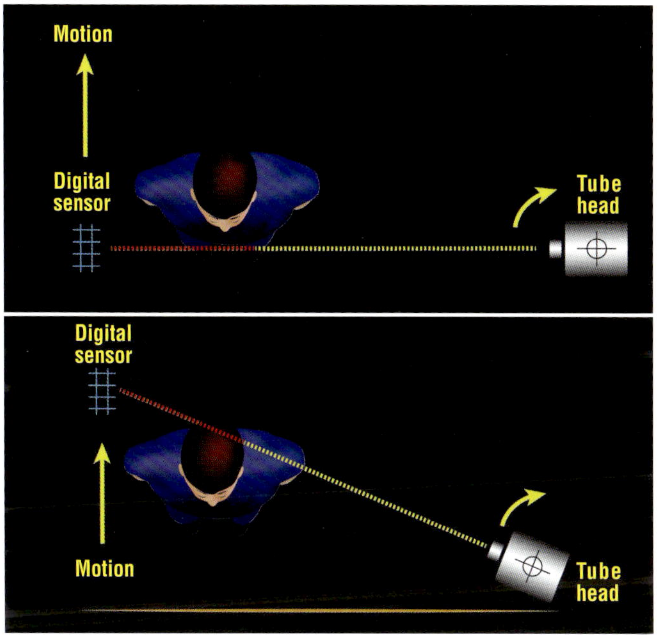

Fig 2-5 Graphic representation of scanning motion for direct digital cephalometric units.

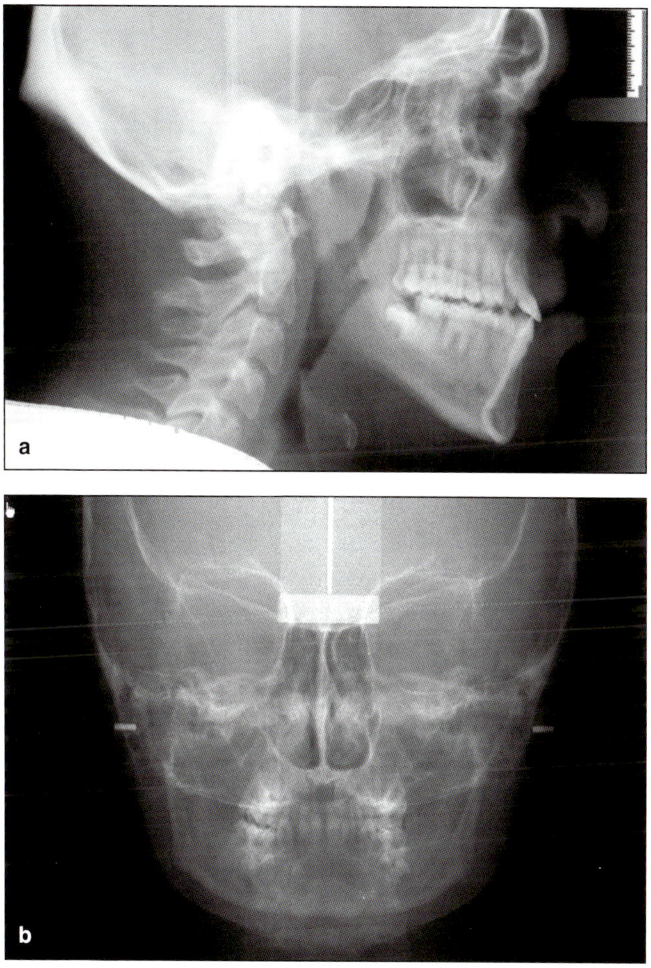

Fig 2-6 Examples of direct digital (scanned) lateral *(a)* and PA *(b)* cephalograms.

tem. However, when one factors in the costs of film, processing chemistry, and lost staff efficiency, the difference in initial cost is recouped rather quickly. The issue of differences in projection geometry is covered in the section entitled "Digital Versus Conventional Cephalometry."

PSP plates

PSP plates are image receptors that convert x-radiation into an electrical charge contained within the imaging plate. PSP plates come in all sizes (from 0 to an 8 × 10–inch plate) for cephalometry. The PSP plate is placed in the 8 × 10–inch cassette with the intensifying screens removed. The imaging plate is coated with europium-activated barium fluorohalide. The electronic information is converted into a visible image by subjecting the phosphor plate to a helium-neon laser. The PSP plate in turn emits a blue-violet light at 400 nm that is captured by the scanner and converted into a digital image. As a final step, the plate must be exposed to white light to remove the latent image; this step is performed in most scanners automatically. PSP plates are considered to be indirect digital images because the x-ray data is captured as analog or continuous data and converted into digital data in the scanner. This is the same reason that film-based images that are scanned as digital images are considered to be indirect digital images.

CCD/CMOS receptors

Direct digital cephalometric x-ray machines use either a CCD or CMOS receptor for image capture. While these two types of digital receptor differ with regard to image capture and data transfer, both generate comparable images. Some panoramic cephalometric combination machines use only one sensor that has to be moved depending on the type of image captured. Other combination machines use two sensors, which is much more efficient and decreases the risk of damaging the sensor by dropping it. The majority of these units capture an image in a scanning motion either horizontally or vertically (Figs 2-5 and 2-6). This type of image capture differs from film-based and PSP imaging, which capture the image in a single exposure. Image capture with the scanning motion requires the patient to remain motionless for up to 10 seconds. The possibility for motion artifact increases as the exposure (or in this case scanning) time increases. At least two companies (Carestream and Vatech) have produced a "one-shot" image capture system that potentially can create the same projection geometry as conventional cephalometry while significantly decreasing the time the patient must remain motionless.

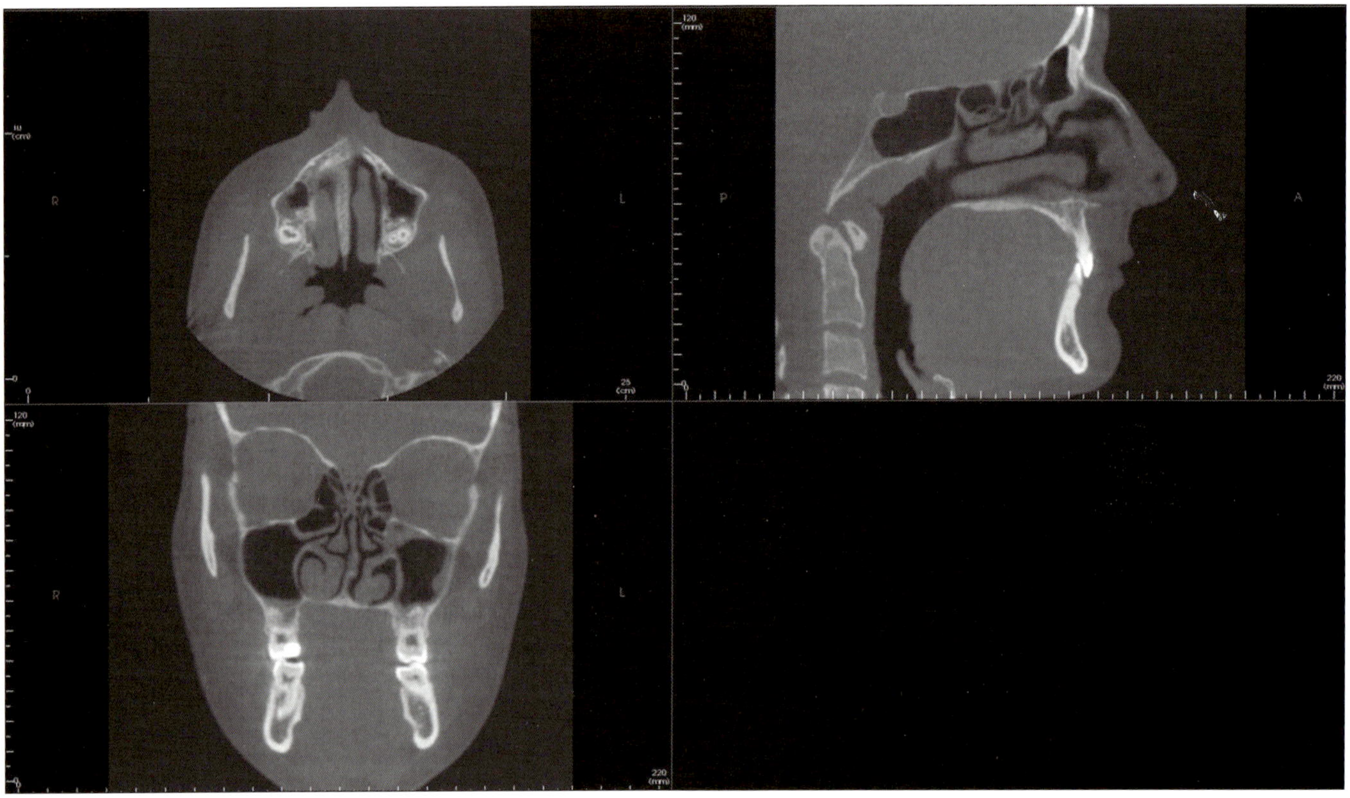

Fig 2-7 Multiplanar reformation.

Digital Versus Conventional Cephalometry

Not all digital cephalometric images are the same. Cephalometric images captured on a PSP plate have the same projection geometry used to capture a film-based image. The majority of digital receptors, however, capture the image with a scanning motion and therefore have different magnification factors than in film-based cephalometry. Chadwick et al reported differences among several different systems that appear to be system dependent and recommended that the magnification factor be experimentally determined prior to any cephalometric analysis.[8] McClure et al compared digital cephalometry with film-based cephalometry and found no differences in linear measurements; however, in their study, pretreatment cephalograms were compared with posttreatment cephalograms.[9] The time frame between pre- and posttreatment images may introduce the confounder of active growth during the orthodontic treatment.

CBCT

CBCT began to appear in the late 1990s. CBCT machines consist of a radiation source shaped like a cone and a solid-state detector that rotates around the patient's head and captures all of the scan data in a single rotation.[10] This raw data is then reconstructed in the coronal, axial, and sagittal planes (also known as *multiplanar reformation*) (Fig 2-7). The data can be further reconstructed to produce either 2D images such as panoramic or cephalometric images (Fig 2-8) or 3D data sets[11] (Fig 2-9). The images produced with CBCT are not magnified, so standard cephalometric analysis must be altered to address this difference in projection geometry.

While the name implies similarity with conventional CT, the two technologies differ in a number of ways. The most important difference for the patient is the difference in dose. Conventional CT produces a four- to tenfold higher dose than CBCT when imaging the maxillofacial region.[6] There are several reasons for this difference in dose, but the fundamental difference is that CBCT captures the entire data set in one rotation, whereas conventional CT requires multiple rotations to capture the data. This single rotation decreases the dose but also is more susceptible to patient motion. If the patient moves during conventional CT imaging, only that slice of data is impacted. However, patient movement affects every voxel during CBCT image capture. Another difference has to do with the imaging of soft tissue. Conventional CT uses a high mA, which contributes to the soft tissue contrast; CBCT uses a fairly low mA, with minimal soft tissue contrast. CBCT will capture soft tissue, but the soft tissue is displayed as a fairly homogenous image.

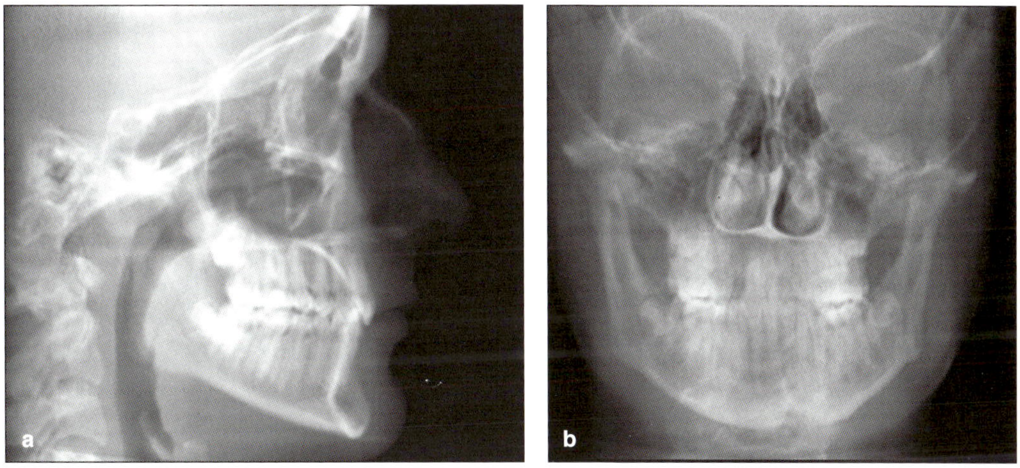

Fig 2-8 Examples of CBCT-derived lateral *(a)* and PA *(b)* cephalograms.

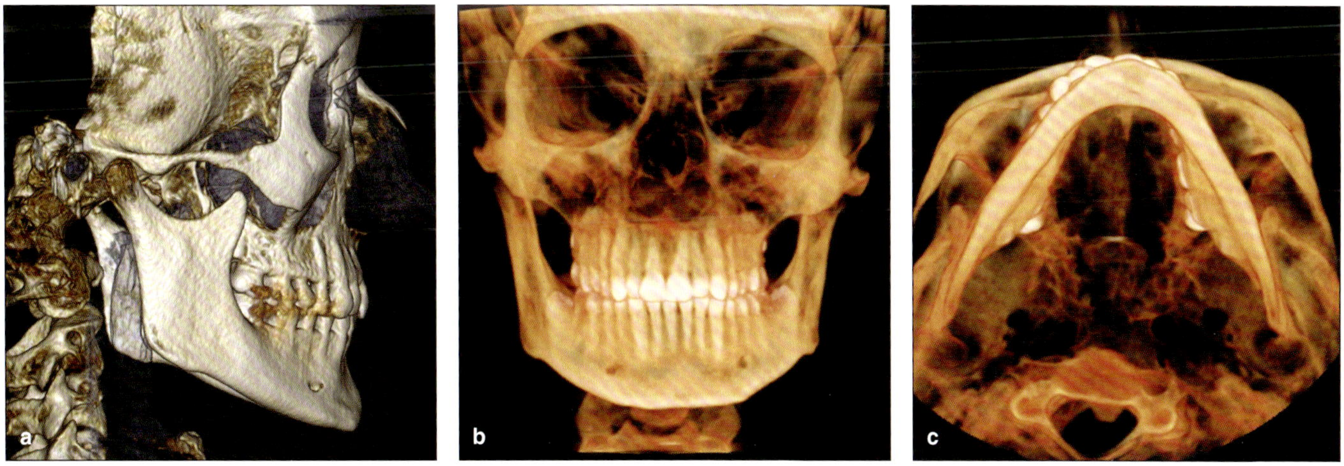

Fig 2-9 Examples of 3D reconstructions. *(a)* Lateral cephalometric rendering. *(b)* PA cephalometric rendering. *(c)* Submentovertex rendering.

Selection criteria

CBCT can provide a wealth of information regarding the maxillofacial regions. The ability to generate 3D images greatly enhances the treatment-planning process for many patients but may be unnecessary for some patients. The decision to scan or not to scan will be dependent on the patient's condition. The delineation of whom to scan is called *selection criteria*. In 2013, the American Academy of Oral and Maxillofacial Radiology published clinical recommendations for the use of CBCT in orthodontics.[12] The first recommendation is to use the appropriate imaging modality based on the patient's clinical presentation and history.[12] The second recommendation pertains to radiation risk assessment, and the third recommendation addresses ways to keep the dose to the patient as low as reasonably achievable (ALARA),[12] such as focusing on resolution, scan time, and field of view (FOV).

Scanning protocol

Because the goal in orthodontic imaging is to get the best data with the lowest dose to the patient, several factors should be included in the scanning protocol. The first consideration is the volume of the scan. Volume will be dictated by the choice of the FOV. The larger the FOV, the higher the dose to the patient. Keeping the FOV as small as possible will minimize the dose to the patient. Determining resolution requirements is another way to diminish dose to the patient. Generally, the higher the resolution, the higher the dose. Using the lowest resolution that still provides adequate diagnostic information is a good way to decrease the dose to the patient. Finally, the last consideration is exposure time. As with any radiographic imaging, the longer the exposure time, the higher the dose. Therefore, the shortest scan time that provides adequate diagnostic information should be used. The imaging protocol should address all of these parameters.

Patient positioning and preparation

The patient should be draped with a lap apron for image acquisition. Patient positioning differs with every commercially available scanner. Some systems capture the image with the patient standing, while others capture the image with the patient seated. Regardless of manufacturer, all units provide some form of head stabilization. It is important to position the patient's head with the Frankfort plane parallel to the floor and the midsagittal plane perpendicular to the floor. While the position of the head can be altered during the image-reconstruction process, the same cannot be said for the cervical spine. Many CBCT scanners provide a bite stick for patient positioning. The bite stick produces an end-to-end occlusion that can alter the width of the airway and the condyle/fossa relationship. The use of the bite stick should therefore be avoided.

Image reconstruction

Once the appropriate scan is captured, the acquisition computer will generate data as a multiplanar reformation (MPR) providing images in the sagittal, coronal, and axial planes. While this data is captured in a 3D matrix, the MPR images are sequential 2D images. Further reconstruction is needed to generate useful 3D data. Additionally, conventional 2D images—cephalograms and panoramic radiographs—can be derived from the 3D data. As previously stated, there is no magnification in the CBCT-derived cephalograms as opposed to conventionally acquired cephalograms. Numerous studies have quantified the differences between landmark identification in conventional versus CBCT-derived cephalograms.[13–15] For the most part, the identification of landmarks has been comparable between the two. Some of the outcomes of these studies suggest that some "landmarks" visualized in two dimensions are not necessarily point landmarks in 3D data. Research is ongoing to better elucidate cephalometric landmarks in 3D data sets.

References

1. Broadbent BH. A new x-ray technique and its application to orthodontia. Angle Orthod 1931;1:45–66.
2. Jacobson A, Jacobson RL (eds). Radiographic Cephalometry: From Basics to 3-D Imaging, ed 2. Chicago: Quintessence, 2006.
3. American Dental Association. Dental Radiographic Examinations: Recommendations For Patient Selection And Limiting Radiation Exposure [PDF]. http://www.ada.org/en/~/media/ADA/Member%20Center/FIles/Dental_Radiographic_Examinations_2012. Accessed 22 May 2017.
4. Brand JW, Gibbs SJ, Edwards M, et al. Radiation Protection in Dentistry [Report 145]. Bethesda, MD: National Council on Radiation Protection and Measurements, 2003.
5. Ludlow JB, Davies-Ludlow LE, White SC. Patient risk related to common dental radiographic examinations: The impact of 2007 International Commission on Radiological Protection recommendations regarding dose calculation. J Am Dent Assoc 2008;139:1237–1243.
6. Ludlow JB, Davies-Ludlow LE, Brooks SL, Howerton WB. Dosimetry of 3 CBCT devices for oral and maxillofacial radiology: CB Mercuray, NewTom 3G and i-CAT. Dentomaxillofac Radiol 2006;35:219–226.
7. Rottke D, Grossekettler L, Sawada K, Poxleitner P, Schulze D. Influence of lead apron shielding on absorbed doses from panoramic radiography. Dentomaxillofac Radiol 2013;42:20130302.
8. Chadwick J, Prentice RN, Major PW, Lam EW. Image distortion and magnification of 3 digital CCD cephalometric systems. Oral Surg Oral Med Oral Pathol Oral Radiol Endod 2009;107:105–112.
9. McClure SR, Sadowsky PL, Ferreira A, Jacobson A. Reliability of digital versus conventional cephalometric radiology: A comparative evaluation of landmark identification error. Semin Orthod 2005;11:98–110.
10. White SC, Pharoah MJ. Oral Radiology Principles and Interpretation, ed 7. St Louis: Mosby/Elsevier, 2014.
11. Swennen G, Schutyser F, Hausamen J. Three-Dimensional Cephalometry: A Color Atlas and Manual. Berlin: Springer-Verlag, 2006.
12. Clinical recommendations regarding use of cone beam computed tomography in orthodontics. Position statement by the American Academy of Oral and Maxillofacial Radiology. Oral Surg Oral Med Oral Pathol Oral Radiol 2013;116:238–257 [erratum 2013;116:661].
13. Park JW, Kim N, Chang YI. Comparison of landmark position between conventional cephalometric radiography and CT scans projected to midsagittal plane. Korean J Orthod 2008;38:426–436.
14. Chien PC, Parks ET, Eraso F, Hartsfield JK, Roberts WE, Ofner S. Comparison of reliability in anatomical landmark identification using two-dimensional digital cephalometrics and three-dimensional cone beam computed tomography in vivo. Dentomaxillofac Radiol 2009;38:262–273.
15. Zamora N, Llamas JM, Cibrián R, Gandia JL, Paredes V. Cephalometric measurements from 3D reconstructed images compared with conventional 2D images. Angle Orthod 2011;81:856–864.

3

Skeletal Landmarks and Measures

Katherine Kula, MS, DMD, MS
Ahmed Ghoneima, BDS, PhD, MSD

In order to determine relative position, size, and changes in size, one has to establish what will be measured and precisely where the measures will start and end. Everyone involved needs to agree upon where and how the object will be measured and at least know how to interpret the measure for the sake of proper diagnosis and treatment planning. This is particularly important for measuring irregular anatomical structures such as the maxilla and the mandible. The relationship of one object to another and their potential changes also need to be defined and accepted by those using the measures. This applies to cephalometric analysis of shape, size, relationships, and changes of bones in the cranium and the face. The definitions of the cephalometric landmarks and the linear and angular measures based on these landmarks have to be understood and accepted globally in order to have a common basis of classification and discussion of growth, development, and treatment effects.

A line requires only two points, whereas area or volume requires more points for accurate measurement. To precisely measure two-dimensional (2D) measurements like length, width, or height, the two places selected for measurement should be points. These points are called *landmarks*, similar to on maps. Three-dimensional (3D) measurements can provide more information about the cross-sectional area and volume of anatomical structures than 2D measurements.

Landmarks should be well-defined points that can be reliably identified. These points should have a relationship with other landmarks that indicates growth or treatment effects.

Many cephalometric landmarks are based historically on anthropometry, the study of skulls. However, the position of the landmarks affects reliable radiographic identification. Some skeletal cephalometric landmarks are internal to the skull, whereas others are surface landmarks. Some are medial or in the center of the skull, whereas others are bilateral, occurring on both sides of the center of the skull. Radiographic identification in any of these areas can be complicated because of overlapping soft tissue and skeletal structures and because of geometry.

Landmarks used in 2D cephalometrics are usually more easily and consistently identified on the profile of the subject.

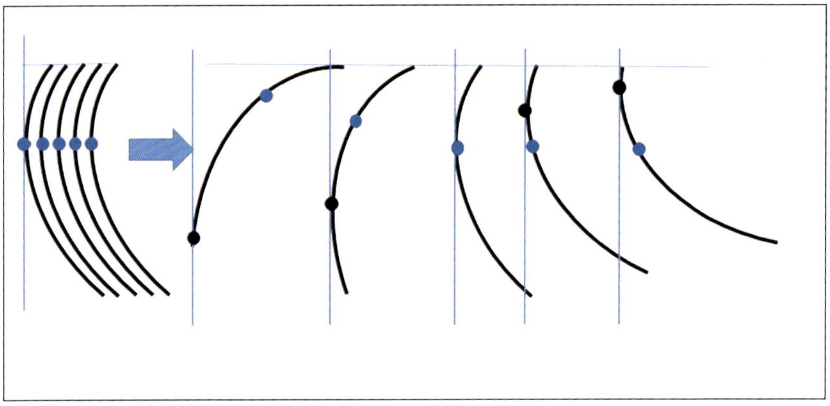

Fig 3-1 A landmark on a curve (eg, A-point) can change position as the head is rotated. Five identical curves with the most posterior point on the curve identified as a *blue dot* are replicated and placed at different angles to a horizontal line. A line perpendicular to the horizontal line touches the most posterior point on the curve, and the *black dot* now identifies that the most posterior point on the curve has changed position. If the lines are viewed from the reverse perspective as being convex, they illustrate a point (eg, pogonion) on a chin and the changes that can occur.

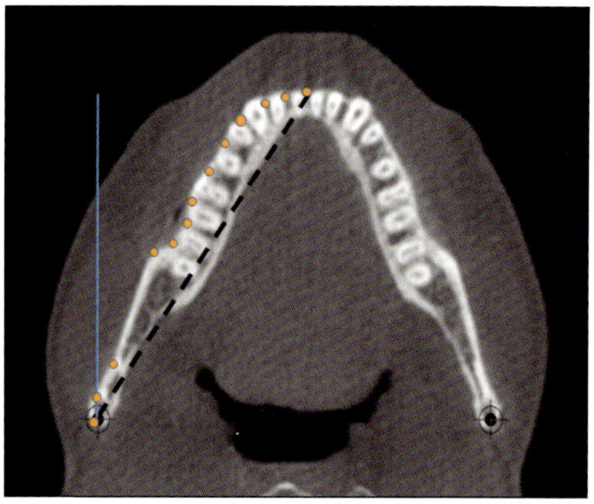

Fig 3-2 A 3D cone beam computed tomography (CBCT) section illustrating the differences in lengths if a 3D object is measured from one posterior lateral landmark to another anterior midline landmark from a 2D lateral perspective *(blue line)* or a 2D axial CBCT perspective *(dashed black line)*. The actual length would be different if the perimeter of the object was measured *(series of orange dots)* because of the curve (3D CBCT perspective).

However, reliability can be minimized if they are on a part of a curve influenced by position of the head or on a straight line.[1] Identification of intracranial 2D cephalometric landmarks is limited by overlying structures that make many landmarks difficult to identify. Magnification and improper head orientation can affect the reliability of bilateral landmark identification in both symmetric and asymmetric subjects. Even the identification of edges of medial structures can be problematic because of asymmetries and rotational mispositioning of the patient.

Changes in head position cause changes in surface geometry that affect reliable identification of various landmarks.[1] Any landmark identified at the most anterior or most posterior position on a curve can change in position by rotating or tipping the head and by nonstandardization of head position during image capture (Fig 3-1). A-point on the anterior outline of the maxilla, B-point on the anterior outline of the mandible, and pogonion on the most anterior portion of the chin are examples of such landmarks.

In 2D, the measures between the landmarks are made linearly as a line or as an angle. Currently, linear measures are frequently made in 3D also. 2D measures are conventionally made in an anteroposterior (AP), vertical, or diagonal direction. Thus, the true size of an object is not always measured. For example, the length of any 3D object that has a curved or a diagonal edge is not truly measured in 2D, just the linear distance between two points (eg, gonion to B-point). A good example is the length of the mandible, which is measured from lateral structures to a medial structure. Many AP measures are made from lateral landmarks to midline landmarks (Fig 3-2) without accounting for the third dimension, which would increase the distances as compared to a straight line. Even in 3D cephalometry, if the standard lateral or frontal view is measured, the measurements are frequently linear and do not take into account the curvature and morphology of the anatomical structures. Not surprisingly, Wen et al[2] found that 3D AP measures were significantly greater than conventional 2D measures and 2D measures derived from 3D images. There were no significant differences in vertical measures. Their conclusions about 3D measures being misleading in cephalometry, however, appear preliminary because the new technology will require additional research and interpretation. An understanding of geometry is also required.

Magnification caused by 2D radiography is not corrected in all published articles, making it difficult to compare values between articles. In comparison, 3D radiography is almost 1:1 with little or no magnification. The lack of magnification could also account for measure differences between 2D and 3D images.

Cephalometry, as used in orthodontics, developed slowly as a clinical tool. In 1953, Steiner[3] recognized the fact that despite being used in research for decades, few orthodontists used cephalometry in clinical practice. Various landmarks (eg, pogonion) have undergone either name changes or definition changes through time that were significant enough to confuse interpretation.[4] Some landmarks and parameters are used heavily in certain treatment philosophies but not in others.

Currently, transition is occurring between 2D and 3D cephalometry. Obviously, the newest technologies will not reach all areas of orthodontic education and practice at the same time throughout the world. Technology is expensive, and there are learning curves involved in incorporating the technologies into schools and practices. This chapter therefore discusses the tracing of 2D conventional radiographs both manually and digitally and then presents the most commonly used landmarks, planes, and angles and their interpretation in practice. Some methods such as mesh diagrams are used primarily in research and are not presented here. Later in this chapter, landmark identification and construction of planes and angles in 3D images are addressed in AP and vertical directions.

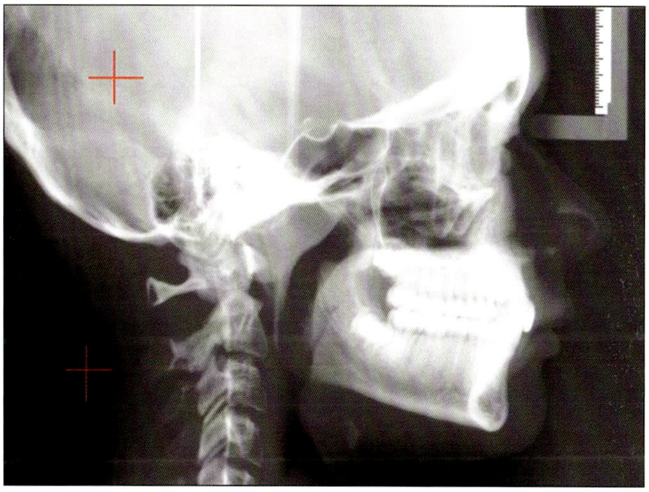

Fig 3-3 Prior to tracing, the cephalogram should be examined to check that head position is correct, that the nose and chin are included, and that resolution and contrast are adequate. Fiducial marks *(red crosses)* should be added to the conventional cephalogram.

As noted in the computerized cephalometric programs, many orthodontists essentially pick and choose the planes and angles based on their training or philosophy of treatment. For example, Tweed[5] gave credit to many of the early cephalometric pioneers for their significant contributions that helped him develop his treatment philosophy. In developing his analysis, Steiner[3] credited multiple individuals (eg, Downs, Riedel, Thompson, Margolis, Wylie, and others) with ideas or some of the measurements. The American Board of Orthodontics (ABO) has required few cephalometric measures for case analysis.[6,7] This chapter is organized to present the planes and angles that are closely related to each other relative to interpretation and tries to minimize use of esoteric landmarks and measures. The main emphasis is clinical cephalometry.

Tracing 2D Cephalometric Radiographs

Prior to taking radiographs at the time of initial records, an initial intraoral examination can help to determine the need for a 3D cone beam computed tomograph (CBCT) rather than 2D radiographs, which would minimize the need for additional radiographs, the cost, and the amount of radiation delivered to the patient. It is easy to become lost in measurements and miss obvious problems, so each radiograph should be reviewed prior to tracing. Both manual and computerized tracings can hide pathology or other problems when they are overlaid on the cephalogram. If the 2D cephalogram shows a questionable structure that was not obvious in the extraoral and intraoral examination, a 3D radiograph could be indicated. Obvious pathology, craniofacial disorders, obvious facial asymmetry, and overall disproportion of the face should not require a retake of a 2D radiograph but are good indications for an initial 3D CBCT. Therefore, preliminary examination will help the orthodontist diagnostically. Some of these issues are addressed in other chapters.

Before tracing any cephalometric radiograph, the cephalometric radiograph should be examined for adequate contrast and resolution, for proper head positioning of the patient, and to ensure that the nose and chin are in the radiograph (Fig 3-3). If these are inadequate, then the radiograph will probably need to be retaken, correcting for these problems, before attempting to identify landmarks that are difficult to find.

Manual tracing of conventional lateral radiographs

Currently, technology allows 2D cephalometric tracing to be performed in several manners. In conventional radiology, the radiographic image is captured on celluloid film. In order to see and trace the image, the celluloid film needs to be placed on a light box. The image is usually traced first onto acetate tracing paper, incorporating hard and soft tissue structures and identifying the landmarks later. Rarely is the tracing performed directly on the film because it destroys the integrity of the record.

Materials for tracing

The following materials should be gathered and placed within an arm's reach: acetate tracing paper, tape, sharp no. 2 carbon pencils, an eraser (although it can cause unsightly smudging that masks landmarks), a protractor with a long straight edge or a ruler with tooth templates incorporated into it, and a light box. If progress or final tracings or superimpositions will be made, then colored pencils will be necessary. Black or charcoal is used for the initial radiograph. Blue standardly is used for progress records, and red is used for final records.

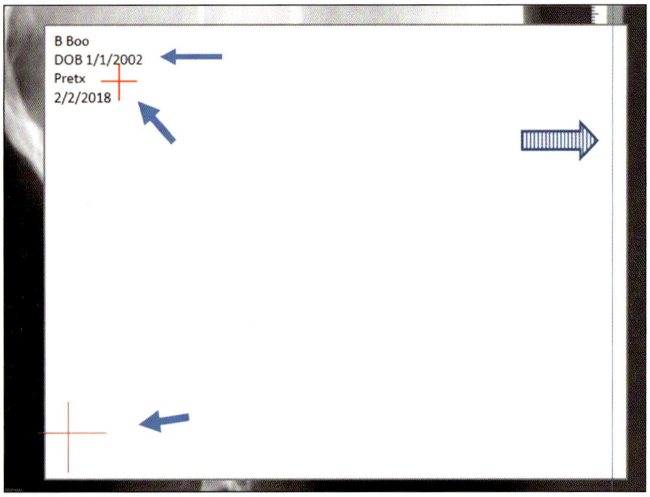

Fig 3-4 The acetate paper should be taped at two contiguous corners to the cephalogram with the image facing to the right. The *small blue arrows* point to fiducial marks traced onto the paper and the patient name, date of birth (DOB), stage of treatment, and date of radiograph. The *large blue arrow* to the right points to the true vertical line drawn onto the tracing.

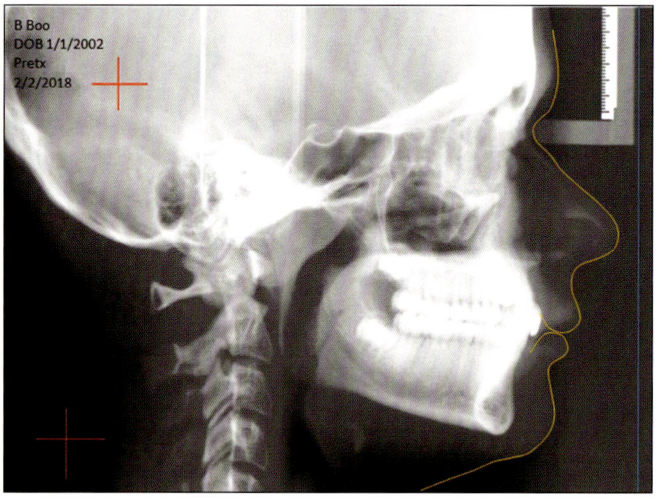

Fig 3-5 The profile is traced as shown in *yellow*.

Acetate tracing paper, which is smooth on one side and somewhat rough (matted) on the other side, is taped to the film at a minimum of two adjoining corners. The smooth side should be placed against the film and the rough side of the acetate tracing paper should face up to allow pencil to adhere. Taping at two corners allows the acetate paper to be lifted as needed in order to properly identify the anatomical structures of the craniofacial region (Fig 3-4). Typically, the image is faced to the right.

Use a sharp no. 2 lead pencil to trace the image. In order to identify the tracing when the acetate paper is separated from the film, the name and age of the patient as well as the date of the radiograph and treatment status (initial, progress, final, retention) is written on a corner of the acetate that will not hold any tracing. At least two fiducial marks (eg, + or X) are added to the initial film and traced onto the acetate to act as guides to realign the film and the acetate paper, if necessary. If the radiograph does not fill the light box screen, use thick paper or cardboard to block light leaking around the radiograph. Extraneous light interferes with cephalometric identification. Overhead lighting and light from windows also interfere with viewing the radiograph, so the room should be darkened while tracing the cephalogram.

Tracing procedure

A vertical reference line should be drawn parallel to the right edge of the film using a ruler or straight edge (see Fig 3-4). This assumes that the film holder is parallel to the floor. If a vertical plumb line is available in the radiograph, that line could be assumed to be true vertical. The vertical indicator on the cephalostat transfers to the radiograph and usually acts also as a magnification gauge. The ABO has required that the magnification gauge be visible in each cephalogram for purposes of superimposition.[6] The true vertical is also used as a reference line to determine soft tissue and skeletal proportions.

Soft tissue. If the soft tissue is indistinct, it would be better to trace the soft tissue first, then the hard tissue. Tracing the hard tissue first can obscure soft tissue identification. If soft tissue is seen easily on the film, then it might not matter which is traced first. Start tracing the soft tissue profile at the hairline and continue tracing the facial soft tissue outline smoothly down the forehead, incorporating the supraorbital ridge, the bridge of the nose, the tip of the nose, the columella of the nose, both lip outlines, the labiomental fold, the chin, and as much of the throat as possible (Fig 3-5). The profile should be traced as accurately as possible. Pulling the pencil down the profile toward you should be easier and more controllable than pushing the pencil away from you and up the profile.

Knowledge of anatomy is important to trace the correct structure and correctly identify a landmark. However, in some cases, the clinician has to make an educated guess because of poor resolution. Figure 3-6 is provided to help identify basic external and internal skull anatomy and its appearance in a 2D rendition of a 3D CBCT. The images showing tracing on conventional 2D radiographs in the sections that follow also provide the anatomical names of the structures to be traced.

Cervical area. Tracing hard tissue can start in either of several places, for example the cervical bones, the cranial base, or the anterior profile starting at the forehead. The choice of the starting point is personal and probably depends on the initial training.

Some clinicians prefer to start their tracings with the cervical bones to minimize the chance of missing important findings such as fused or missing cervical bones (see chapter 12). Be-

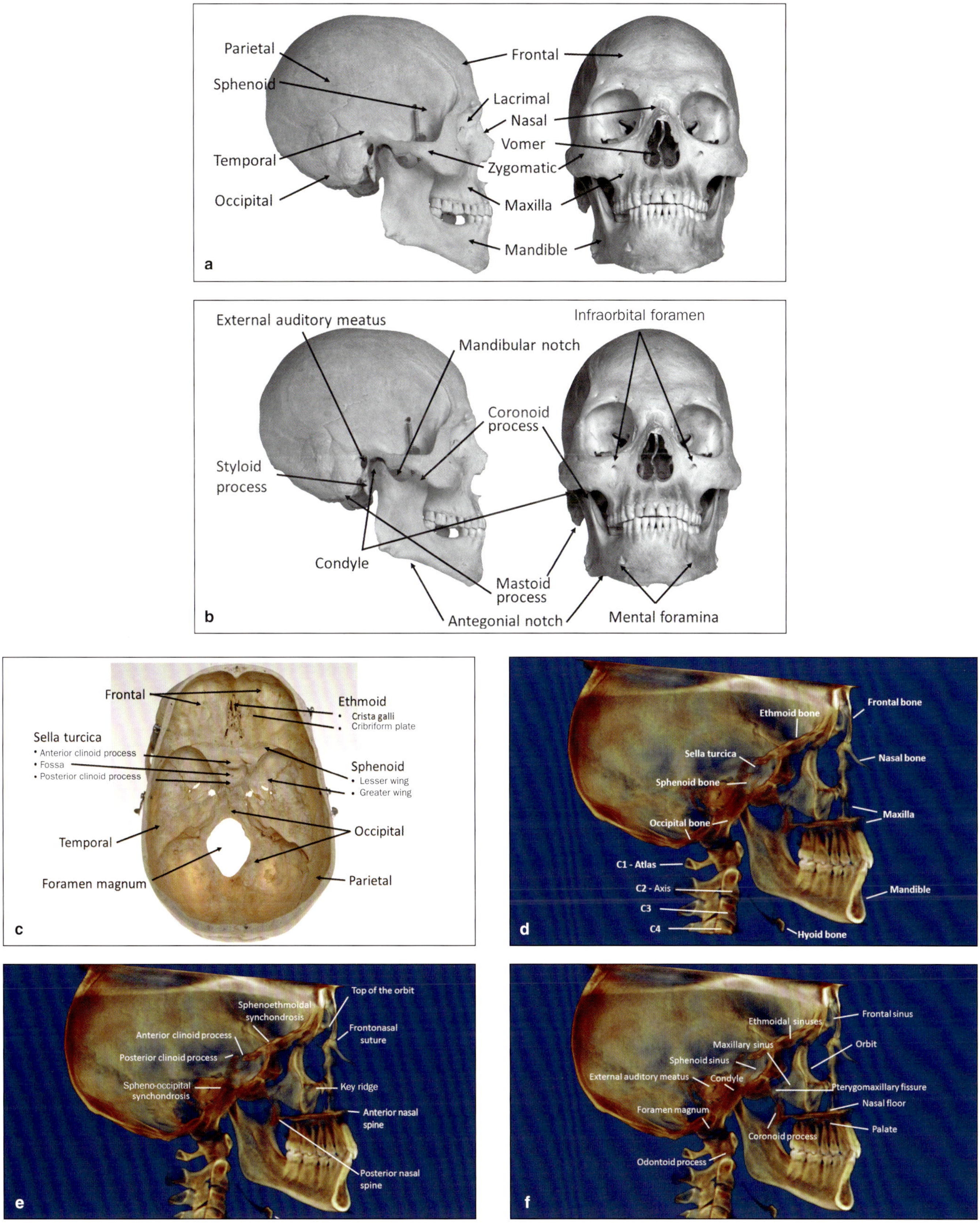

Fig 3-6 External and internal skull anatomy. *(a)* The bones of the face and the cranium are identified laterally and frontally. *(b)* Cranial and facial structures used in 2D and 3D cephalometry are identified on a skull. *(c)* Intracranial structures related to cephalometry are identified on the skull. *(d)* Cranial, facial, and cervical bones identified on a 2D rendition of a 3D CBCT. *(e)* Extracranial structures identified on a 2D rendition of a 3D cephalogram. *(f)* Additional structures that need to be identified on a lateral cephalogram.

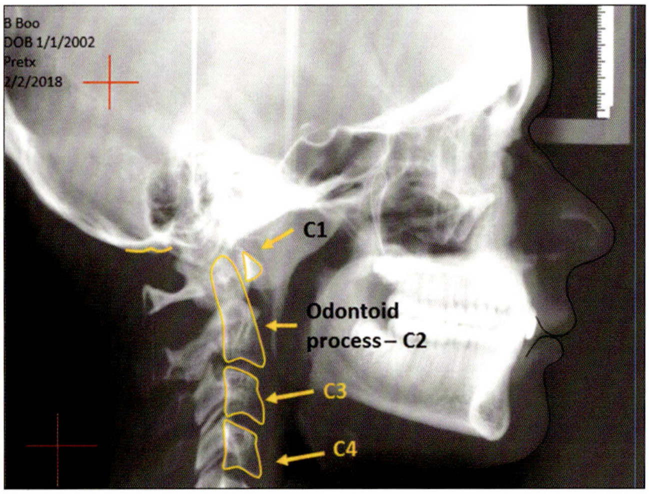

Fig 3-7 The cervical bones (C1, odontoid process of C2, C3, and C4) are traced as well as the external outline of the occipital bone posterior to the foramen magnum.

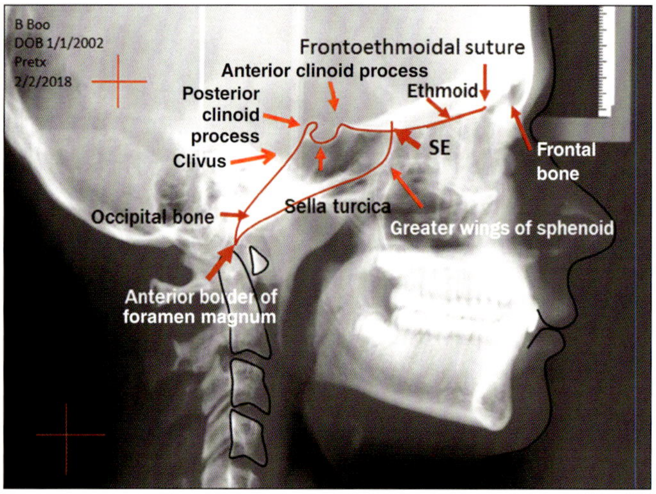

Fig 3-8 The tracing of the cranial base includes the occipital, sphenoid, and ethmoid bones and the frontoethmoidal suture. SE, ethmoid registration point.

cause the odontoid process of C2 is usually more obscure than the other bones, trace it first. It usually looks like a finger pointing superiorly on the spinal column to the skull and will help identify the position of basion (Fig 3-7). Trace the most inferior portion first, then up one side to the point and then down the other side.

Trace the first, second, third, and, if visible, fourth vertebrae, being sure to follow any inferior curvature and the length of each side as accurately as possible (see Fig 3-7). Tracing the vertebrae will help to determine the growth potential of the patient. At this time, clinicians who use landmarks posterior to the foramen magnum trace the outer aspects of the posterior skull base as well as the most consistent intracranial outline of the posterior skull. Identification of some landmarks (eg, Bolton point) is dependent on viewing the skull posterior to the foramen magnum.

Cranial base. Following the tracing of the posterior skull, the anterior cranial base tracing can start at the posterior clinoid process, moving anteriorly to outline the sella turcica (pituitary gland fossa), up the anterior clinoid process, across the superior portion of the sphenoid bone, and across the ethmoid bones to the posterior portion of the frontal bone (Fig 3-8). The superior portions of the sphenoid and ethmoid bones form the planum sphenoidale. This area is often poorly demarcated because the ethmoid is almost radiographically translucent. Be careful not to include the superior outlines of the orbits, which can be more apparent than the ethmoid bone.

Complete the posterior cranial base by starting at the most inferior point traced on the posterior clinoid process and tracing posteriorly and inferiorly down the back of the sphenoid and the occipital bones to the anterior portion of the foramen magnum. The smooth surface from the posterior clinoid process to the foramen magnum is called the *clivus*. The junction between the sphenoid and the occipital bones is called the *spheno-occipital synchondrosis* because it is cartilaginous. This is a growth site. The junction will appear open radiographically until the average age of 13 years, when it ossifies and appears closed. An open junction is an indication of potential for growth vertically and anteroposteriorly depending on the angle of the posterior cranial base.

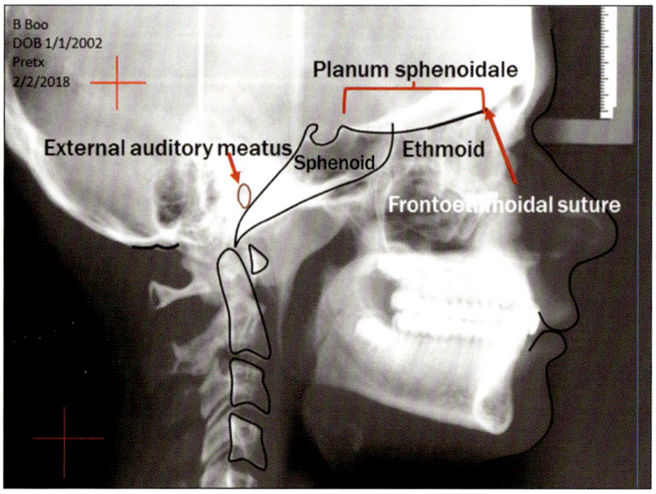

Fig 3-9 The external auditory meatus is traced. It is about the same height as the top of the condyle. Planum sphenoidale is identified as the top of the sphenoid and ethmoid bones.

The most inferior point of the occipital bone at the anterior portion of the foramen magnum is called *basion*, and identification of it is made somewhat easier by identifying the top portion of the odontoid process, which tends to point to it. Trace the anterior portion of the occipital bone and the sphenoid bone to the planum sphenoidale (see Fig 3-9). If the greater wings of the sphenoid show as double, trace between them (average them). Consistency is important in tracing these outlines in the initial, progress, and final tracings for standardization purposes.

Identify the external opening of the external auditory meatus in the temporal bone and trace it (Fig 3-9). The external audito-

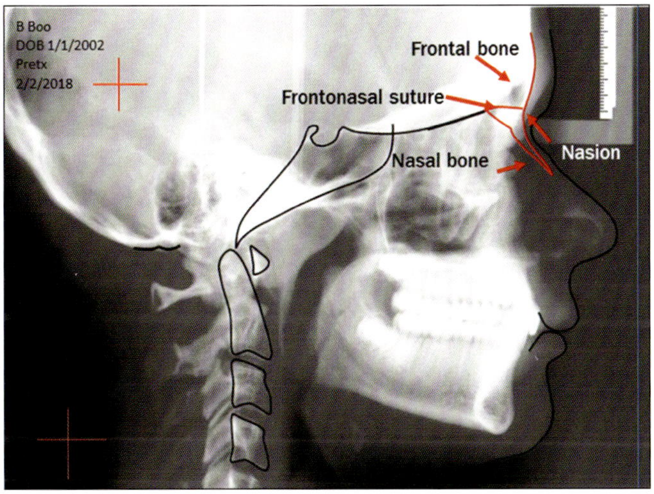

Fig 3-10 The outer cortical plate of the frontal bone and the entirety of the nasal bone, including the frontonasal suture, are traced.

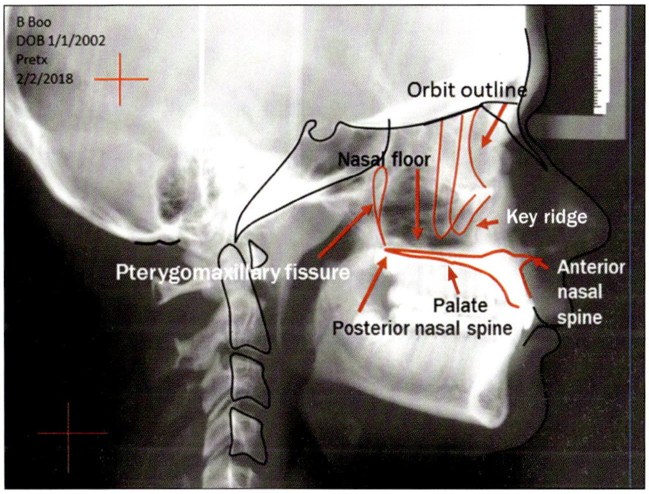

Fig 3-11 The orbits and maxillary structures are traced.

ry canal is frequently identified as a rounded radiolucency posterior to the condyle and vertically at about the same height. Some patients show two radiolucencies in this area, making identification of the correct one to trace difficult. One radiolucency could be the internal auditory meatus at the tympanic membrane, with the other being the external auditory canal opening, or bilateral meatuses are showing. Some cephalometric machines, particularly early machines, have radiopaque ear rods that hide the external auditory canal opening. In that case, the ear rod is traced and labeled as machine porion. The assumption is that the ear rod was placed properly in the external auditory meatus and that the ear rod and its accessories will not extend beyond the meatus.

Frontal and nasal bones. Trace the hard tissue profile starting from the uppermost portion of the forehead, along the supraorbital ridge, and along the entire outline of the nasal bones (Fig 3-10), marking the suture between the frontal bone and the nasal bone. The most anterior portion of the frontonasal suture is nasion.

Maxilla. Identify and trace the pterygomaxillary fissure, a teardrop-shaped radiolucency that is between the posterior of the maxillary bone and the sphenoid bone (see Fig 3-11). Trace from the pterygomaxillary fissure along the nasal floor of the maxilla to the anterior nasal spine; then trace the profile of the anterior maxilla ending at the neck of the most anterior maxillary incisor. Identify the oral side of the palate starting at the cervical portion of the maxillary incisors and trace it to the pterygomaxillary fissure, if tracing 2D images. In 3D, the actual posterior nasal spine can be traced. Frequently, unerupted teeth will obscure the posterior palate, but the pterygomaxillary fissure is used to identify the end of the maxilla. Be aware that the pterygomaxillary fissure denotes the posterior portion of the lateral surface of the maxilla and that the palatine bone, which is the posterior bone of the hard tissue palate, might not extend that far in all subjects. Identify and trace the orbits, being sure to trace the lowermost portion.

Trace the posterior side of the zygoma, including the radiodense base, proceeding anteriorly and connecting with the lowermost portion of the orbit. This area is also called the *key ridge*. Trace the posterior orbital outlines inferiorly and across the inferior border of the orbits and the anterior curve upward (Fig 3-11). Orbits are bilateral structures and often show as two asymmetric structures or shadows. Usually both are traced as dotted structures, and a solid line between them represents the halving of the two structures.

Mandible. The mandibular anterior outline starting at the cervical portion of the most forward mandibular incisor should be traced down the mandible to the chin and up the posterior portion of the symphysis to the inner cortical plate (see Fig 3-12). Trace the lower border of the mandible and the posterior portion of the ramus. If the lower border of the mandible shows up as two shadows, trace the average line between both shadows. This is either an indication of asymmetry between the sides or because of magnification, provided that the patient's head is properly oriented. The condyle should be traced as well as the sigmoid notch and, if possible, the coronoid processes and the anterior portion of the ramus. When finishing tracing the ramus, identify and trace an unerupted molar crown, preferably the third, and the inferior alveolar canal (Fig 3-12). A traced unerupted molar crown and the inferior alveolar canal can be useful for orienting superimpositions.

Teeth. Either trace the teeth directly or use a template to draw the maxillary and mandibular first molars and most forward incisors, making sure the tracing of the incisal tips and inclination of all teeth match the radiographic image as closely as possible (Fig 3-13). Some clinicians trace all erupted permanent teeth.

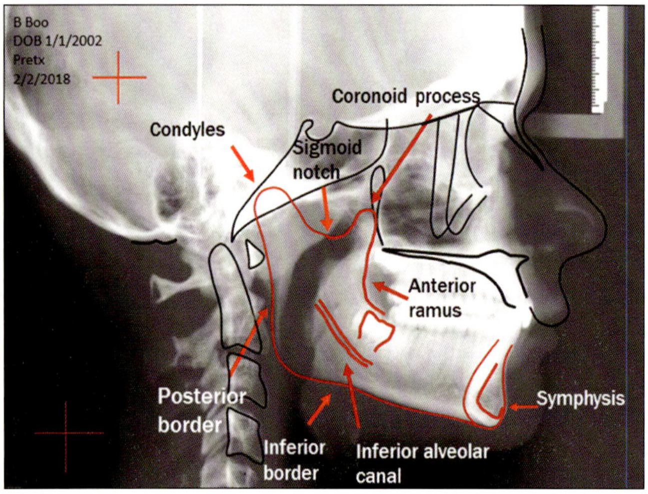

Fig 3-12 The mandibular symphysis, body, ramus, condyles, and coronoid processes are traced. If present, an unerupted molar crown without a root and the inferior alveolar canal should be traced to help with superimpositions.

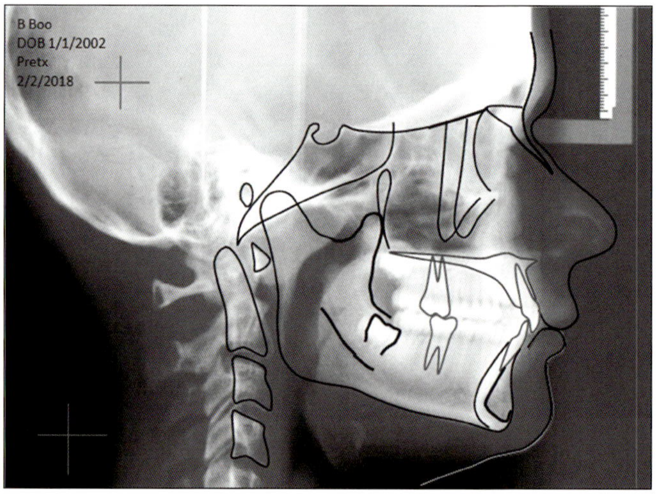

Fig 3-13 Tracing the maxillary and mandibular first molars and the most forward incisors completes the basic tracing process.

Asymmetry. Magnification or asymmetry can cause bilateral structures to show both borders of a bone (eg, mandible) or of teeth. If it appears that magnification causes the borders to be different, some clinicians trace both borders as dashed lines and halve the difference between the borders with a solid line. Other clinicians trace only one border (eg, the right mandible), thinking it is the closest and is least magnified. Whichever way a clinician decides to trace borders should remain consistent to allow reliable interpretation. However, if definitive asymmetry exists, both borders should be traced to be sure that the asymmetry is identified and addressed, if necessary. Also consider the need for a 3D CBCT.

Tracing digital radiographs

Conventional radiographs need to be scanned without distortion and imported as a DICOM (Digital Imaging and Communications in Medicine) file into the computer if computer programs are intended to be used for cephalometric digitization and analysis.

Cephalograms from digital radiographic machines can be imported directly into the cephalometric software. Computerized cephalometric programs generally oblige the clinician to identify landmarks in a specific order, and the program's algorithm curve constructs the tracing based on landmark identification. The clinician must still identify the landmarks. Each software offers choices of cephalometric parameters for the clinician to use and automatically provides the patient values for those parameters. Depending on the software and the person entering the landmarks, there may be errors in a particular measure, so a clinician should always review and correct as necessary.

The computerized tracing will be superimposed over the radiographic image by the software and can be stored in the hard drive for future review separately from the radiographic image. The norms, patient values, and tracing can be printed. The benefits and the problems associated with each method and computer program are topics outside the domain of this chapter.

Identification of Landmarks

Following manual tracing, landmarks are identified[8–10] (Fig 3-14 and Tables 3-1 to 3-3). Then lines and angles are drawn onto the acetate tracing and measured using rulers and cephalometric protractors. Although many lines and angles are used in research to determine changes in various bones or soft tissue and can be found in atlases on craniofacial growth,[8,9,11–13] clinicians tend to use far fewer measures to determine diagnosis and treatment. For utility's sake, only those landmarks associated with measures frequently used in clinical practice are described in this chapter.

The history of cephalometry is so extensive that it is not conceivable to remark on every publication within a single chapter. The reader is referred to the *A Syllabus in Roentgenographic Cephalometry* by Drs Krogman and Sassouni,[4] who reviewed cephalometry from its origin to 1957. This chapter reviews landmarks and parameters (lines, planes, and angles) that the authors feel are pertinent to clinical orthodontics. The information discussed by Krogman and Sassouni[4] is still pertinent today. Some of the discussion is about the inability to accurately identify a bilateral landmark (eg, condyle) on a lateral cephalogram because of the overlying structures and the potential difference in magnification between the right and left condyle.

Given that measurements are objective, the decision as to what is being measured is the question. In addition to the problems of seeing the structure on a cephalogram and reliably identifying a point on the structure, a problem also lies with the definition of the landmark.[4] During the history of cephalometry, various authors have defined landmarks differently enough to question comparison of measures derived in one study with

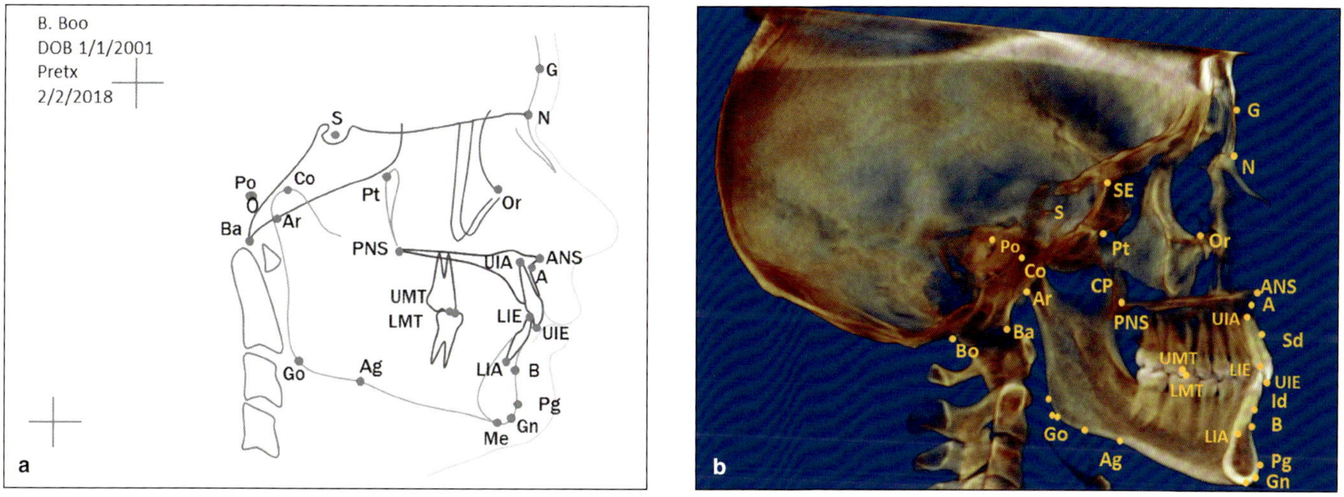

Fig 3-14 Identification of landmarks. *(a)* 2D cephalometric tracing identifying *(dots)* and labeling (acronyms) landmarks. Labeling usually is not needed when the clinician is familiar with the landmarks. *(b)* Identification of landmarks on a 2D rendition of 3D CBCT. Computer programs do not usually label the landmarks. Because the 2D rendition is the internal aspect of a 3D CBCT, the condyle is hidden by the temporal bone, and porion is the internal auditory meatus.

Table 3-1 **2D cephalometric skeletal landmarks listed alphabetically with abbreviation and definition**

Landmark	Abbreviation	Definition
Antegonion	Ag	Highest point of the notch or concavity of the lower border of the ramus where it joins the body of the mandible[8]
Anterior border of the ramus	AB	The intersection of the functional occlusal plane with the anterior border of the ramus[9]
Anterior Downs point	ADP	The midpoint of the line connecting landmarks LIE and UIE; this represents the anterior point through which Downs occlusal plane passes[9]
Anterior nasal spine	ANS	Sharp median process formed by the forward prolongation of the two maxillae at the lower margin of the anterior aperture of the nose[8]
	ANS	The tip of the median, sharp bony process of the maxilla at the lower margin of the anterior nasal opening[9]
Articulare	Ar	Intersection of the lateral radiographic image of the posterior border of the ramus with the base of the occipital bone (Bjork)[8] On the lateral cephalometric tracing, the point of intersection of the posterior border of the condyle of the mandible with the Bolton plane (Bolton)[8]
	Ar	The point of intersection of the inferior cranial base surface and the averaged posterior surfaces of the mandibular condyles[9]
	AA	The point of intersection of the inferior surface of the cranial base and the averaged anterior surfaces of the mandibular condyles[9]
Basion	Ba	Point where the median sagittal plane of the skull intersects the lowest point on the anterior margin of the foramen magnum[8]
	Ba	The most inferoposterior point on the anterior margin of the foramen magnum[9]
Bolton point	Bo	Point in space, about the center of the foramen magnum, that is located on the lateral cephalometric radiograph by the highest point in the profile image of the postcondylar notches of the occipital bone[8]
	BP	The highest point in the retrocondylar fossa in the midline[9]
Condyle	C1	A point on the condyle head that contacts the ramus plane[10]
Condylion	Co	The most posterosuperior point on the curvature of the average of the right and left outlines of the condylar head, determined as the point of tangency to a perpendicular constructed to the anterior and posterior borders of the condylar head; the Co point is located as the most superior axial point of the consular head rather than as the most superior point on the condyle[9]
Coronoid process	CP	The most superior point on the average of the right and left outlines of the coronoid processes[9]

(cont)

Table 3-1 (cont) 2D cephalometric skeletal landmarks listed alphabetically with abbreviation and definition

Landmark	Abbreviation	Definition
Ethmoid registration point	SE	Intersection of the sphenoidal plane with the averaged greater sphenoid wing[9]
Functional occlusal plane point	FPP	Point used to define the posterior location of the functional occlusal plane, and consequently its value is related to the presence (or absence) of molars; if second molars are present, the point is marked at their distal contact points; if second molars are absent, the posterior cusp tip of the maxillary first molar is used[9]
Glabella	G	The height of curvature of the bone overlying the frontal sinus; in cases where this point is not readily apparent, the overlying soft tissue is used to locate it
Gnathion	Gn	Lowest, most anterior midline point on the symphysis of the mandible[8]
	Gn	Most anteroinferior point on the contour of the bony chin symphysis, determined by bisecting the angle formed by the mandibular plane and a line through pogonion and nasion[9]
Gonial intersection	GoI	The intersection of the mandibular plane with the ramal plane[9]
Gonion	Go	External angle of the mandible, located on the lateral radiograph by bisecting the angle formed by tangents to the posterior border of the ramus and the inferior border of the mandible (a line from menton to the posteroinferior border of the mandible)[8]
	Go	Midpoint of the angle of the mandible, found by bisecting the angle formed by the mandibular plane and a plane through articulare, posterior and along the portion of the mandibular ramus inferior to it[9]
Infradentale	Id	The anterosuperior point on the mandible at its labial contact with the mandibular central incisor[9]
Lingual symphyseal point	Sym	A constructed point used to determine symphyseal width at pogonion, located at the intersection of a constructed line that runs through pogonion and is parallel to the posterior border of the mandibular symphysis[9]
Lower first molar	LMT	Mandibular first molar mesial cusp
Lower incisor apex	LIA	The root tip of the mandibular central incisor[9]
Lower incisor incisal edge	LIE	The incisal tip of the mandibular central incisor[9]
Lower incisor lingual bony contact	LIB	The lingual contact of alveolar bone with the mandibular central incisor; generally corresponds with the lingual cementoenamel junction (CEJ)[9]
Menton	Me	Most inferior point on the symphysis of the mandible in the median plane, seen in the lateral radiograph as the most inferior point on the symphyseal outline when the head is oriented in Frankfort relation[8]
	Me	The most inferior point on the symphyseal outline[9]
Nasal bone	NB	The tip of the nasal bone
Nasion	N	Craniometric point where the midsagittal plane intersects the most anterior point of the frontonasal suture[8]
	N	The junction of the frontonasal suture at the most posterior point on the curve at the bridge of the nose[9]
Opisthion	Op	The posterior midsagittal point on the posterior margin of the foramen magnum[9]
Orbitale	Or	In craniometry, the lowest point on the inferior margin of the orbit (left orbit)[8]
	Or	The lowest point on the average of the right and left borders of the bony orbit[9]
Pogonion	Pg	Most anterior point on the symphysis of the mandible in the median plane when the head is viewed in Frankfort relation[8]
	Pg	The most anterior part on the contour of the bony chin, determined by a tangent through nasion[9]
Point A (subspinale)	A	Point in the median sagittal plane where the lowest front edge of the anterior nasal spine meets the front wall of the maxillary alveolar process (Downs point A)[8]
A-point	A	The most posterior point on the curve of the maxilla between the anterior nasal spine and supradentale[9]

(cont)

Table 3-1 (cont) 2D cephalometric skeletal landmarks listed alphabetically with abbreviation and definition

Landmark	Abbreviation	Definition
Point B (supramentale)	B	Deepest midline point on the mandible between infradentale and pogonion (Downs point B)[8]
B-point	B	The point most posterior to a line from infradentale to pogonion on the anterior surface of the symphyseal outline of the mandible; B-point should lie within the apical third of the incisor roots[9]
Point R (Bolton registration point)	R	Center of the Bolton cranial base; a point midway on a perpendicular erected from the Bolton plane to the center of the sella turcica (S)[8]
Porion	Po	Point on the upper margin of the porus acusticus externus[8]
	Po	The midpoint of the line connecting the most superior point of the radiopacity generated by each of the two ear rods of the cephalostat[9]
	Pr	A point located at the most superior point of the external auditory meatus, tangent to the Frankfort plane[10]
Anatomical porion	Apo	The midpoint of a line connecting the most superior points of anatomical poria[9]
Machine porion	Po	Most superior point on the machine ear rod
Posterior border of the ramus	PB	The intersection of the functional occlusal plane with the posterior border of the mandibular ramus[9]
Posterior nasal spine	PNS	Process formed by the united projecting medial ends of the posterior borders of the two palatine bones[8]
	PNS	The most posterior point at the sagittal plane on the bony hard palate[9]
Prosthion	Pr	The most anterior point of the alveolar portion of the premaxillary bone, usually between the maxillary central incisors
Protuberance menti (suprapogonion)	Pm	Point selected at the anterior border of the symphysis between B-point and pogonion where the curvature changes from concave to convex[10]
Pterygoid point	Pt	Intersection of the inferior border of the foramen rotundum with the posterior wall of the pterygomaxillary fissure as viewed in a lateral head film[10]
Pterygomaxillary fissure	PTM	Inverted, elongated, teardrop-shaped area formed by the divergence of the maxilla from the pterygoid process of the sphenoid[8]
Pterygomaxillary fissure inferior	PTMI	The most inferior point on the average of the right and left outlines of the pterygomaxillary fissure[9]
Pterygomaxillary fissure superior	PTMS	The most superior point on the average of the right and left outlines of the pterygomaxillary fissure[9]
Sella turcica	S	Hypophyseal or pituitary fossa of the sphenoid bone, lodging the pituitary body; the landmark S is the center of the sella, as seen in the lateral radiograph and located by inspection[8]
	S	The center of the pituitary fossa of the sphenoid bone, determined by inspection[9]
Supradentale	Sd	The most anteroinferior point on the maxilla at its labial contact with the maxillary central incisor[9]
Suprapogonion	Pm	Point selected at the anterior border of the symphysis between B-point and pogonion where the curvature changes from concave to convex[10]
Upper first molar	UMT	Maxillary first molar mesial cusp
Upper incisor apex	UIA	The root tip of the maxillary central incisor[9]
Upper incisor incisal edge	UIE	The incisal tip of the maxillary central incisor[9]
Upper incisor lingual bony contact	UIB	The lingual contact of alveolar bone with the maxillary central incisor; this point generally corresponds with the lingual CEJ[9]
Labial of the upper incisor	UIL	The most labial aspect of the maxillary incisor[9]
Zygion	Zy	Craniometric points at either end of the greatest bizygomatic diameter or width on the outer surface of the zygomatic arch[8]

Table 3-2 Additional landmarks for Ricketts analysis[10]

Landmark	Abbreviation	Definition
Center of cranium	CC	Point formed from intersection of basion-nasion (BaN) and pterygoid-gnathion
Center of face	CF	Point formed by intersection of Frankfort horizontal and a perpendicular through pterygoid
DC point	DC	Point representing the center of the condylar neck on the BaN line
Gonion	Go	Most lateral point on the mandibular angle close to the bony gonion
Protuberance menti (suprapogonion)	PM	Point selected at the anterior border of the symphysis between B-point and pogonion where the curvature changes from concave to convex
	R1	Deepest point on the curve of the anterior border of the ramus about half the distance between the inferior and superior curves
	R2	Point on the posterior border of the ramus
	R3	Point at the center and most inferior aspect of the sigmoid notch of the ramus
	R4	Point on the lower border of the mandible directly inferior to the center of the sigmoid notch of the ramus
Xi point	XI	Point at the geometric center of the ramus
Distal of maxillary first molar	A6	Horizontal position of the maxillary first molar
Distal of mandibular first molar	B6	Horizontal position of the mandibular first molar

those of other studies. Some authors have only identified landmarks on a figure but did not define them.

Landmarks are selected to identify the vertical or AP position of the various parts of a craniofacial structure. In 3D, these points require definitions that include a third dimension to best define a position or volume of the structure; these are addressed at the end of the chapter. The following sections describe 2D landmarks that define the limits/boundaries of the primary structures of the face—the cranial base, the maxilla, the mandible, and the dentition—and their clinical use. This method, however, leaves out glabella (G), the most anterior point on the frontal bone.

Cranial base landmarks

The cranial base divides the bony face (maxilla, mandible, and teeth) from the cranium and is used to compare the positions of the parts of the face to the cranium. In a lateral cephalogram, the cranial base consists of several bones of cartilaginous origin: the ethmoid, the sphenoid, and the occipital bones (Fig 3-15). The sphenoid and the occipital bones are large transversely and prone to magnification error, whereas the ethmoid is relatively narrow but has multiple sinuses, making visualization difficult (see Fig 3-6c). The easiest way of identifying the ethmoid on a lateral cephalogram is by its junction with the sphenoid and the frontal bones.

The superior portion of the sphenoid (see Fig 3-15) contains a bony structure called the *sella turcica* (Turk's saddle) that surrounds the pituitary gland. The shape of the sella turcica is quite similar to a Turkish saddle, with bony extensions both anterior (anterior clinoid process) and posterior (posterior clinoid process) surrounding a somewhat circular space in which the pituitary gland resides. A major landmark is a point in the center of sella turcica called *sella* (S) (see Table 3-1). The anterior cranial base extends from sella anteriorly to the suture demarcating the ethmoid and the inner cortex of the frontal bone, a portion of the cranium. During development, the anterior portion of the sphenoid bone has a cartilaginous junction, the sphenoidethmoidal synchondrosis, with the ethmoid bone. The synchondrosis gradually ossifies and becomes known as the *sphenoidethmoidal suture* (SE). This sutural landmark is identified by the bilateral greater wings of the sphenoid touching the ethmoid bones. Even though SE could be considered a medial landmark, the width and height of the ethmoid bones makes SE a relatively wide junction. Frequently, two distinct greater wings of the sphenoid are seen touching the ethmoid bones, indicating asymmetry, magnification, or positional error.

Depending on definitions, the most anterior portion of the suture of the frontal bone with the nasal bone is included in the anterior cranial base, although it is really external to the cranial base. That most anterior portion on the frontonasal suture is called *nasion* (N) (see Table 3-1). This landmark can be difficult to identify if the nasal bone grows superiorly over the frontal bone. Pneumatization of the frontal sinus causes expansion of the anterior cortex of the frontal bone. The forward remodeling of the cortex of the frontal bone moves nasion forward, although the junction between the frontal and the ethmoid bones does not appear to move. The inclusion of nasion in the anterior cranial base could explain why the position of the maxilla relative to the anterior cranial base does not change appreciably throughout life when a measure called SNA is used.

Table 3-3 2D cephalometric planes and angles

Parameter	Abbreviation	Definition
AP growth axis		Transverse zone delineated by a plane running through the coronal suture superiorly, passing down through the pterygomaxillary fissure near the posterior termination of the hard palate and then through the junction of the horizontal and vertical component of the mandible[8]
A to N perp to FH		Distance on a straight line from A-point to a line from nasion perpendicular through Frankfort horizontal (FH)[9]
Pg to N perp to FH		Distance on a straight line from pogonion to a line from nasion perpendicular through FH[9]
Bolton plane	BoN	Line joining the Bolton point and nasion on the lateral radiograph[8]
Basion-nasion	BaN	Dividing line between the face and the cranium[10]
Facial angle	FH-NPg	Angle formed by the junction of a line connecting nasion and pogonion (facial plane) with the horizontal plane of the head (FH plane)[8,10]
Facial axis	PtGn-NPg	Expected direction of growth of the chin and the relative height to the depth of the face (pterygoid-gnathion to nasion-pogonion)[10]
Total facial height		Distance between nasion and gnathion when projected on a frontal plane[8]
Facial plane	NPg	Line from nasion to pogonion for measure of facial height and other measures[10]
Frankfort horizontal plane	PoOr	Porion-orbitale[9]
Lower facial height		Distance between anterior nasal spine (ANS) and gnathion when projected on a frontal plane (frontal cephalogram)[8]
Upper facial height		Distance between ANS and nasion when projected on a frontal plane (frontal cephalogram)[8]
Internal angle of the mandible		Located on the lateral radiograph by bisecting the angle formed by tangents to the anterior border of the ramus and the superior border (alveolar crests) of the mandible[8]
Mandibular planes		Tangent to the lower border[8]
	GoGn	Line joining gonion and gnathion[8]
	GoMe	Line joining gonion and menton[8]
	Me	Line from menton tangent to the posteroinferior border[8]
	MeGoI	Menton–gonial intersection[9]
Functional occlusal plane	PMC-FPP	Premolar mesial contact point–functional occlusal plane point[9]
Downs occlusal plane	ADP-PDP	Anterior Downs point–posterior Downs point[9]
Nasion perpendicular	N perp-FH	A line through nasion perpendicular to the FH plane[9]
Upper facial height	N-ANS	Line from nasion to ANS on a lateral cephalogram[9]
Lower facial height	ANS-Me	Line from ANS to menton on a lateral cephalogram[9]
Total facial height	NMe	Line from nasion to menton[9]
Occlusal plane		Line passing through one-half the cusp height of the permanent first molars and one-half the overbite of the incisors[8]
Palatal plane		Line connecting the tip of ANS with the tip of posterior nasal spine (PNS) as recorded on the lateral radiograph[8]
	ANS-PNS	Anterior nasal spine–posterior nasal spine[9]
PTM vertical	PTMI-SE	Pterygomaxillary fissure, interior–ethmoid registration point[9]
Pterygoid vertical	PTV	Perpendicular to FH plane through the distal of the pterygopalatine fissure[10]
Ramal plane	ArGoI	Articulare, posterior–gonial intersection
Sella-nasion plane	SN	Sella-nasion[9]
Sella-nasion/Frankfort plane	SN-PoOr	Sella-nasion plane to porion-orbitale plane[9]
Sella-nasion/palatal plane	SN/ANS-PNS	Sella-nasion plane to ANS-PNS[9]
Sella-nasion/ ramal plane	SN-ArGoI	Sella-nasion plane to posterior articulare–gonial intersection
Sella-basion	SBa	Line from sella to basion to measure the posterior cranial base
y-axis		Line joining sella turcica center (S) and gnathion, which subtends a measurable angle with FH[8]

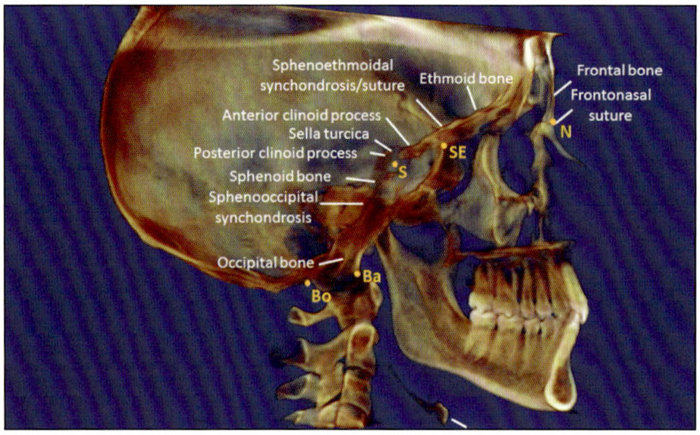

Fig 3-15 The cranial base landmarks are identified on a 2D rendition of a 3D CBCT.

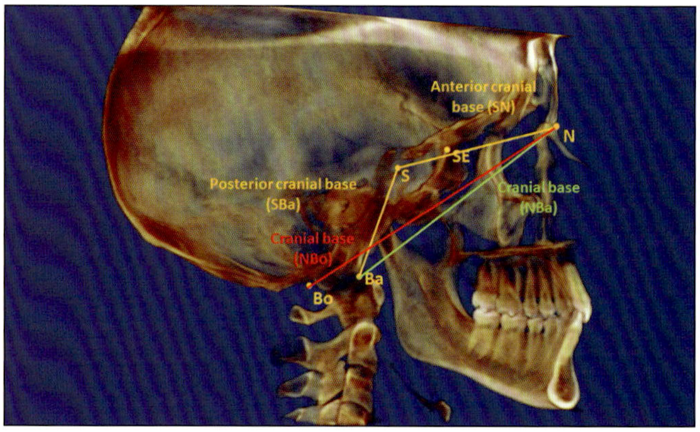

Fig 3-16 Four cranial bases are illustrated: anterior (SN) and posterior (SBa) cranial base parameters are shown in *gold*, nasion to Bolton point (NBo) in *red*, and nasion to basion (NBa) in *green*.

The posterior cranial base extends from sella in the sphenoid bone to the most inferior point of the occipital bone at the anterior base of the foramen magnum. The most inferior point of the occipital bone on the anterior foramen magnum is called *basion* (Ba) (see Table 3-1). The most inferior portion of the sphenoid bone interdigitates with the anterior portion of the occipital bone in a cartilaginous junction called the *spheno-occipital synchondrosis* that frequently is seen on lateral cephalograms until about 13 years of age, when ossification is usually complete. Visual evidence of an open synchondrosis indicates the potential for growth, although an unknown amount of growth.

There is some discrepancy among clinicians and orthodontists as to which landmarks to include in the cranial base (Fig 3-16). Whereas some clinicians consider sella to nasion (SN) to be the anterior cranial base and sella to basion (SBa) to be the posterior cranial base, some clinicians (eg, Bolton) identify landmarks on the portion of the occipital bones posterior to the foramen magnum in the cranial base. Bolton point (Bo), the highest midline point in the retrocondylar fossa, is external to the cranium (see Fig 3-15). It is identified on the exterior portion of the cranium as an indentation on the retrocondyles. Some investigators consider nasion to Bolton point as the cranial base cephalometrically. Bolton point was selected by the Brush Bolton group because Broadbent wanted to better understand the total cranial base and because many of the early cephalostats masked basion.[8] Others (eg, Ricketts) use nasion to basion as the cranial base (see Fig 3-16). Discussion concerning cranial base measures should clarify which parameters are being discussed or measured.

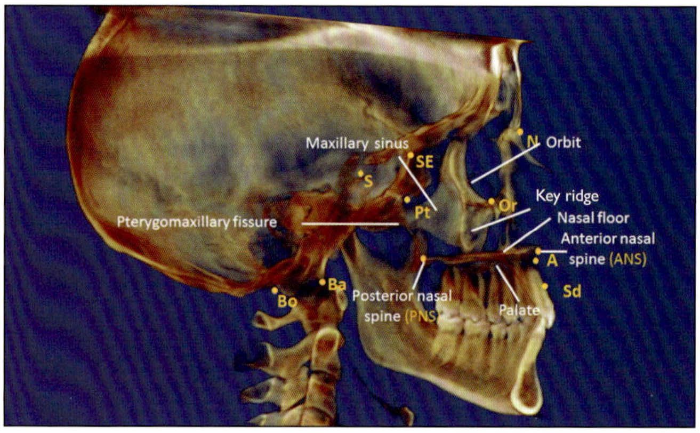

Fig 3-17 Maxillary structures and landmarks are illustrated on a 2D rendition of a 3D CBCT.

Maxillary landmarks

There are several landmarks along the 2D anterior maxillary profile (Fig 3-17). Superiorly, the anterior maxilla is identified cephalometrically as the most inferior edge of the orbital rims, orbitale (Or) (see Fig 3-17 and Table 3-1). Inferior to orbitale, the anterior nasal spine, a thin midline structure supporting the nose, projects anteriorly. The tip of the nasal spine is a landmark called the *anterior nasal spine* (ANS). It is the anteriormost portion of the base of the maxillary nasal cavity. The most anteroinferior portion of the maxillary alveolar bone that touches the most forward maxillary incisor is called *supradentale* (Sd) (see Table 3-1). This landmark is affected by tooth eruption and presence. The thinness of the bone over the incisors makes exact measurement of Sd on CBCTs difficult depending on the resolution of the radiograph. The profile of the maxillary bone is usually concave between ANS and Sd. Another very similar landmark is prosthion (Pr), which is the most anterior point of the alveolar portion of the premaxillary bone, usually between the maxillary central incisors. The most posterior point on the concavity between ANS and Sd currently is called *A-point* (A). A-point is frequently used to define AP skeletal relationships between the maxilla and either the cranial base or the mandible. However, recently, a study[14] comparing 2D lateral cephalograms derived from 3D CBCT images with the same 3D images themselves has shown that in Caucasians, the actual maxillary bone surface is usually posterior

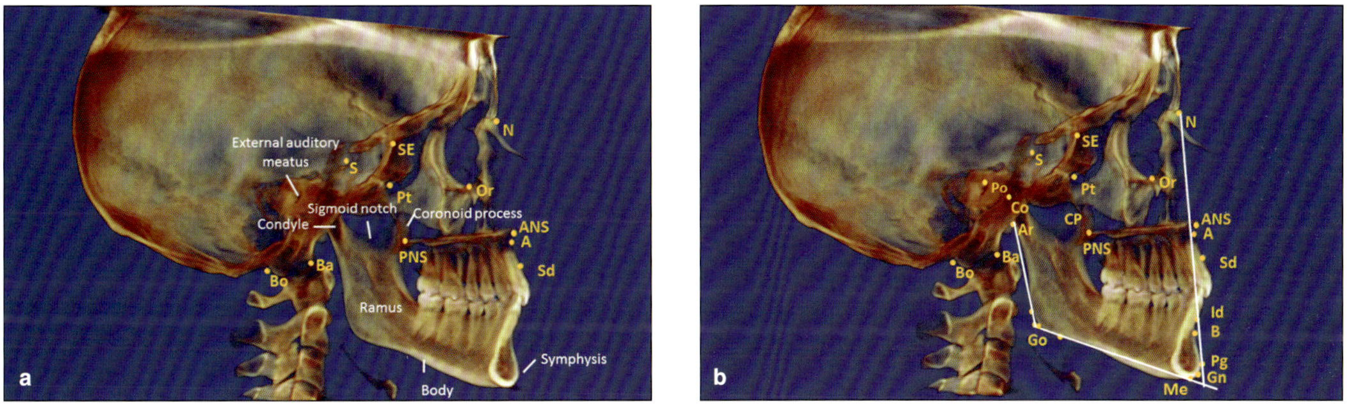

Fig 3-18 Mandibular structures and landmarks. *(a)* Mandibular structures illustrated on a 2D rendition of a 3D CBCT. *(b)* Mandibular landmarks identified on a 2D rendition of a 3D CBCT. The lines drawn as tangents to identify various mandibular landmarks are constructed by the software.

to A-point, questioning the relevance of A-point as a landmark to determine the anterior position of the maxilla. This distance from A-point to the maxillary surface could explain the minimal changes in A-point after various treatments.

Identifying the most anterior landmark of the maxilla depends on the individual and ethnic characteristics of the patient. In some patients, ANS could be considered the most anterior portion of the maxilla, but it is usually just a minor midline projection on the maxilla and is easily obscured by the soft tissue. A-point is defined by the curve between ANS and Sd, which can vary based on the position of the head or the incisor angulation (see Figs 3-1 and 3-17). In some cases, upright incisor roots positioned at the cortical plate mask the position of A-point.

The posterior portion of the maxilla is demarcated by the pterygomaxillary fissure between the maxilla and the sphenoid bone. The most posterior portion of the maxilla at the point that the inferior portion of the palate touches the pterygomaxillary fissure is the landmark called *posterior nasal spine* (PNS), which represents the most distal medial point on the palate. However, PNS is actually on the palatine bone, not the maxilla. In 2D, structures interfere with the identification of the actual PNS. The pterygomaxillary fissure denotes the terminal end of the maxillary alveolar bone. The midpoint of the palatine bone (PNS) usually extends as far distally as the alveolar bone, making the pterygomaxillary fissure a reasonable landmark in 2D for the end of the palate. At the most posterosuperior point of the pterygomaxillary fissure is a maxillary landmark called *pterygoid point* (Pt), which marks the foramen rotundum.

Mandibular landmarks

The most superoanterior portion of the mandible can be noted as the outer cortical plate of the alveolar bone at the anterior of the most forward incisor, *infradentale* (Id) (Fig 3-18; see also Table 3-1). Tooth eruption or loss will affect this landmark. Similar to the maxilla, some landmarks on the profile of the mandible are determined by their projection or retrusion on curves. The most anterior point on the mandibular symphysis or chin is called *pogonion* (Pg). The most posterior point on the curve between Id and Pg is call *B-point* (B). Similar to A-point, B-point and Pg are affected by head position. B-point is also affected significantly by the proclination of the mandibular incisors. In cases where the mandibular incisors are extremely proclined, little or no curve exists between Id and Pg, making identification of B-point difficult and unreliable. In some cases, Pg is also difficult to identify because no chin (distinct outward curve) is apparent. Ethnic characteristics affect the identification of both B-point and Pg.

The most inferior point of the anterior mandibular symphysis is *menton* (Me) (see Table 3-1). Between Pg and Me on the anterior aspect of the symphysis is a constructed landmark called *gnathion* (Gn), which occurs at the intersection of two tangents and another intersecting line. Both tangents, one tangent touching N and Pg and the other tangent touching Me and gonion (a landmark on the most inferior border of the body of the mandible), are extended beyond the borders of the mandible until they intersect each other. Then a line connecting S and the intersection of the two tangents is drawn. Gn has also been defined as the point halfway between Pg and Me.

The landmarks on the inferior border of the mandible seem simple to identify, but the variable anatomy of the mandibular border can complicate landmark identification. If a tangent is drawn contacting Me and the most posterior point on the border of the mandible, that point is called *gonion* (Go) or gonion inferiorus. The inferior border of the mandible can vary in shape from convex to extremely concave. If the border is concave, the most superior point on the curve is antegonion (Ag).

The condyle is the most superior structure of the posterior mandible and is usually rather circular in shape. The landmark condylion (Co) (see Table 3-1) is usually identified as the most posterosuperior point on the condyle, but it has also been defined as the most superior point on the condyle. Unfortunately, in 2D cephalometry, the bilateral condyles are often difficult to see because the temporal bone runs across them on both sides and cranial bones are between them. One key to identifying the condyles is that the top of the condyles is frequently at

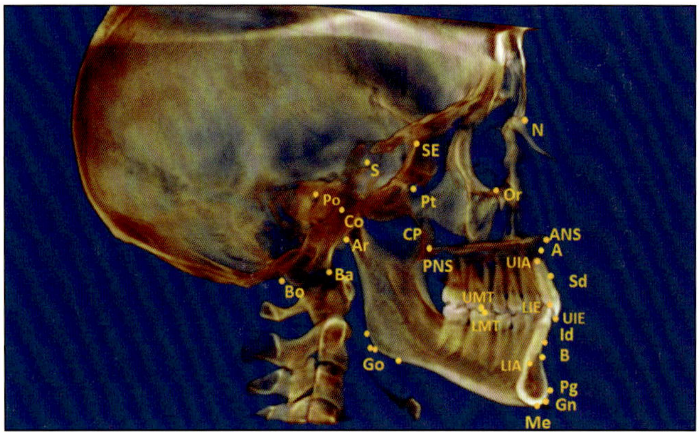

Fig 3-19 Dental landmarks identified on a 2D rendition of a 3D CBCT.

about the height of the top of the external auditory meatus. The most superior point on the external meatuses is called *porion* (Po). The angle of the external auditory canal is relatively flat in young children and gradually angles inferiorly with age and growth,[15] possibly making the outline of the external auditory meatus less distinct.

As the mandibular outline is traced to the angle of the mandible, the ramus intersects the outline of the temporal bone. The point at which the posterior border of the ramus intersects the inferior border of the temporal bone is easily identified and is called *articulare* (Ar). If a tangent is dropped from Ar inferiorly along the posterior border of the ramus to the point that touches the tangent, this ramal point is gonion superiorus (Go superiorus). The tangent should continue until it intersects the tangent touching the lower border of the mandible. The intersection of the two tangents is called *gonion intersectus*. If the angle is bisected and the bisecting line carried to the border of the mandible, that point on the mandibular angle is called *constructed gonion*. So technically four gonions are identified in the literature, and measures using gonion need to identify which landmark is being used.

The coronoid process (CP) is probably one of the most difficult landmarks to identify because of the overlying tissues. CP is the most superior point on the averaged coronoid processes (see Table 3-1). In order to identify the processes, the coronoid notches and the anterior borders of the rami need to be traced. Many times, a dashed line is used to portray the coronoid processes because it cannot be identified exactly.

Dentition

Usually the incisal/cuspal and apical tips of the first molars and the most forward maxillary and mandibular permanent incisors are used as landmarks to show current AP positions of the dentition. By using a straight line to connect the incisal or cuspal tips of each molar or incisor with its apical root tips, the inclination of the tooth relative to a reference plane or another structure can be determined as an angle. The incisal or cuspal tip can be measured linearly to another plane or structure. The upper incisor tip or edge (UIE) and the lower incisor tip or edge (LIE) are usually much easier to discern than the upper incisor root apex (UIA) and the lower incisor root apex (LIA) (Fig 3-19; see also Table 3-1). The root of the most forward incisor can be particularly difficult to identify during the mixed dentition when the canines could be overlying the incisor roots or the roots are not fully formed.

The maxillary first molar mesial cusp tips (UMT) are frequently interdigitated with the mandibular first molar mesial cusp tips (LMT) or another tooth's cusp tips, making them difficult to identify. The root apices of the maxillary first molars and the mandibular first molars are more difficult to identify reliably. Because these teeth are usually bilateral, slight magnification differences and particularly asymmetry make identification of molar landmarks unreliable. Reviewing the patient's dental cast or image of the mouth can be helpful while tracing these teeth.

3D Landmarks

The same landmarks can be identified in 3D images as either a 2D rendition, which has some of the same problems as a regular 2D image, or as a totally 3D image. If the actual 3D image is used, each landmark must be identified in three dimensions—anteroposteriorly, vertically, and transversely[16] (Figs 3-20 to 3-30). In addition, the measures may need to be interpreted differently depending on the curvature of the structures.

Reliability of landmark identification is important because it affects the measures that are demarcated by those landmarks. The reliability of landmarks varies both in 2D and in 3D. Lagravère et al[16] compared the reliability of landmark identification using digitized 2D cephalograms and 3D reconstructed CBCTs. Intraexaminer reliability was high for most landmarks except porion, basion, and condylion on 2D lateral cephalograms in both the x and the y coordinates. Interexaminer reliability for those three landmarks was less so. In contrast, both intraexaminer and interexaminer reliability for all landmark identification was high in the x, y, and z coordinates using 3D reconstructed CBCTs. Landmarks on flat or curved surfaces showed lower reliability as did landmarks (eg, condylion) located on structures with lower radiodensity. Other structures (ie, root apices) are difficult to identify in 3D because of the small distance between two radiodense structures, the root and cortical bone. They suggested that new landmarks should be considered for 3D CBCT analysis.

3D CBCT images could be considered reliable in terms of landmark identification, but the lack of a standardized 3D cephalometric analysis, inconsistent use of 3D landmark definitions, the variability of 3D image acquisition and reconstruction, and the use of different software programs and scanning settings could question the reliability of the 3D cephalometric analysis. In addition to the aforementioned factors, bilateral landmarks should be identified and measured on both sides, which makes the 3D cephalometric process more complicated. Similar to 2D analysis, it has been found that the 3D landmarks located on the median sagittal plane and dental landmarks are more reliable than landmarks located on a curvature such as condyle, porion, and orbitale.

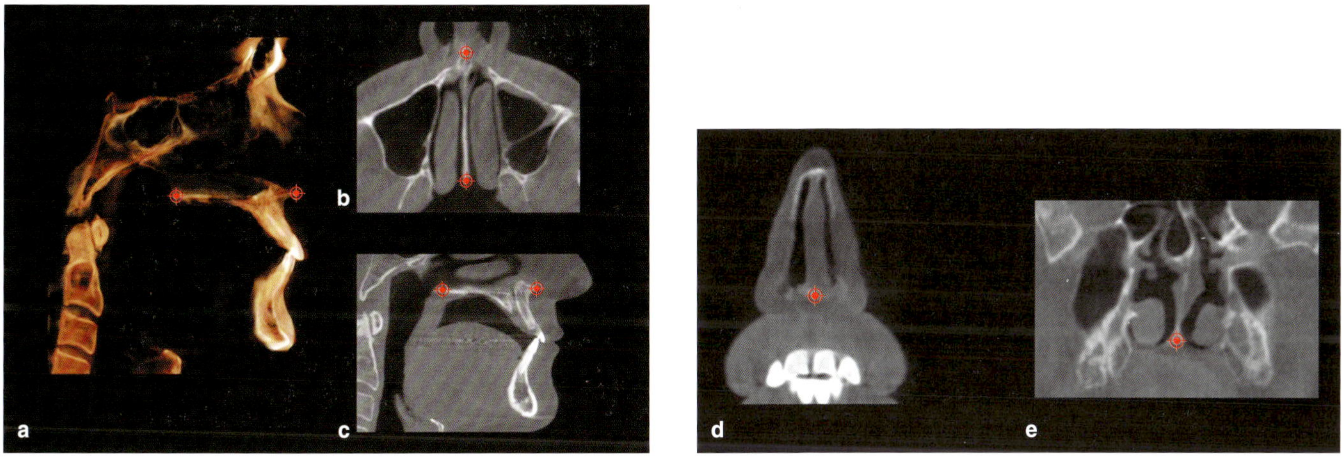

Fig 3-20 ANS and PNS located on multiple images. *(a)* 3D image, midsagittal view. *(b)* Axial section oriented with the palatal plane parallel to the floor. *(c)* Sagittal section oriented with the palatal plane parallel to the floor. *(d)* Coronal section showing the tip of the bony ANS and oriented with the palatal plane perpendicular to the true vertical. *(e)* Coronal section showing the most posterior point along the palatal plane and oriented with the palatal plane perpendicular to the true vertical plane.

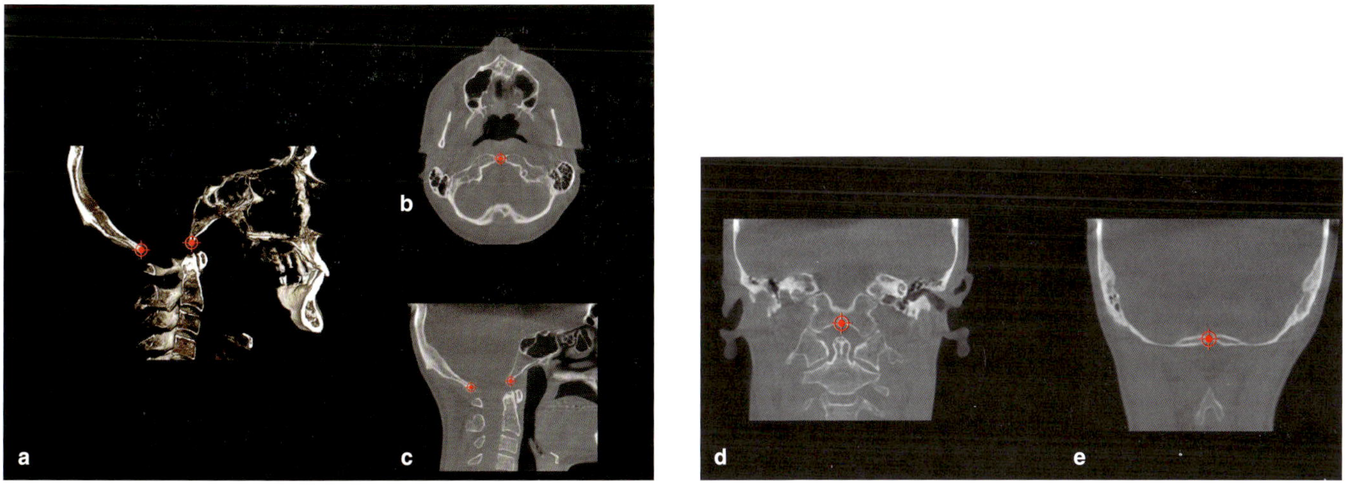

Fig 3-21 Ba and opisthion (Op) located on multiple images. *(a)* 3D image, midsagittal view. *(b)* Axial section oriented with the palatal plane parallel to the floor. *(c)* Sagittal section at the level of the midsagittal plane, oriented with the palatal plane parallel to the floor. *(d)* Coronal section showing Ba point and oriented with the palatal plane perpendicular to the true vertical. *(e)* Coronal section showing Op point and oriented with the palatal plane perpendicular to the true vertical plane.

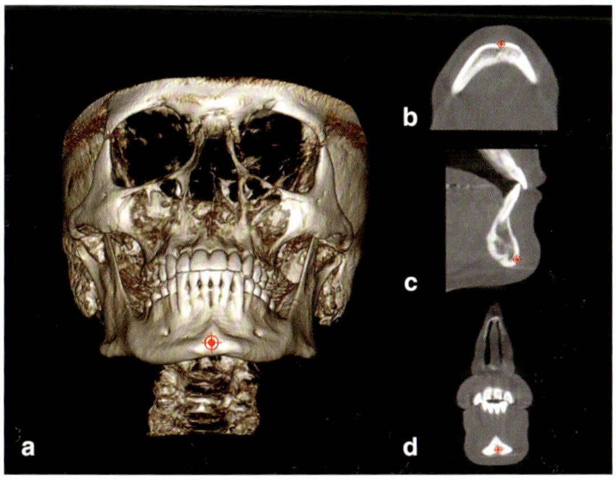

Fig 3-22 Gn, the most anteroinferior point on the symphysis, located on multiple CBCT images. *(a)* 3D reconstruction. *(b)* Axial section. *(c)* Sagittal section at the level of the midsagittal plane. *(d)* Coronal section.

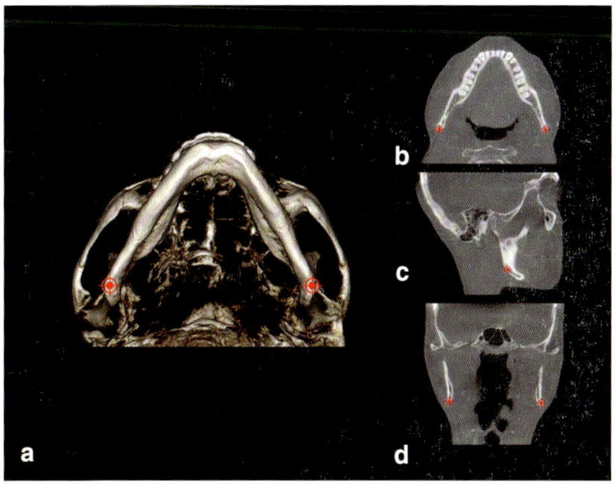

Fig 3-23 Go (right and left sides) located on the curvature of the mandibular angle on multiple CBCT images. *(a)* 3D reconstruction. *(b)* Axial section at the level of the angle of the mandible. *(c)* Sagittal section at the level of the right Go. *(d)* Coronal section at the level of right and left Go points.

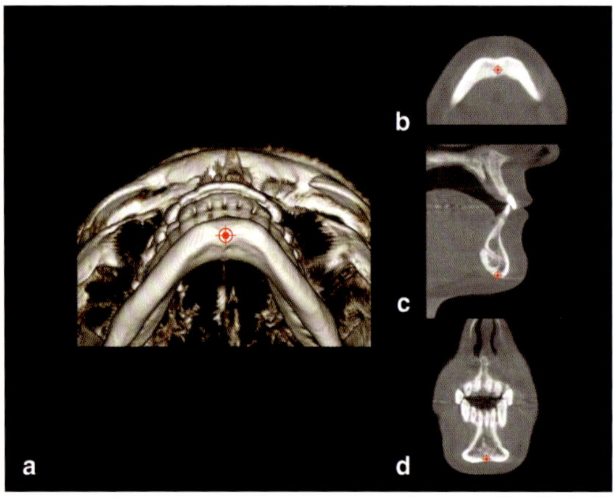

Fig 3-24 Me, the most inferior point on the symphysis of the mandible, located on multiple CBCT images. *(a)* 3D reconstruction. *(b)* Axial section. *(c)* Sagittal section oriented at the midsagittal plane. *(d)* Coronal section.

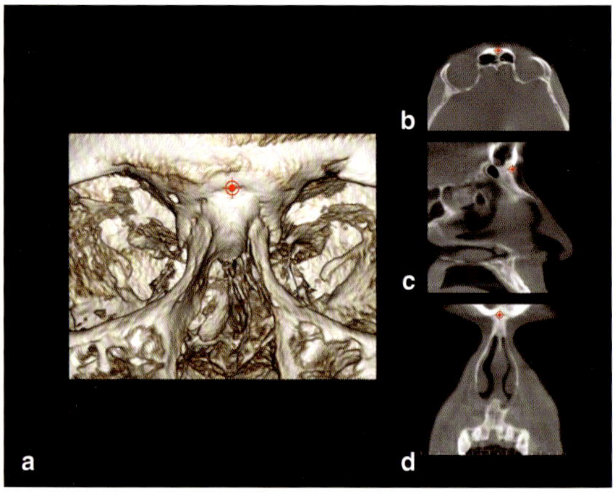

Fig 3-25 N, the most anterior point on the frontonasal suture, located on multiple CBCT images. *(a)* 3D reconstruction. *(b)* Axial section. *(c)* Sagittal section at the level of the midsagittal plane. *(d)* Coronal section.

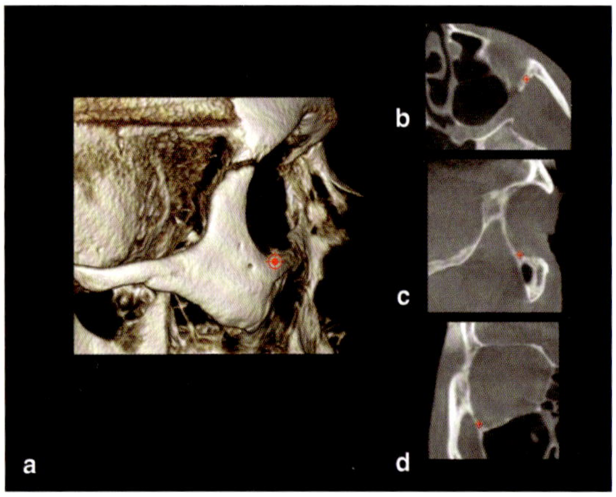

Fig 3-26 Or, the most inferior point on the inferior margin of the orbit, located on multiple CBCT images. *(a)* 3D reconstruction at the level of the right Or. *(b)* Axial section at the level of the right Or. *(c)* Sagittal section at the level of the right Or. *(d)* Coronal section at the level of the right Or.

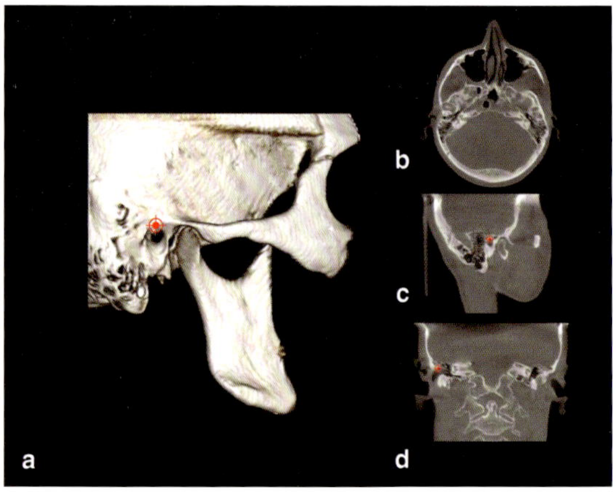

Fig 3-27 Po, the most superior point at the border of the external auditory meatus, located on multiple CBCT images. *(a)* 3D reconstruction, right Po. *(b)* Axial section. *(c)* Sagittal section at the level of the right Po. *(d)* Coronal section.

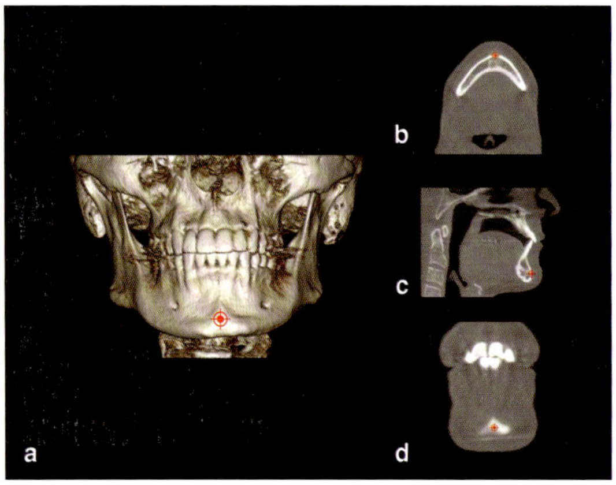

Fig 3-28 Pg, the most anterior point on the bony chin, located on multiple CBCT images. *(a)* 3D reconstruction. *(b)* Axial section. *(c)* Sagittal section at the level of the midsagittal plane. *(d)* Coronal section.

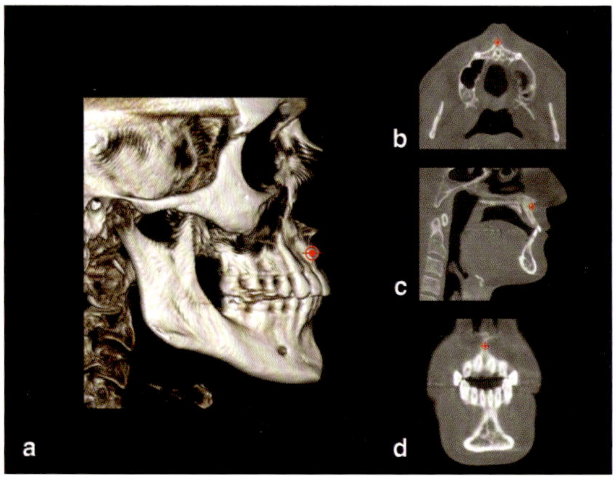

Fig 3-29 A-point, the most posterior point on the concavity between ANS and prosthion (see Table 3-1), located on multiple images. *(a)* 3D reconstruction. *(b)* Axial section. *(c)* Sagittal section at the level of the midsagittal plane. *(d)* Coronal section.

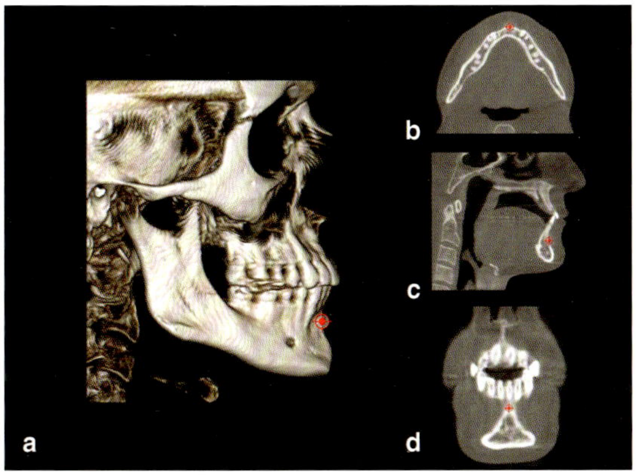

Fig 3-30 B-point, the most posterior point on the concavity between pogonion and the mandibular alveolar process (see Table 3-1), located on multiple CBCT images. *(a)* 3D reconstruction. *(b)* Axial section. *(c)* Sagittal section at the level of the midsagittal plane. *(d)* Coronal section.

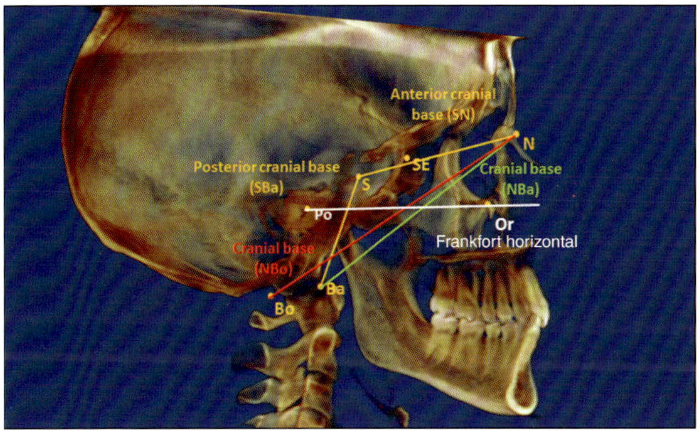

Fig 3-31 FH (PoOr) is compared to four cranial base cephalometric measures: anterior (SN) and posterior (SBa) cranial base parameters are shown in *gold*, nasion to Bolton point (NBo) in *red*, and nasion to basion (NBa) in *green*.

Reference Planes

Connecting the dots (landmarks) now becomes important in the interpretation of the cephalogram. A line is the connection of two landmarks. In 2D cephalometry, a plane is really just a straight line connecting two landmarks. A line is only one dimension, whereas a plane is two dimensions. Although definitions of such planes as the Frankfort horizontal (FH) plane include identifying landmarks on both sides of the skull, in actuality, the points are averaged in 2D to a single point and connected by a line. In other words, a plane used in 2D cephalometry is usually a misnomer, being just a line. For the sake of continuity, we will maintain the same jargon. Actual planes can be constructed in 3D.

The FH plane, for example, is a reference plane transferred from craniometry. The top of the external auditory meatus (porion) and the inferiormost portion of the orbit (orbitale) are connected using a straight line in 2D cephalometry (Fig 3-31). If the right and left porion and the right and left orbitale are each identified as separate landmarks, the bilateral points are usually averaged in 2D and the averaged portion and orbitale connected with a line.[4] It is impossible in 2D to construct a plane between the four landmarks and then measure linearly or angularly from other landmarks to them. So a line is actually constructed using the average of the landmarks. A plane can be constructed in 3D.

This can be confusing though when determining symmetry on a 2D frontal cephalogram using the midsagittal plane, for example, which is in actuality just a vertical line through various landmarks on the front of the face without assurance that the posterior portion of the head is in alignment (on the same plane) with the anterior face. The midsagittal plane is more easily defined and constructed in 3D.

In 2D cephalometry, a plane is frequently a reference from which other measures are made. For example, the position of the maxilla, the mandible, the teeth, and other craniofacial structures are determined relative to planes, eg, the sella-nasion (SN) plane or the FH. These planes can divide the face vertically or anteroposteriorly. Historically,[4] multiple planes have been created by authors trying to measure growth, development, and treatment effects. Some of the planes are still used in modern cephalometry and have been transferred to 3D cephalometry. Figure 3-31 provides an example of three planes used to study growth, development, and treatment effects. Various orthodontic camps reference one plane more than another based on their rationale of head position and landmark reliability.

Cephalometric reference planes can be AP or vertical. Krogman and Sassouni[4] suggest that planes can be used for orientation or for superimposition but that not all planes are effective in both roles. The role of a plane in determining orientation of the facial structures to each other is important in determining prognathism as well as in static situations. A plane used for superimposition is more important for growth studies and to compare treatment effects. The following sections relate facial structures to each other first in an AP direction and then in a vertical direction.

Frankfort horizontal plane

The FH plane (see Fig 3-31) is based on an agreement by anatomists in the 1800s to establish a common reference plane for the study of skulls. The bilateral external auditory meatuses (Po) and the lowest point on the right orbital rim (Or) were easily identifiable on the 3D external skull. The transfer of these landmarks to a 2D lateral cephalogram (Fig 3-32) is more complicated due to the 2D nature of the radiographs, magnification of bilateral landmarks, asymmetry, the confounding presence of soft and hard tissue, and the size and radiopacity of various ear rods, particularly those used in early cephalometric machines. The mean average of the FH plane according to Downs[17] was closely related to the natural balance of the head

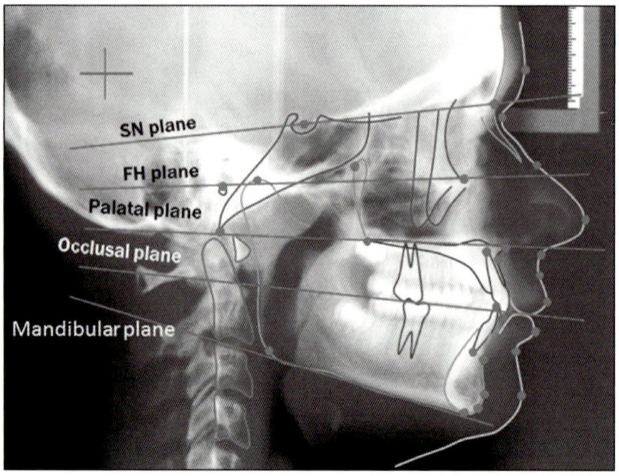

Fig 3-32 Planes used in cephalometry (SN, FH, palatal, occlusal, and mandibular) illustrate the slight convergence of the lines posterior to the cranium in a reasonably well-balanced face. No plane is intersecting another within the cranium.

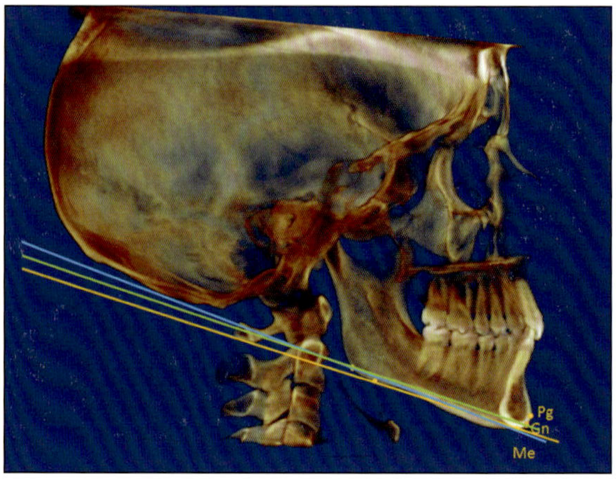

Fig 3-33 Three mandibular planes are illustrated to show potential differences in measures depending on the landmarks used (Me versus Gn, mandibular border versus constructed Go).

(difference = 0.9 ± 5 degrees). In 2D cephalometry, the identification of porion and orbitale can be unreliable, especially when ear rods mask porion. In 3D, these landmarks should be much more reliably identified. FH has also been a useful reference for standardizing cephalometric head position during imaging. Tweed[5] believed FH to be a practical basis for comparing patient profiles and radiographs.

Bolton plane

Broadbent chose the landmarks nasion and Bolton point to anchor the Bolton plane (see Fig 3-31). The ear rods of early cephalostats made it difficult to determine anatomical porion and basion. Broadbent also wanted to examine the entire cranial base and chose Bolton point as a reference.

Nasion-basion plane

Although many horizontal planes have been developed in cephalometric history,[4] only a few remain. In some cases, the names might have been changed. For example, the plane extending from nasion to basion has also been called *Huxley's plane*, but it has been used extensively by Ricketts and the bioprogressive camp as a substitute for SN (see Fig 3-31).

Mandibular plane

The landmarks establishing the mandibular plane vary. One definition by Downs[17] is a tangent to the lower border of the mandible extending from the lowest point on the mandibular symphysis (Me) through the lowest posterior point on the gonial angle (Go) (Fig 3-33; see also Fig 3-32). Downs measured the angle between FH and the mandibular plane. The norm for 20 children with excellent occlusions was 21.9 degrees, with a range of 17 to 28 degrees.[17] The lower the angle, the more a tendency to Class II, division 2 malocclusion with a deep bite exists. The higher the angle, the more hyperdivergent is the patient profile, and potentially the greater is the tendency to open bite.

Tweed[5] called the angle between FH and the mandibular plane the Frankfort mandibular angle (FMA) and used this angle as a part of a triangle to help determine the needs for extractions and the prognosis of the case. If FMA is 16 to 28 degrees, the prognosis is excellent and the treatment option would include ±5-degree variation of the mandibular incisor. If FMA is 28 to 32 degrees, the prognosis is good to fair, but the treatment option indicates extraction. If FMA is 32 to 35 degrees, the prognosis is fair to not favorable, and the patient will not benefit from orthodontic treatment. An FMA between 35 and 45 degrees indicates that the prognosis is not favorable. Prognosis is very poor if FMA is greater than 45 degrees. Visually, either cephalometrically or clinically, if the mandibular plane is extended posteriorly in a case with a favorable growth pattern, the mandibular plane intercepts FH approximately 3.5 to 3.8 inches posterior to tragion. As the mandibular plane angle increases, the mandibular plane will intercept FH closer and closer to the tragus (projection of the outer ear tissue that points to the external auditory meatus). As the mandibular plane angle decreases, interception of the two planes occurs quite far behind the head. Today, the options would include orthognathic surgery when the prognosis is not favorable.

Other clinicians such as Steiner[3] compared the mandibular plane to SN and various planes. Steiner constructed a mandibular plane based on a line from the constructed gnathion (Gn) to constructed gonion (Go). His rationale was that the border of the mandible varied significantly among patients.

Behrents showed that the mandibular plane (MeGoI) to SN angle was significantly greater for adult women than for men.[9] Cephalometric software uses 32.9 ± 5.2 degrees as the norm for Caucasian adults.

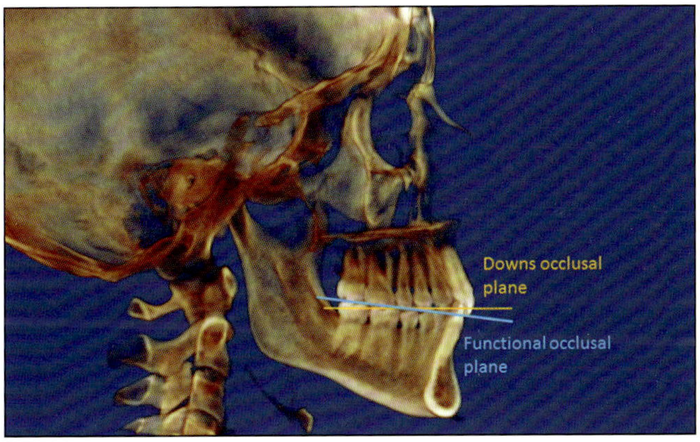

Fig 3-34 Difference in occlusal planes (Downs and functional occlusal plane) can occur in patients with deep bites.

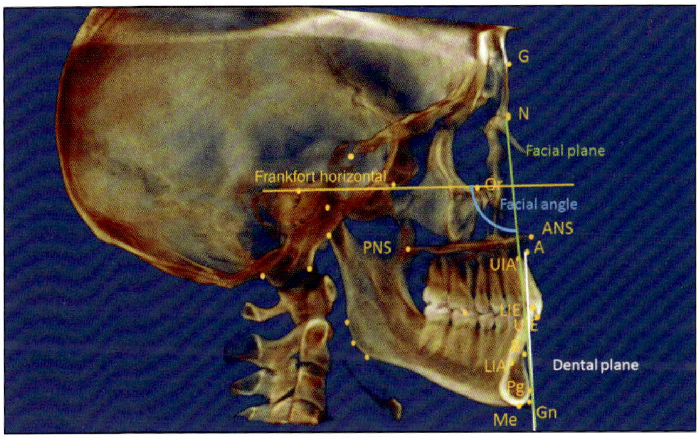

Fig 3-35 Frontal planes: facial plane, NPg *(green)*; dental plane, APg *(white)*; and facial angle, the angle between FH and NPg *(blue)*.

Occlusal plane

Downs defined the *occlusal plane* as the bisection of the points denoting the intersections of the first permanent molars and of the incisors[18] (Fig 3-34). He also drew another occlusal plane that followed a line between the first permanent molars and the premolars that is known as the *functional occlusal plane* in patients with severe malocclusions. The functional occlusal plane can differ from the other occlusal plane in cases with supraeruption of the mandibular incisors and in open bite cases. Linear measures can be made to or along this plane, although the occlusal plane is often compared as an angle to other planes. The average angle between the occlusal plane and FH in adolescents with excellent occlusions was 9.3 degrees with a range of 14.0 to 1.5 degrees. Behrents reported that the mean angle for the occlusal plane to SN varied slightly among adult males and females depending on age.[9] Adult women had significantly larger angles than men, indicating more anterior divergence in this area.

Palatal plane

The palatal plane is the AP line from ANS to PNS (see Fig 3-32) and represents the vertical orientation of the maxilla. The length can be measured linearly or compared to other reference planes. For example, the norm for the angle between SN and ANS-PNS is 8.0 ± 2.5 degrees, and the norm for the angle between GoGn and ANS-PNS is 25.0 ± 6.0 degrees. A decreased angle between GoGn and ANS-PNS could indicate lack of maxillary molar eruption or a decreased mandibular plane. In this case, a deeper bite could be expected. An increased angle between GoGn and ANS-PNS could indicate a maxilla tipped anteriorly or an increased mandibular plane. Both could be indicative of an open bite.

Dental plane

The dental plane extends vertically from A-point to Pg and is used to determine protrusion of the incisors to the apical bases of the maxilla and the mandible (Fig 3-35).

Facial plane

The facial plane (NPg) provides a reference for the convexity or concavity of the profile based on the cranium and the mandible (see Fig 3-35).

According to Downs,[18] the facial angle is the internal angle between NPg and FH (see Fig 3-35). This plane represents the AP position of the mandible. Although the means were different, Downs found little difference in the range when he compared the values of the facial angle to the values for NPg to SN and to BoPg (Bolton plane) in cases with excellent occlusions. The mean value for the facial angle is 87.8 ± 3.6 degrees.

Maxilla to Cranial Base

Anteroposteriorly

The protrusion of the maxilla relative to the cranial base can either be measured as an angle or as a distance of a landmark to a plane using any of several measures. Protrusion can be measured as the angle between SN and A-point to nasion (SNA) (Fig 3-36a). The norm is 82 ± 3.8 degrees for Caucasians with excellent occlusion[19] and changes minimally with age. There are ethnic differences, which are discussed in chapter 6.

Protrusion of the maxilla can also be measured as the distance between A-point and N perpendicular to FH[20] (see Fig 3-36a). In a well-balanced, mixed-dentition face, the measurement averages 0 mm and increases slightly in the adult face. An adult female measurement averages 0.4 ± 2.3 mm, and an adult male measurement averages 1.1 ± 2.7 mm. A measurement of A-point anterior to N perpendicular is given a positive value, whereas a measurement posterior to N perpendicular is

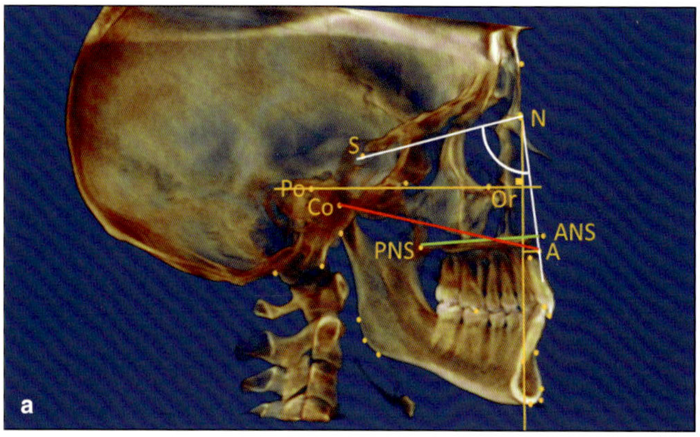

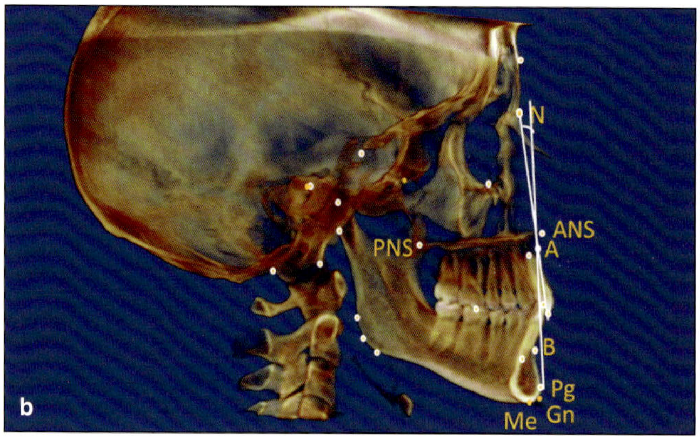

Fig 3-36 *(a)* Maxillary relationships: SNA *(white)*; A (mm) to N perpendicular to Frankfort horizontal *(gold)*; length of maxilla, ANS to PNS (mm) *(green)*; and relative maxillary length, Co to A (mm) *(red)*. *(b)* Angle of convexity, maxilla to cranium and chin (angle between NA and APg) (degrees) *(white)*.

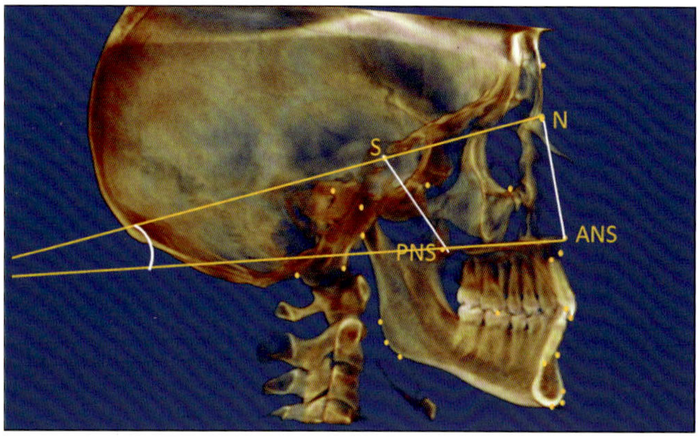

Fig 3-37 Vertical maxillary measures to the cranial base: anterior upper facial height, N-ANS (mm) *(white)*; posterior maxillary height, S-PNS (mm) *(white)*; and relative maxillary height, angle between SN and ANS-PNS (degrees) *(gold)*.

given a negative value. The larger the positive value, the more protruded the maxilla is compared with the cranial base; the larger the negative number, the more retruded the maxilla. A retrusive cranial base is corrected by constructing a parallel line to N perpendicular passing through A-point.

The length of the maxilla can be measured as ANS-PNS (see Fig 3-36a), with a norm of 51.6 ± 4.3 mm (used in cephalometric software).

The angle of convexity (NA-APg) relates the protrusion of the maxilla to both the cranium and the chin (Fig 3-36b). In teenagers with excellent occlusion, the two lines would merge and there would be no angle (0 degrees). The lines would merge to form a single straight line. In other words, the angle of convexity would be the same as the facial plane. However, the range is +10 degrees (convex) to –8.5 degrees (concave). If A-point is distal to the facial plane, the angle would be negative, and if A-point is mesial to the facial plane, the angle would be positive. The more negative the angle, the more concave the face, and the more positive the angle, the more convex the face.

Vertically

The significance of the following measures should not be considered as absolutes but as related to other vertical measures (ie, facial proportions). Large faces can have larger measures than small faces but still be proportional. Measures of the anterior face can be proportional to each other but not to posterior measures.

The distance from N to ANS provides the measure of the distance from the anterior cranial base to the base of the nose, that is, the upper face (norm of –50 ± 2.5 mm) (Fig 3-37). A smaller number can indicate a proportionally smaller face or a tipped-up maxilla. A larger number can indicate maxillary excess or a large face. The measure changes with age.

S-PNS (see Fig 3-37) provides information about the height of the posterior face and can help to explain whether over-eruption of the molars or possible anterior pressure contributed to an open bite. These numbers must be considered with the length of the rest of the face to determine their significance.

The angle between the palatal plane (ANS-PNS) and SN (see Fig 3-37) is not a truly vertical measure but could be considered a relative vertical measure. The measure should be slightly positive (norm = 8.0 ± 3.0 degrees). A smaller number indicates that the anterior portion of the maxilla is tipped more upward than the posterior, indicating either a developmental skeletal/dental discrepancy or significant sustained pressure in the anterior from a digit or tongue habit. A larger number than the norm indicates a potential deep bite.

Mandible to Cranial Base

The position of the mandible to the cranial base has usually been emphasized in esthetics and orthodontic treatment because of the difficulty of modifying it by orthodontics alone. The interpretation of the anterior position of the mandible compared to the cranial base depends on the reference point and the landmark being measured. As discussed previously, various planes have been used as references to measure skeletal and dental positions. Also, the landmarks B-point and Pg have both been used to describe the AP position of the mandible. B-point has been considered the junction of the alveolar bone and the basal bone. The alveolar bone supports the dentition and is dependent on the presence of the dentition. The basal bone remains if the dentition is lost and is the actual skeletal bone that supports the chin point. The profile is dependent on the position of both landmarks, but treatment can vary depending on the interpretation of the landmarks.

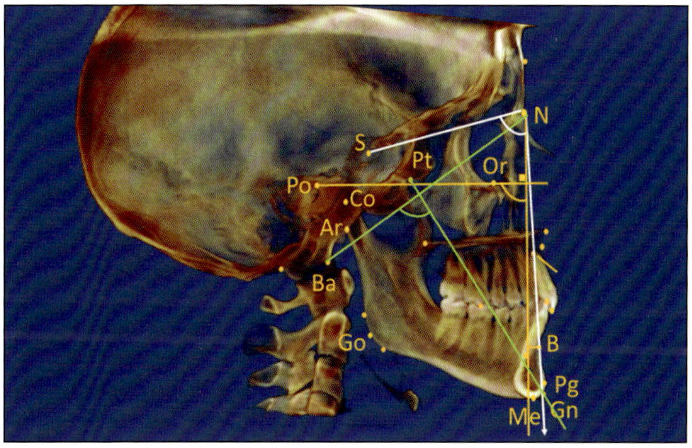

Fig 3-38 Mandibular protrusion measures: SNB (degrees) *(white)*; B to N vertical, B to N vertical to FH (mm) *(yellow)*, and facial axis angle, posterior angle between PtGn and NBa (degrees) *(green)*.

Anteroposteriorly

The angle SNB indicates the relative position of the mandible to the cranial base (Fig 3-38). Riedel[19] indicated that the adult norm is 80 ± 3.9 degrees, and Steiner[3] concurred. The norm for this angle varies with age, sex, and with ethnic groups. A large angle means that the mandible is relatively protrusive compared to the cranial base, whereas a small angle means the opposite. Because this measure is from landmarks from the profile, it indicates relative position, not size. An unusual tipping or length of the SN plane also influences the interpretation of this angle.

The protrusion of the mandible can also be compared to the cranial base by measuring the distance of pogonion to N perpendicular (see Fig 3-38). This measure varies by sex and age. In a well-balanced adult face, the average measure is −1.8 ± 4.5 mm for females and −0.3 ± 3.8 mm for males.[20] A negative number is given to a landmark distal to N perpendicular, and a positive number means the landmark is anterior. As the mandible grows forward, pogonion moves forward also.

The facial axis is the angle between the NBa plane and a plane from Pt (foramen rotundum) to Gn (see Fig 3-38). Ricketts indicated that this angle is usually 90 degrees. A larger-than-normal angle indicates a more protrusive mandible than normal, whereas a smaller-than-normal angle indicates a more retrusive mandible.

The facial angle is the angle between the facial plane (NPg) and FH (see Fig 3-38), and the norm is 87.8 ± 3.6 degrees in teenagers with excellent occlusion.[18] It changes with age, and the norm is different based on sex and ethnic group. The facial angle provides another means of establishing the relative position of the mandible. Similar to all angles, the interpretation depends on the reliability of the landmarks comprising the planes. A larger-than-normal angle means the chin is relatively protrusive, and a smaller angle means the chin is relatively retrusive.

Vertically

The angle FMA, formed by the mandibular plane (MP) to FH, can indicate the relative proportion of the anterior facial height to posterior height (Fig 3-39a). The values between 16 and 22 degrees are considered good to favorable in prognosis. The lower the angle, the more closely the posterior facial height approximates the anterior facial height. This can indicate that the patient has a deep bite, and some clinicians do not like to include extractions as their optimal treatment plan. The higher the angle, the steeper the mandibular plane and the less likely the posterior facial height will approximate the anterior facial height.[5] Downs[18] called this angle the *mandibular plane angle* and reported that in a group of teenagers with good occlusion the mean was 21.9 ± 3.2 degrees.

The angle of the mandibular plane to SN (MP-SN) provides similar information, although the angle of SN can also be discrepant (see Fig 3-39a). Depending on the definition of mandibular plane (GoGn versus MeGoI), the values for adults vary by age and sex.[9] The values for GoGn were approximately 1 degree greater than for MeGoI. The values all showed anterior divergence.

A rule of thumb is that the extension of the mandibular planes to the back of the head in a well-balanced face will not enter the cranium. Although this is not always true, the mandibular plane in a well-balanced face will tend to converge with the other anteroposterior planes of the face at a distance behind the skull (see Fig 3-33). The convergence of a plane (eg, mandibular plane) over the others indicates a dysmorphic situation.

The mandibular angle (ArGo-GoMe) (see Fig 3-39a) also provides similar information. The values for men decreased slightly with age. This measure can help to explain morphologically the mandibular plane, especially if used in conjunction with the length of the ramus, ArGo. Behrents[9] showed that adult men had significantly smaller angles than women, which could explain their more forward growth of the mandible than women. The average angle for age and sex varied between 16.8 ± 6.6 (the lowest) and 122.7 ± 6.7 (the highest) degrees.

The y-axis shows the resultant of the horizontal and vertical directions of mandibular growth. It is the anterior angle between SGn and FH (Fig 3-39b). The mean is 59.4 ± 3.8 degrees. A larger number indicates that the mandibular growth is more vertical than horizontal, and a smaller number indicates more horizontal than vertical growth.

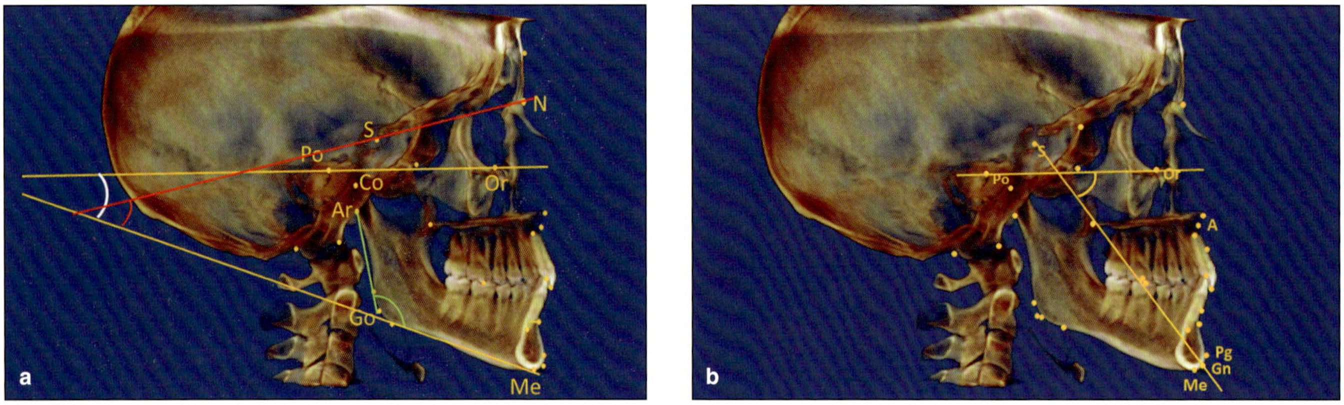

Fig 3-39 *(a)* Relative vertical position of the mandible: FMA, angle between FH (PoOr) and the lower border of the mandible (GoMe) (degrees) *(gold)*; mandibular plane angle, angle between SN and GoMe (degrees) *(red and gold)*; and mandibular angle, angle between ArGo and GoMe (degrees) *(green and gold)*. *(b)* The y-axis, or the anterior angle between SGn and FH (PoOr) (degrees).

Maxilla to Mandible

Anteroposteriorly

The ANB angle relates the maxillary and mandibular skeletal bases to each other (Fig 3-40). Riedel[19] first proposed this measure as a means of relating the maxilla to the cranium in 1952. The norm for Caucasian adults is 2 degrees. A large positive number is interpreted as a Class II skeletal discrepancy, and a negative number is interpreted as a Class III skeletal discrepancy. Steiner[3] developed a method of relating the ANB angle to incisor position for clinical use.

Wits appraisal is the difference in the distance between vertical lines from A-point and B-point to the functional occlusal plane (see Fig 3-40). The measure is positive if A-point is anterior to B-point and negative if A-point is posterior to B-point. Studies suggest that the measure is not affected by age. Males with excellent occlusions have a more negative measurement (–1.17 ± 1.9 mm) than females (–0.10 ± 1.77 mm). A large negative number suggests a Class III discrepancy, and the greater the negative number, the greater the skeletal discrepancy. A positive number suggests a Class II discrepancy, and the greater the positive number the greater the skeletal discrepancy. Jacobson[21] strongly supports the concept that the Wits appraisal can identify a severe skeletal discrepancy better than the ANB angle but suggests that multiple cephalometric measures might be needed.

The position of the mandible and the maxilla can also be measured based on the distance from the most posterosuperior point on the mandible.[20] The maxillary position is measured from condylion to A-point and compared with the mandibular length measured from condylion to gnathion (CoGn) (see Fig 3-40). In a well-balanced face, the relationship is linear. The measures are reduced to small, medium, and large and compared with the differential between the maxillary and the mandibular lengths. An individual with a smaller face would have a smaller difference (eg, 20 to 24 mm) between the maxillary and mandibular lengths, whereas the difference for an individual with a medium face would be 25 to 28 mm, and the difference for a large face would be 29 to 33 mm. Diagnostic discrepancies are solved by interpreting A-point to N perpendicular. Because this measure is based on the position of the mandibular condyle on the cranium, it does not actually measure maxillary length. It measures the maxillary position based on A-point compared with a method of measuring the length of the mandible.

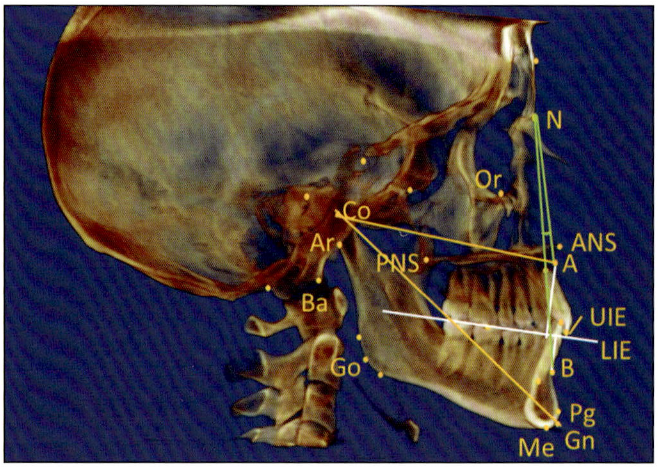

Fig 3-40 Maxillary to mandibular relationships: ANB, angle between NA and NB (degrees) *(green)*; lengths of CoA versus CoGn (mm) *(gold)*; and Wits analysis, distance along the occlusal plane between vertical lines from A-point and B-point (mm) *(white)*. If B line is anterior to A, the measure is negative; if B line is distal to A, the measure is positive.

Vertically

The relationship of the maxilla to the mandible can be measured vertically from ANS to Me to establish the lower facial height (Fig 3-41). According to McNamara,[20] the lower facial height of a well-balanced face should correlate with the effective length of the maxilla. If the mandibular plane increases or decreases beyond normal (22.7 ± 4.3 mm for a well-balanced face), the length of the lower facial height changes accordingly. A decreased mandibular plane can occur as a result of a vertically or an anteroposteriorly deficient maxilla. An increased mandibular plane can occur as the result of excessive molar eruption or an increased antegonial notch in the lower border of the mandible. The average for women is 66.7 ± 4.1 mm and for men is 74.6 ± 5.0 mm. This measure is not the length of ANS and Me along a true vertical, so the frontal appearance could change dramatically if the same measure from ANS-Me occurs but at different angles from true vertical. This will produce a different diagnostic outcome. The significance of the vertical lengths of facial structures is not as absolutes but as related to other vertical measures (ie, facial proportions). As McNamara[20] indicated, the size of the lower anterior facial height in a well-balanced face is related to the total size of the face. The knowledge that a triangle with three angles that equal 180 degrees and three sides allows one to know easily the size of one angle (eg, FH to mandibular incisor [FMIA]) by knowing the other two (eg, the mandibular plane angle [FMA] and the mandibular incisor to mandibular plane [IMPA]). Knowing the length of two sides of a triangle (effective length of the maxilla [CoA] and the effective length of the mandible [CoGn]) and one angle (mandibular plane to CoA) allows one to estimate the anterior facial height (ANS to Me) by using geometry and estimates of the differences between ANS and A-point and between Gn and Me.

Anterior facial height can also be measured as a vertical line from the palatal plane to Me (see Fig 3-41). This eliminates the geometric effect of measuring diagonal lines. The Tweed analysis indicates that this measure should be about 65 mm for 12-year-olds but will increase with age.

Posterior facial height is the ramal length and is measured from articulare on a tangent to the posterior ramus to the mandibular plane (see Fig 3-41). By itself, it is just a measure, but when compared to the anterior facial height, it can help to explain vertical discrepancies related to the mandibular plane.

The facial height index (FHI) is the ratio of the posterior facial height to the anterior facial height. This index was developed as an adjunct to the Tweed analysis.[22] The anterior facial height is usually much greater than the posterior facial height in a patient with a high mandibular plane angle. Deficient ramal growth can cause a short posterior height. Normal range would be between 0.65 and 0.75. As the ratio decreases (eg, to 0.4), the patient has a tendency to an open bite; as the ratio increases (eg, to 0.9), the patient has a tendency to a deep bite. A small ratio suggests that extractions should be treatment planned, whereas a large ratio suggests extractions would be problematic.

The relative ratio of the anterior maxillary height to the mandibular height can also be compared by measuring the height of ANS to stomion and from stomion to Me on a true vertical

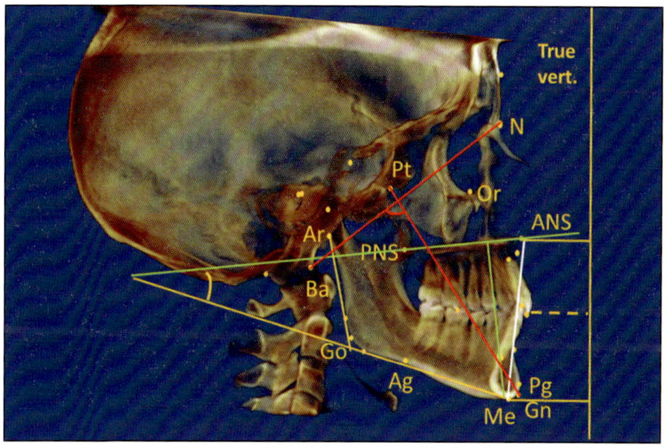

Fig 3-41 Various mandibular height measures: posterior mandible height, ArGo (mm) *(gold)*; lower anterior facial height, ANS-Me (mm) *(white)*; lower anterior facial height, distance on a true vertical between ANS and Me (mm) *(solid gold)*; upper lower facial height, distance on a true vertical between ANS and stomion (mm) *(dashed and solid gold)*; lower lower facial height, distance from stomion to Me on a true vertical (mm) *(dashed and solid gold)*; anterior mandibular height, distance between the palatal plane and Me (mm) *(green)*; and the angle between the palatal plane *(green)* and the mandibular plane *(gold)* (mm).

(see Fig 3-41). Although soft tissue is not included on this cephalogram, it was assumed that the intersection of the incisor tips could demonstrate stomion. The ratio of a well-balanced maxillary to mandibular height should be about 60%. A smaller ratio indicates a disproportionately smaller maxillary height or a disproportionately larger anterior mandibular height. A larger ratio indicates a disproportionately larger maxillary height or a disproportionately smaller anterior mandibular height. This measure does not provide absolute measures, just proportions.

The mandibular plane angle (FH-GoMe) is 22.7 ± 4.3 degrees for women and 21.3 ± 3.9 degrees for men. Although an increased mandibular plane angle by itself suggests increased anterior mandibular height, many morphologic variations can occur that negate that premise. For example, increased anterior maxillary height causing a deep bite can occur. The posterior ramal height can be decreased, allowing the increased mandibular plane angle to produce a normal anterior mandibular height. An increased mandibular plane angle does not necessarily mean that an open bite exists. Other values need to be considered to determine the problem.

The facial axis angle, which is the anterior angle between BaN and a line from Pt through Gn, is used to indicate the direction of growth of the mandible (see Fig 3-41). A large angle indicates downward growth, and a small angle indicates forward growth. The norm for 20 individuals (the number of males and females were about equally divided) aged from 12 to 17 years with excellent occlusion was 87.8 degrees with a range of 82 to 95 degrees.[10]

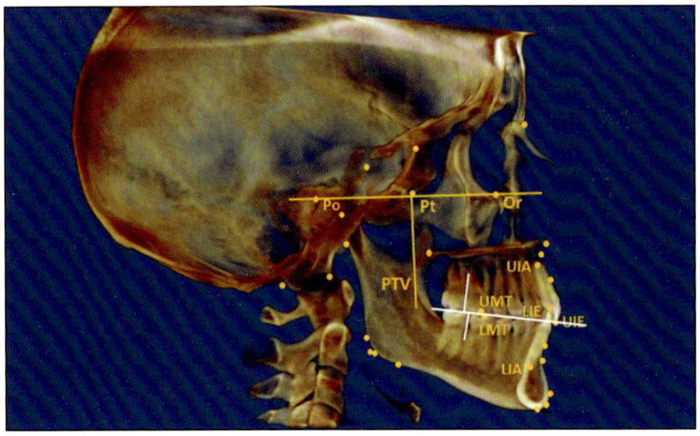

Fig 3-42 Molar relationships: the distance along the occlusal plane between the distal of the mandibular first molar to the distal of the maxillary first molar (mm) *(white)*; the distance between LMT (mesial cusp of the mandibular first molar) and UMT (mesial cusp of the maxillary first molar) *(gold dots)*; and the distance between the distal of the permanent first molars and Pt vertical (PTV) through FH (mm) *(gold)*.

Dentition

Anteroposteriorly

Molars

Molar relationships are often difficult to determine cephalometrically because of the overlap of structures. It is strongly suggested that trimmed dental casts be available when tracing to help determine symmetry of the right and left molar relationships and the actual relationships themselves. Identification of molar outlines is much easier prior to the eruption of the second premolars and second molars.

One measure for molar relationships uses the difference between vertical lines from the distal of the maxillary first molar and the distal of the mandibular first molar to the occlusal plane to (Fig 3-42). The mean difference is 3 mm. If the mandibular molar is mesial to the maxillary molar, the number is positive, whereas a negative number indicates that the mandibular molar is distal to the maxillary molar. Thus, a small positive number indicates Class I, a large positive number is Class III, and a negative number is Class II. This does not account for small maxillary molars relative to the mandibular molars.

The distance from the distal of the maxillary first molars to a perpendicular line from Pt through FH (PTV; see Fig 3-42) is used to indicate whether there will be adequate room for eruption of the second and third molars. The norm of this measurement is the age of the patient plus 3 mm but seems to discontinue this formula by age 24 years, with a distance of 30 mm.[10] If the measure is small, there might not be adequate room for eruption of the maxillary second or third molars, depending on tooth size or unexpected growth. This measure can help the clinician make decisions concerning extractions, particularly if moderate to severe crowding exists mesial to the first molars.

Incisors

Incisor inclination and protrusion are two separate but related concepts that describe the AP position of the incisors based on the incisal edges. Inclination is an angle measured based on a straight line drawn through the apical and incisal tips of the most forward mandibular or maxillary incisor relative to a reference line or plane. Protrusion is the distance of the incisal tip of the most forward mandibular or maxillary incisor to a reference line or plane. Inclination and protrusion are usually used to interpret measurements larger than the norm, and retroclination and retrusion are usually interpreted based on measures smaller than the norm. Proclination and protrusion are obviously related but influence treatment decisions differently based on the amount of alveolar support, crowding, lip support, and intercuspation with opposing teeth.

Several AP cephalometric measures help with diagnosis and treatment planning. The protrusion and proclination of the incisors are important because they affect the soft tissue drape of the lips, the part of the profile that orthodontics without surgery can affect the most. The inclination of the incisors also affects the amount of arch space. Prior to measuring incisor protrusion and proclination, the clinician should assess the quality and quantity of alveolar bone around the incisor roots.

Overjet is the horizontal distance of the maxillary incisal tip to the mandibular incisal tip (Fig 3-43). The norm is 2 to 3 mm. A large positive value can indicate a skeletal Class II discrepancy or proclined maxillary incisors caused by crowding or a digit or tongue habit. Overjet has also been defined clinically as the horizontal distance of the maxillary incisal tip to the most forward position along the mandibular crown when a deep bite is present because the mandibular incisal tip cannot be seen.

The protrusion of the mandibular incisors can be evaluated several ways, all of which identify the balance of the profile. The protrusion of the mandibular incisors relative to both maxillary and mandibular bases can be determined by measuring the distance of the mandibular incisal tip to the AB line (Fig 3-44).

If the chin (Pg) is considered the limit of the mandibular base, another method compares the distance of the mandibular incisal tip to a line extending from A-point to pogonion.[10] The ideal norm is 1.0 ± 2.5 mm mesial to the APg line. The APg line is also called the *dental plane*. McNamara[20] reported an average of 2.7 ± 1.7 for women and 2.3 ± 2.1 for men.

The protrusion of the mandibular incisors can also be compared to the cranium and mandible by measuring the distance from the mandibular incisal tips to the NB line[3] (see Fig 3-44). The ideal measure is 4 mm. The protrusion of the mandibular incisors can also be compared relative to the chin. The distance of pogonion and the distance of the forward surface of the mandibular incisor to the NB line are ideal when both are 4 mm. As the discrepancy between the two measures increases, the esthetics decrease.

The protrusion of the maxillary incisors can be compared to several reference points. The distance of the maxillary incisal

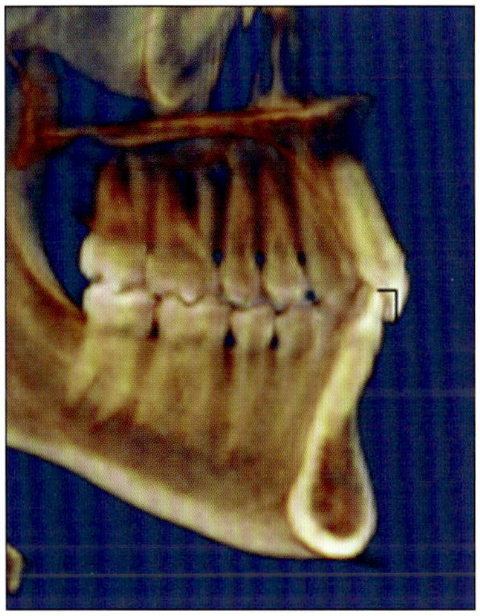

Fig 3-43 Incisor relationships: overbite, vertical distance between the cusp tips of the most forward maxillary and mandibular incisors (mm); overjet, horizontal distance between the cusp tips of the most forward maxillary and mandibular incisors (mm).

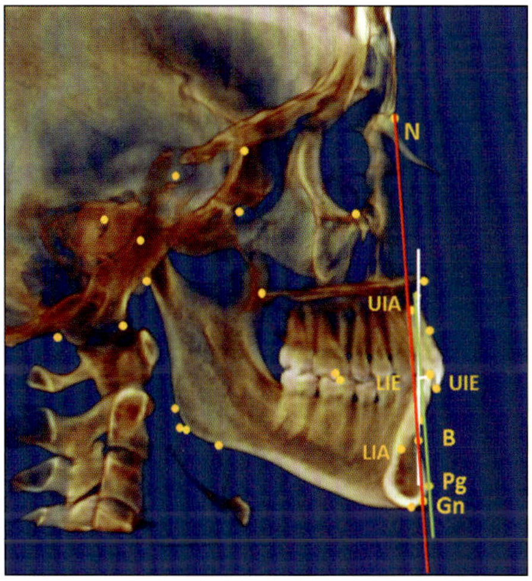

Fig 3-44 Protrusion of the mandibular incisor: the distance of the mandibular incisor tip (LIE) to the NB line (mm) *(red)*; the distance of the mandibular incisor tip to the APg line (mm) *(white)*; and the distance of the mandibular incisor tip to the AB line (mm) *(green)*.

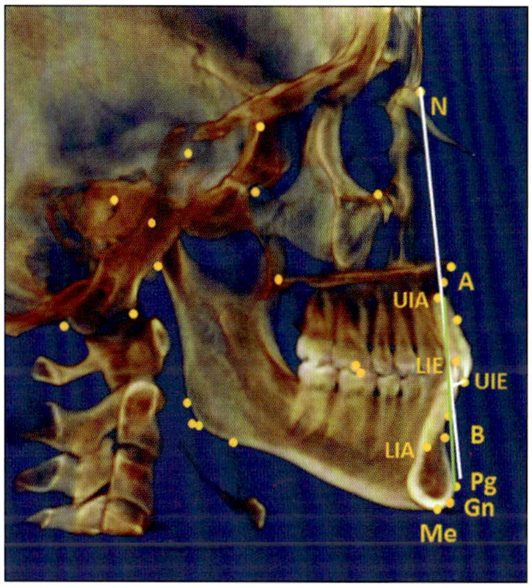

Fig 3-45 Protrusion of the maxillary incisor: the distance of the maxillary incisor tip (UIE) to NA (mm) *(white)*, and the distance of the maxillary incisor tip to APg (mm) *(green)*.

tip to the line NA (UIE-NA) (Fig 3-45) compares the maxillary incisor to the cranial base.[3] The norm for adults is 4 mm.

The distance of the maxillary incisal tip to APg (UIE-APg) compares the protrusion to the denture bases (see Fig 3-45). Downs[18] reported 2.7 ± 3.1 mm in a group of teenagers with excellent occlusions. Landmarks anterior to APg are positive; posterior are negative.

The protrusion of the maxillary incisor has also been compared to a constructed NA by McNamara[20] (see Fig 3-45). In this parameter, a line parallel to N perpendicular to FH is reconstructed but through A-point. The distance from the facial surface of the maxillary incisor to the reconstructed N perpendicular should be 4 to 6 mm, with an average of about 5.4 ± 1.8 mm for men and women. The distance anterior to the reconstructed line is positive, whereas the distance posterior to the reconstructed line is negative.

Inclination of the incisors is important because it affects arch space and the support of the lip.

The angle of the mandibular incisor to APg compares the mandibular incisor to the denture bases (Fig 3-46). The norm is 22 degrees.

Comparison of the angle of the mandibular incisor to NB provides the relation to the cranium (see Fig 3-46). The norm is 25 degrees. The inclination of the mandibular incisor is also related to the mandibular base by measuring the angle of the mandibular incisor (L1) to MP[5] (see Fig 3-46). The norm is 90 ± 5 degrees for subjects with acceptable mandibular planes (16 to 25 degrees). Tweed realized that if the L1-MP angle stayed the same but the FMA angle changed, the incisor angle would not support an esthetic lip. So the acceptable measures vary with the angle of the mandibular plane to FH. For example, as the angle of the mandibular plane to FH increases, the angle of L1-MP can be decreased to minimize lip protrusion. Otherwise, the incisor would procline relative to the face and place the lip in an unesthetic position. Reciprocally, as the mandibular plane angle decreases, more proclination of the incisor is acceptable to close the overjet. However, it is important that the mandibular incisors are over the bone as much as possible. Tweed stated that these standards do not apply to all patients.[5]

Downs[18] also measured the angle between the mandibular incisors and the occlusal plane. The range of values for children with clinically excellent occlusions was 3.5 to 20 degrees, with a mean of 14.5 degrees. These values are based on the difference between a right angle (90 degrees) and the value measured. Positive numbers indicated proclination, while negative numbers indicated retroclination of the incisors. Most clinicians currently using this measure express it as the full number.

The proclination of the mandibular incisors could also be compared to APg. The average used by Ricketts[10] was 22 ± 4 degrees.

All of these measurements must be used with the understanding of the reference lines. For example, a mandibular incisor to MP measurement can be ideal, but if the mandibular plane is steep, the incisor can be quite proclined relative to the profile and produce an unesthetic lower lip. In that case, Tweed[5] suggested that as the mandibular plane (FMA) increased, the incisor angle to mandibular plane (IMPA) could be decreased to prevent incisor and lip protrusion. Proclination of mandibular incisors can be increased to close the overjet and mask skeletal discrepancies.

The inclination of the maxillary incisors is compared to the cranial base using the parameter UIE-UIA to SN (Fig 3-47). The ABO has used this measure also in their testing procedures.[6,7]

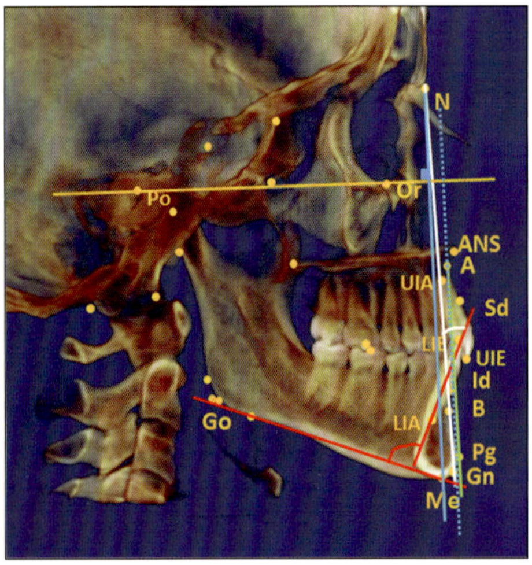

Fig 3-46 Inclination of the mandibular incisor: the angle between the mandibular incisor (LIA-LIE) and NB (degrees) *(white)*; the angle between the mandibular incisor and the mandibular plane (IMPA) (degrees) *(red)*; the angle between the mandibular incisor and APg (degrees); and the angle between N perpendicular to FH modified to pass through A-point (degrees).

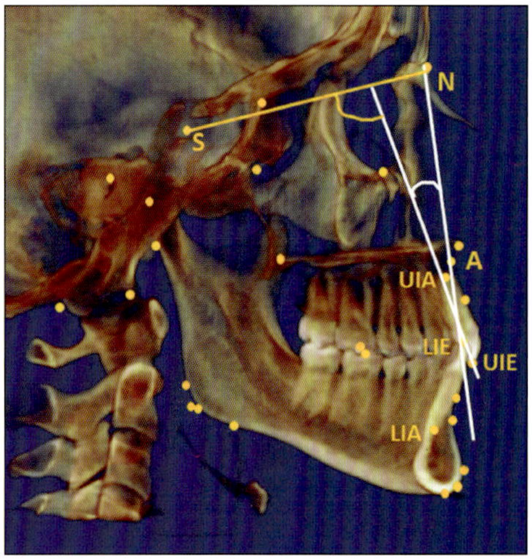

Fig 3-47 Inclination of the maxillary incisor: the angle between the maxillary incisor (UIA-UIE) and NA (degrees) *(white)*, and the angle between the maxillary incisor (UIA-UIE) and SN (degrees) *(gold)*.

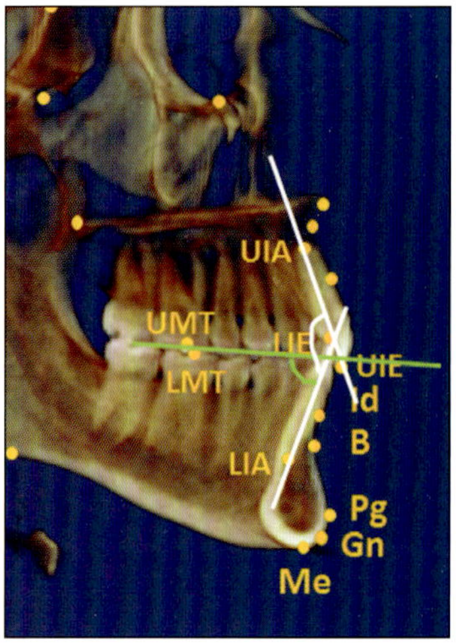

Fig 3-48 Incisal angle between the maxillary incisor (UIA-UIE) and the mandibular incisor (LIA-LIE) (degrees) *(white)*; inclination of the mandibular incisor (LIA-LIE) to the occlusal plane (degrees) *(green)*.

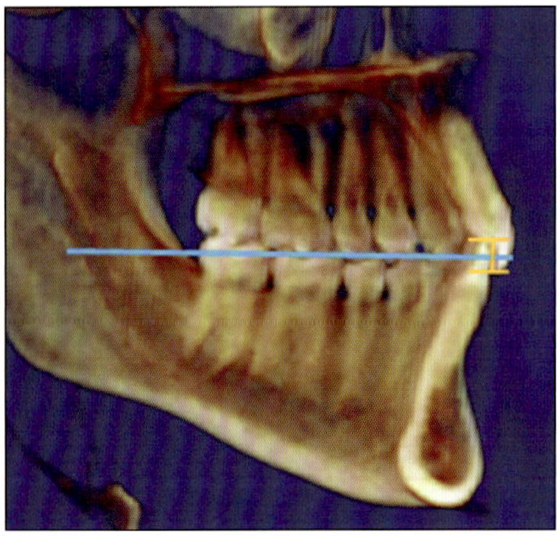

Fig 3-49 Overbite (vertical distance between the incisal tips of the most forward mandibular and maxillary incisors) illustrated as the distance between two horizontal *gold lines*. Extrusion of the mandibular incisor is the vertical distance from the occlusal plane *(blue line)* to the mandibular incisor tip.

The norm for adults with excellent occlusion was reported by Riedel[19] as 104.0 ± 5.8 degrees. A larger number indicates the incisor is more proclined, whereas a smaller number indicates retroclination.

Steiner[23] used the angle between UIE-UIA to NA to determine the inclination of the maxillary incisors (see Fig 3-47). The ideal measure is 22 degrees. As the ANB angle increases from the standard of 2 degrees, the maxillary incisors can recline and the mandibular incisors can procline to close the dental discrepancy. As the ANB angle decreases from 2 degrees, the maxillary incisor can procline and the mandibular incisors can recline to provide an adequate overjet and an esthetic face. Steiner recognized that the particular numbers that he used did not work in all cases.

The incisal angle (Fig 3-48) indicates the relationship of the maxillary and mandibular incisors to each other. The norms for this measure are influenced by ethnic characteristics, and many ethnic groups exhibit smaller incisal angles than Caucasians. The norm for Caucasians is 135 ± 5.8 degrees. The smaller the angle, the more proclined the teeth and the more protruded the lips. The teeth and the lips are more reclined when the angle is larger. One arch can also affect the angle significantly, suggesting that measures of each arch be measured against another reference to determine the potential problem.

Vertically

Overbite is the vertical relationship of the incisors to each other and is measured as the vertical distance between the maxillary and the mandibular incisal tips (Fig 3-49). The norm is 0 to 2 mm. A positive measure means that the incisor tips overlap, whereas a negative measure means the incisor tips do not overlap. Overlaps that are more than half the length of the mandibular incisor are called *deep bites*, whereas a negative measure is called an *open bite*. Some clinicians prefer a slightly greater overbite than normal upon finishing an open bite case because of the potential for relapse. Many clinicians also prefer to finish a deep bite case with only a slight overbite to minimize the effects of relapse, whereas some prefer a greater overbite to allow anterior incisor disocclusion.

The distance of the mandibular incisor tip to the functional occlusal plane (LIE-FOP) indicates the extrusion of the mandibular incisors (see Fig 3-49). Measurement of the mandibular incisor tip to the Downs occlusal plane is not as helpful because that overlap is usually not as great, due to the fact that one end of that occlusal plane is a bisection of the overlap of the maxillary and mandibular incisors.

Conclusion

Numerous parameters are used to measure facial structures cephalometrically. Clinicians should be aware that single measures do not always indicate where the specific problem exists nor how to treat the case. Most cases require additional clinical information for the best possible treatment plan. However, more studies need to be done to determine which provide the most reliable and valid measures for clinical use.

Treatment of a case is dependent on all the factors that affect the case, not just numbers on a cephalogram. Indeed, individuals with excellent occlusions show large variations in their cephalometric values. Not all patients can be treated to norms, although cephalometry provides information for treatment.

Although 2D cephalometry has provided information for the orthodontist for decades, 3D cephalometry will provide more information for better diagnosis and treatment. In addition to providing area and volume, 3D cephalometry can provide the information similar to having the skull in hand.

References

1. Baumrind S, Frantz RC. The reliability of head film measurements. 1. Landmark identification. Am J Orthod 1971;60:111–127.
2. Wen J, Liu S, Ye X, et al. Comparative study of cephalometric measurements using 3 imaging modalities. J Am Dent Assoc 2017;148:913–921.
3. Steiner CC. Cephalometrics for you and me. Am J Orthod 1953;39:729–754.
4. Krogman WM, Sassouni V. A Syllabus in Roentgenographic Cephalometry. Philadelphia: College Offset, 1957.
5. Tweed CH. The Frankfort-mandibular plane Angle in orthodontic diagnosis, classification, treatment planning, and prognosis. Am J Orthod Oral Surg 1946;32:175–230.
6. American Board of Orthodontics website. https://www.americanboardortho.com/orthodontic-professionals/about-board-certification/clinical-examination/case-record-preparation/lateral-cephalogram-requirements/. Accessed 6 March 2018.
7. American Board of Orthodontics website. https://www.americanboardortho.com/media/5024/ceph-tracing.pdf. Accessed 6 March 2018.
8. Broadbent BH Sr, Broadbent BH Jr, Golden WH. Bolton Standards of Dentofacial Developmental Growth. St Louis: Mosby, 1975.
9. Behrents RG. Growth in the Aging Craniofacial Skeleton, monograph 17, Craniofacial Growth Series. Ann Arbor: University of Michigan, 1985.
10. Ricketts RM. Perspectives in the clinical application of cephalometrics. The first fifty years. Angle Orthod 1981;51:115–150.
11. Riolo ML, Moyers RE, McNamara JA Jr, Hunter WS. An Atlas of Craniofacial Growth, monograph 2, Craniofacial Growth Series. Ann Arbor: University of Michigan, 1974.
12. Basyouni AA, Nanda SK. An Atlas of the Transverse Dimensions of the Face, monograph 37, Craniofacial Growth Series. Ann Arbor: University of Michigan, 2000.
13. Richardson ER. Atlas of Craniofacial Growth in Americans of African Descent, monograph 26, Craniofacial Growth Series. Ann Arbor: University of Michigan, 1991.
14. Kula TJ 3rd, Ghoneima A, Eckert G, Parks ET, Utreja A, Kula K. Two-dimensional vs 3-dimensional comparison of alveolar bone over maxillary incisors with A-point as a reference. Am J Orthod Dentofacial Orthop 2017;152:836–847.e2.
15. Sirikci A, Bayazit YA, Bayram M, Kanlikama M. Significance of the auditory tube angle and mastoid size in chronic ear disease. Surg Radiol Anat 2001;23:91–95.
16. Lagravère MO, Low C, Flores-Mir C, et al. Intraexaminer and interexaminer reliabilities of landmark identification on digitized lateral cephalograms and formatted 3-dimensional cone-beam computerized tomography images. Am J Orthod Dentofacial Orthop 2010;137:598–604.
17. Downs WB. The role of cephalometrics in orthodontic case analysis and diagnosis. Am J Orthod 1952;38:162–182.
18. Downs WB. Variations in facial relationships; their significance in treatment and prognosis. Am J Orthod 1948;34:812–840.
19. Riedel RA. The relation of maxillary structures to cranium in malocclusion and in normal occlusion. Angle Orthod 1952;22:142–145.
20. McNamara JA Jr. A method of cephalometric evaluation. Am J Orthod 1984;86:449–469.
21. Jacobson A, Jacobson RL (eds). Radiographic Cephalometry: From Basics to 3-D Imaging, ed 2. Chicago: Quintessence, 2006.
22. Horn AJ. Facial height index. Am J Orthod Dentofacial Orthop 1992;102:180–186.
23. Steiner CC. The use of cephalometrics as an aid to planning and assessing orthodontic treatment. Am J Orthod 1960;46:721–735.

4

Frontal Cephalometric Analysis

Katherine Kula, MS, DMD, MS
Ahmed Ghoneima, BDS, PhD, MSD

Obvious facial asymmetries as well as less noticeable asymmetries and transverse discrepancies that are noted during extraoral examination or on the lateral cephalogram should be evaluated using three-dimensional (3D) cone beam computed tomography (CBCT) images (Fig 4-1) or two-dimensional (2D) frontal or posteroanterior (PA) radiographs (Fig 4-2). Almost everyone, even people considered attractive, has some degree of facial asymmetry[1,2] that does not require clinical treatment. However, some have asymmetries that are associated with malocclusion, for example midline and molar asymmetries[3] (Fig 4-3), or that could compromise the orthodontic treatment outcome unless identified and addressed adequately.

Preliminary identification of these asymmetries or transverse discrepancies allows adequate treatment planning, particularly when multidisciplinary treatment is involved. While some asymmetries can be relatively minor, others are major and require significant treatment planning. 3D CBCTs can be more diagnostic than 2D frontal radiographs because the patient can be examined from many directions to evaluate soft and hard tissue asymmetries, effects of trauma, transverse discrepancies,

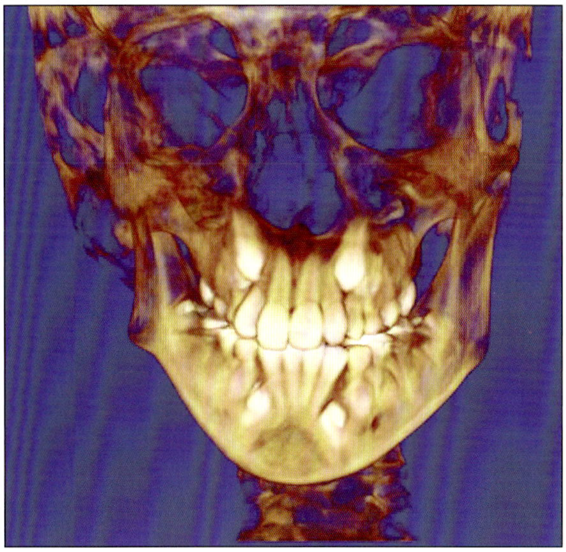

Fig 4-1 CBCT image of a patient with an asymmetric cranium, maxilla, mandible, and dental components.

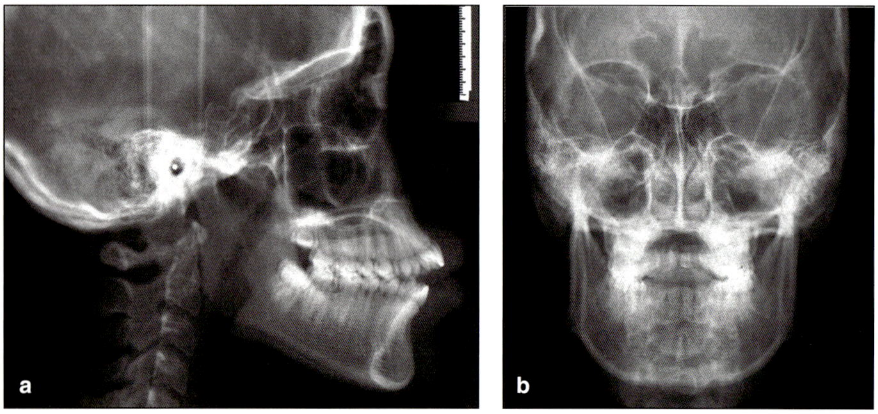

Fig 4-2 Examples of lateral *(a)* and frontal *(b)* cephalograms of the same patient. Note the vertical asymmetry of the mandibular plane and slight anteroposterior asymmetry of the posterior teeth in the lateral cephalogram. The frontal cephalogram shows a slight vertical asymmetry in the mandibular height of the rami and a slight lateral asymmetry in the width at the mandibular angle.

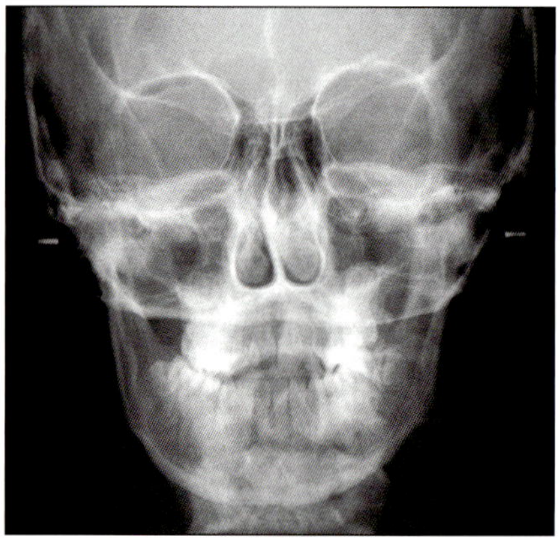

Fig 4-3 Frontal cephalogram of a patient with transverse discrepancies of the maxillary and mandibular posterior teeth and asymmetries of dental and skeletal components.

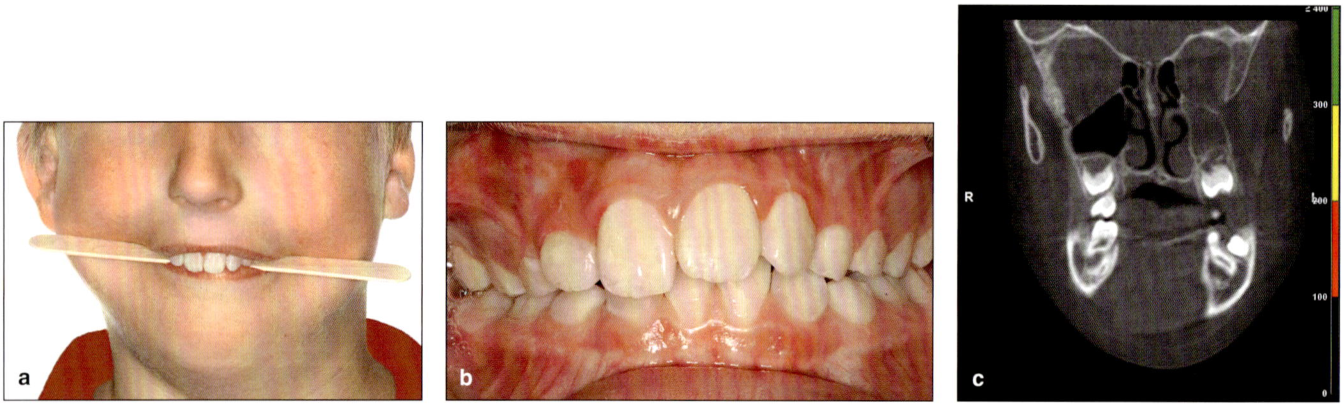

Fig 4-4 Initial extraoral and intraoral examination. *(a)* Extraoral view of the occlusal cant. *(b)* Intraoral view of cant. *(c)* A coronal slice through the molar area of the same patient shows cranial and soft tissue asymmetry. The reconstructed 3D CBCT is shown in Fig 4-1.

or craniofacial anomalies. Internal structures can be evaluated using slices through the CBCT that overlying structures in 2D radiographs make difficult to see.

An initial extraoral and intraoral examination (Fig 4-4) of a patient can provide clues to the existence of underlying skeletal or dental asymmetry, transverse discrepancies, impacted teeth, or other problems that require treatment. The use of a frontal radiograph or a CBCT can confirm the existence and site of a hard or soft tissue asymmetry, a transverse discrepancy, or the position of an impacted tooth (Fig 4-5). In some cases, 2D radiographs could be adequate, but other cases require 3D CBCTs for either additional information or as the initial radiograph. One tenet to follow in the case of trauma is to complete a medical and dental history, including symptoms, followed by an organized and detailed extraoral and intraoral examination with appropriate radiographs to minimize the chance of missing significant findings (Fig 4-6). Adequate preliminary information makes selection of the proper radiograph easier.

Facial asymmetry accompanied by a history of facial trauma, particularly in children, should be examined using a CBCT. Asymmetries noted in children can become more noticeable with growth. Although orthodontists tend to focus more on the facial structures, facial asymmetry can reflect asymmetric cranial structures (eg, craniosynostosis), not necessarily just asymmetries of the maxilla or the mandible. Relative to Class II malocclusion subdivisions, the glenoid fossa can be more distal on one side than on the other, causing asymmetry of molar position and a midline deviation.[4] The role of tooth position and angulation (Fig 4-7) in transverse discrepancies and asymmetry and the potential for unwanted side effects from treatment need to be evaluated as well as condylar size and morphology.

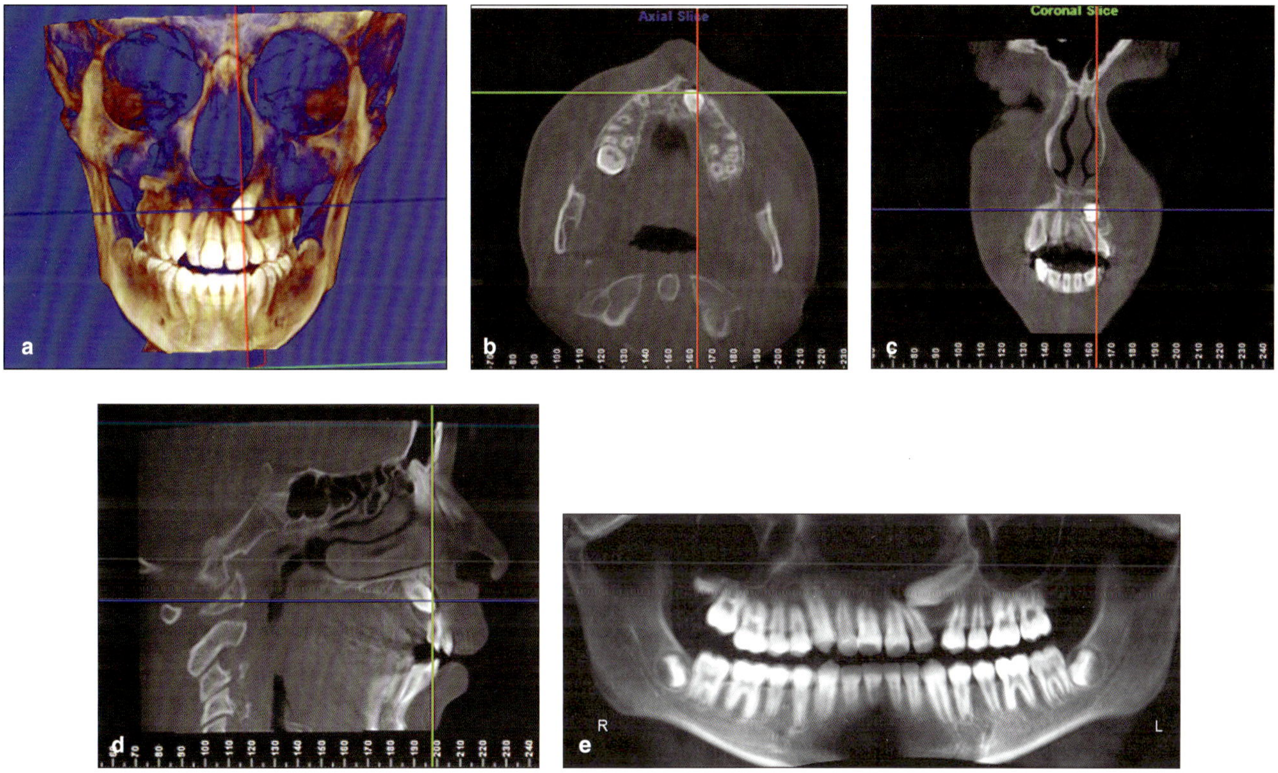

Fig 4-5 *(a)* Reconstructed 3D CBCT showing an impacted canine. *(b)* Axial slice through the impacted canine crown, which is against the labial alveolar plate. *(c)* Coronal slice showing the impacted canine against the root of the lateral incisor. *(d)* Sagittal section showing the canine possibly resorbing the root of the lateral incisor. *(e)* Reconstructed CBCT panoramic view of the patient showing the impacted canine.

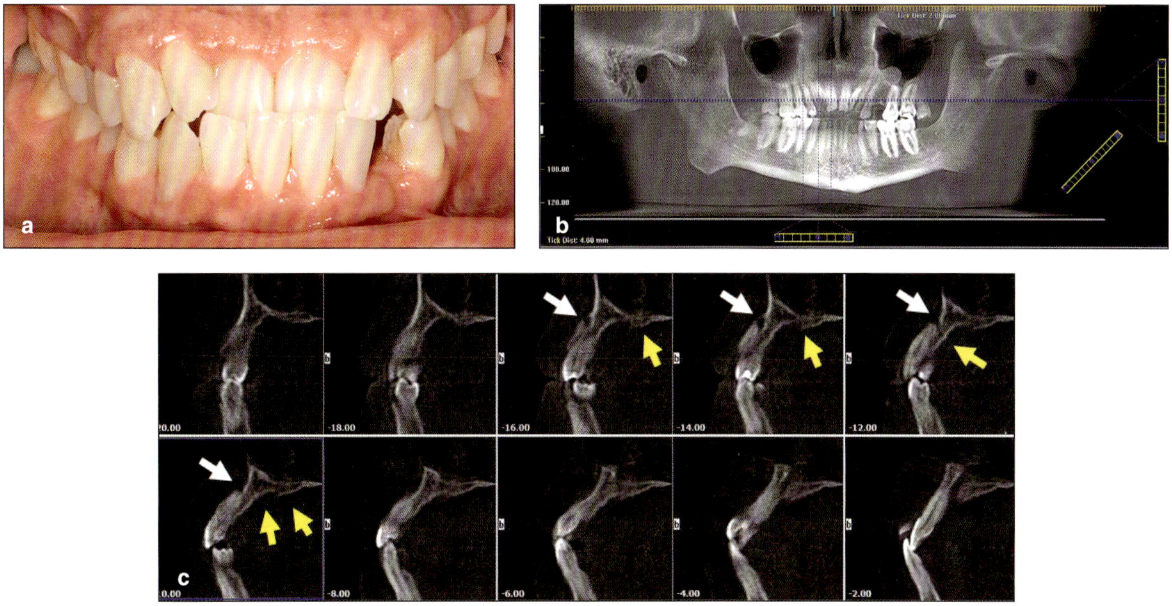

Fig 4-6 This orthodontic patient's medical and dental history indicated previous treatment 6 months ago for a three-site mandibular fracture and loss of two teeth, general dental treatment for fractured and decayed teeth 3 months ago, and current sensitivity in the maxillary right lateral incisor when blowing his nose. According to the patient, only a 2D panoramic radiograph was taken by the oral surgeon. *(a)* An intraoral orthodontic examination revealed erythematous tissue in the maxillary arch, particularly around the right canine, and retroclined central incisors. *(b)* Reconstructed CBCT panoramic view shows inflammatory changes in the maxillary sinuses and two missing teeth. *(c)* Sagittal CBCT sections of the maxillary arch show that the right canine root has ejected through the cortical plate, with a periapical radiolucency *(white arrows)* and possible fractures of the palatal cortical plate *(yellow arrows)*.

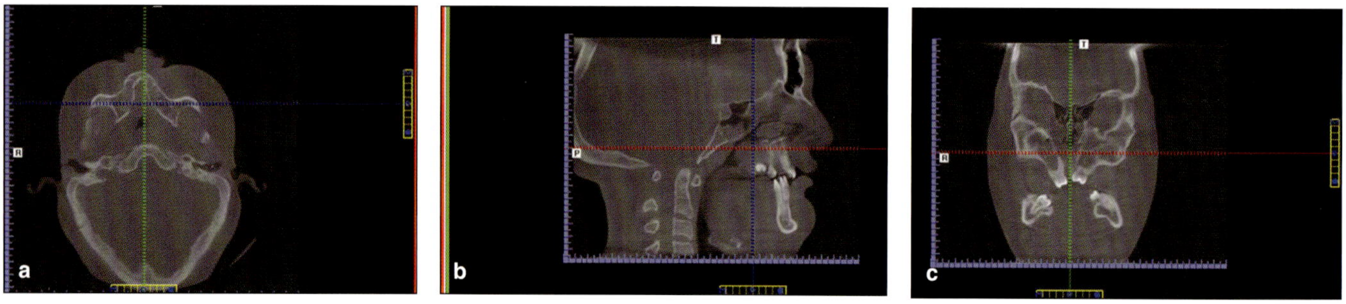

Fig 4-7 Three 3D CBCT views of a patient with undiagnosed cleft palate. *(a)* Axial slice showing a misshapen cranium and mandible. *(b)* Sagittal slice showing retroclined and retrusive incisors, a large frontal sinus, and an unusual configuration of the cranial base. *(c)* Coronal slice showing a collapsed cleft palate, extreme inclination of mandibular molars, and posterior open bites.

Standardizing Head Position

Standardization of image orientation for both lateral and frontal analysis is important for both 2D and 3D cephalometry. Orientation in both 2D and 3D is usually performed prior to image acquisition. Investigators[5,6] have suggested that natural head position should be used during cephalometric acquisition because it is less variable than the Frankfort horizontal plane or sella-nasion. However, this reference plane is not adequate for all patients even in 2D.[5] To minimize the motion distortion that can occur during the lengthy period required for 3D CBCT acquisition, most machines have chin rests or other structures set to stabilize the head. Realizing the difficulty of positioning patient heads for CBCT acquisition, Kumar and Ludlow[7] reported no statistically significant difference in measurements using phantoms in multiple positions during CBCT acquisition. They found that intracranial reference positions were slightly more reliable than natural head position.

The orientation of the CBCT for measurement purposes does not appear to be a major problem for hard tissue measurements, although standardization of head position is recommended. Studies[8] suggest that there are no significant differences in measurements between hard tissue landmarks identified on dry skulls versus nonoriented 3D CBCTs of the skulls. Cevidanes et al,[9] in using CBCTs of patients with unknown head orientations during CBCT acquisition, reported that measurements taken in simulated natural head position and in three intracranial head positions all had acceptable to excellent reliability. However, those measures taken on images oriented on the intracranial head positions were somewhat more reliable than those taken on simulated natural head positions.

Nonetheless, there are limited studies[10] actually determining the difference in frontal landmark identification between a gold standard (dry skull) and a 3D CBCT of the skull. In conventional cephalometry, landmark definitions are based on an x,y orientation. Some landmarks defined on a lateral cephalogram (eg, constructed gonion) cannot be identified accurately on a frontal cephalogram and require a new definition. In 3D, the image is turned and sliced to identify the landmark in all three dimensions (x, y, z). Landmark identification is reliable, although similar to 2D images, those landmarks on a curve, particularly if they are bilateral, are less reliable because of different orientations. There is limited information on the reliability of soft tissue landmarks or measures on 3D CBCTs acquired using oriented versus nonoriented patient positions.

For both modalities, the x, y, and z orientation of the image should be standardized to allow diagnosis of true asymmetry (Fig 4-8). For example, in cases of plagiocephaly, ear rods placed into external auditory meatuses that are vertically or sagittally asymmetric can cause an incorrect assessment of the asymmetry, resulting in the wrong treatment. Slight differences in position of the midsagittal plane can result in a significant appearance of asymmetry.

For 3D CBCTs, orient the Frankfort horizontal plane using the right porion and orbitale and left orbitale to standardize the x- and z-axes (see Fig 4-8a). Then establish the head position of the image so that a vertical line can be drawn through the midsagittal plane using crista galli and the bridge of the nose as the reference points for the y-axis (see Fig 4-8b). Note that some patients are so asymmetric that it is difficult to develop 90-degree angles in all three dimensions.

2D Tracing

Conventional cephalograms

Prior to manual tracing of a conventional frontal radiograph, prepare the necessary materials for tracing similar to manual tracing of a conventional lateral cephalogram. It is best to evaluate the film visually prior to any tracing in order to identify any problem, either quality of the film or pathology. In 2D, the entire craniofacial complex frequently obscures the frontal cephalogram, making landmarks difficult to identify. Knowing the anatomy of the skull (Fig 4-9) helps with identification of the landmarks.

Similar to tracing the lateral cephalogram, orthodontists pick different structures to trace first. However, most trace the same

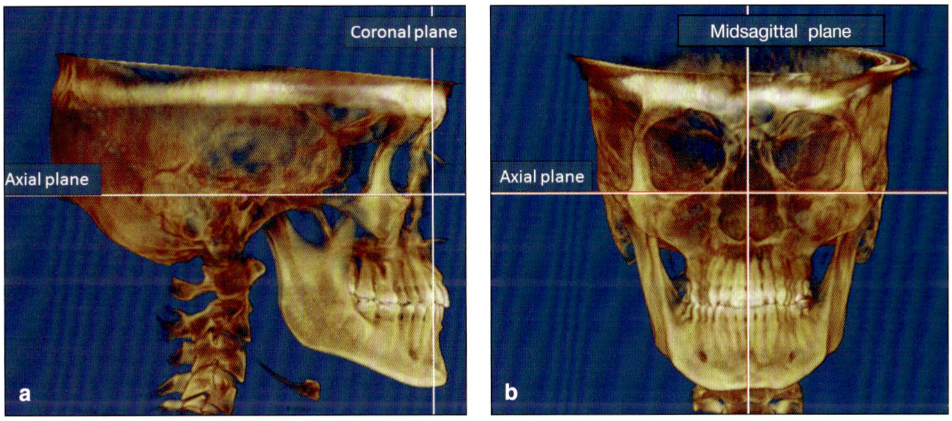

Fig 4-8 3D CBCT views of a reconstructed skull aligned along the Frankfort horizontal plane *(a)* and along the midsagittal plane *(b)*.

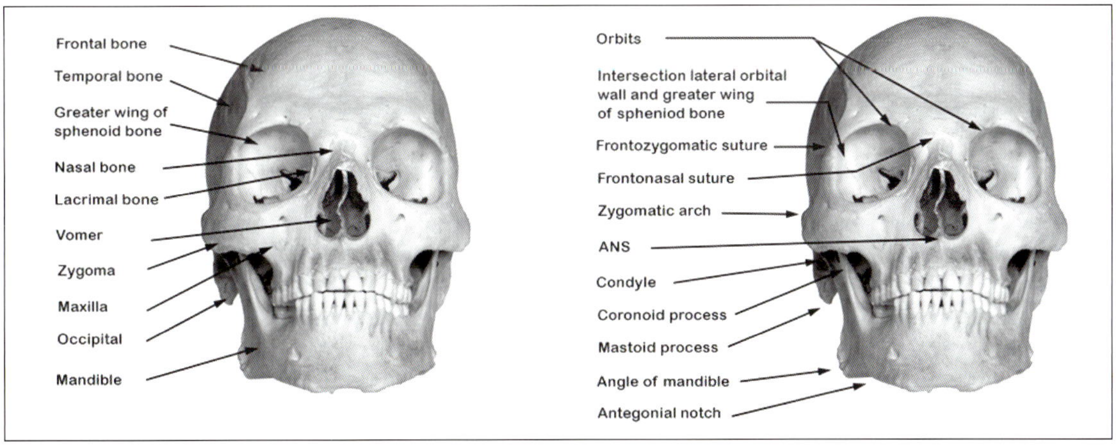

Fig 4-9 Anatomy of the frontal skull.

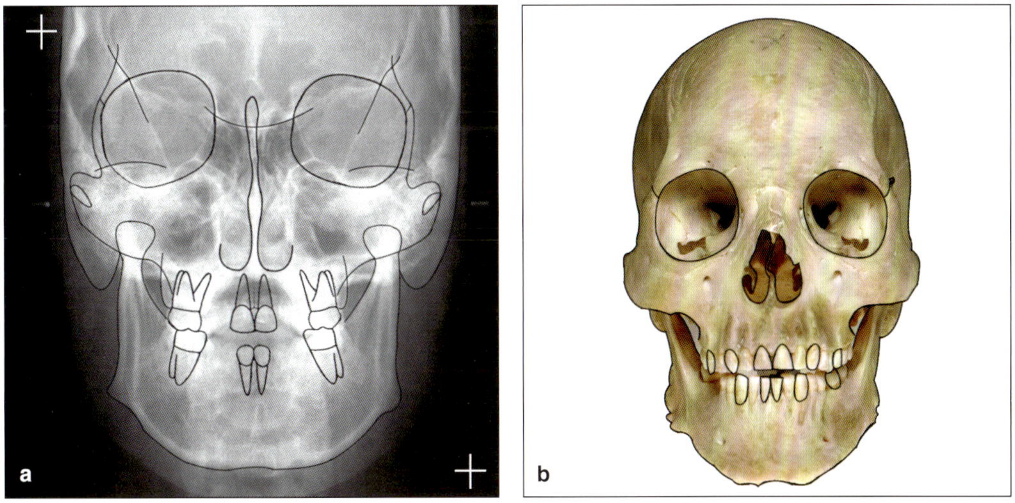

Fig 4-10 Tracing of orbits and zygomaticofrontal suture on a radiograph *(a)* and on a dry skull *(b)*.

structures. The following procedure will provide an introductory protocol for tracing the entire structure. Later, the order in which you prefer to trace can be modified as desired. Make fiducial marks (eg, crosses or Xs) on three corners of the radiograph and then trace the marks onto the acetate paper to help reorient the tracing to the radiograph, if necessary (Fig 4-10).

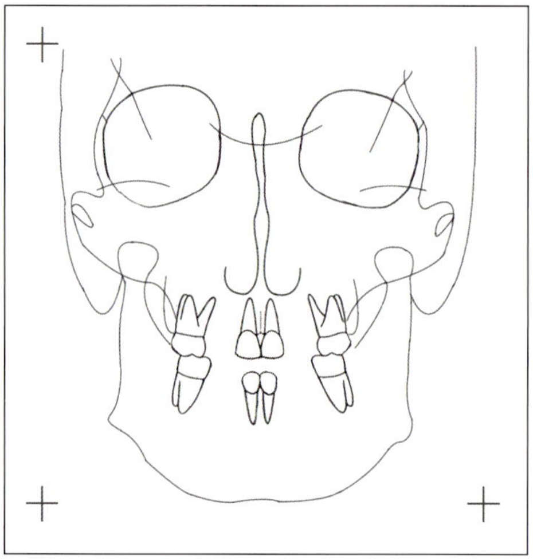

Fig 4-11 Manual tracing of the frontal cephalogram prior to landmark identification.

First, trace the outer aspects of the skull, including the mandible. The skull traced from the frontal aspect usually includes the outlines of the temporal and parietal bones. Include the mastoid processes in the tracing. Depending on the field of view (FOV) and the head shape and size, the frontal bone could be included in the outline. Trace the outline of the maxilla on both sides of the cranium and trace the palatal outline. Trace the outer and inner borders of the rami and around the condyles. The condyles can be difficult to identify because the zygomatic arch overlays it. Identify and outline the radiodense jugal processes on both sides. The jugal process is the "corner" of the zygomatic bone where it turns posteriorly. The mass of bone is more radiopaque at this corner than the rest of the bone and presents as a shape similar to a kidney bean.

Identify and trace the orbits. The orbits will be encircled by the maxilla, frontal, and zygomatic bones with the lacrimal and sphenoid bones apparent in the sockets. Identify and trace the zygomaticofrontal sutures on the lateral sides of the orbits and the greater wing of the sphenoid that cross the lateral orbital rim.

Then trace crista galli (part of the ethmoid bone) and the outline of the nasal apertures, septum, and conchae. Identify anterior nasal spine (ANS), which might have a small radiodense point to it depending on the angle at which the frontal cephalogram was taken. Because ANS is at the level of the inferior floor of the nasal passages on lateral cephalograms, it can be placed on a frontal cephalogram midway between the right and left nasal aperture floors. Identify and trace the crowns and roots of the maxillary and mandibular central incisors and, if visible, the canines. Trace the buccal and occlusal aspects of the permanent first molars in both arches. Missing or impacted teeth are not traced. Tracing all the teeth is not necessary and makes it difficult to identify other landmarks.

Lastly, remove the manual tracing of the 2D conventional cephalogram from the radiograph (Fig 4-11) and identify the landmarks. Removal of the tracings minimizes the chance of scratching the radiograph.

Digital

In order to analyze conventional cephalograms using cephalometric software, the conventional frontal cephalogram has to be converted into a digital format. Similar to the lateral cephalogram, scan the conventional frontal cephalogram, save it with an acceptable file extension for the software, and import the file into cephalometric software for analysis. However, distortion and magnification errors must be eliminated, or the analysis will be inaccurate.

Digital frontal cephalograms can be imported directly into software as a DICOM (Digital Imaging and Communications in Medicine) file for analysis. 3D CBCTs are extremely helpful in identifying the area of asymmetry because they can be used to analyze the face and skull from various aspects with only one radiograph.

Digital frontal cephalograms and 3D CBCTs require landmark identification but not a manual tracing. The algorithms of the software provide the numerical analysis on the screen and, in some software programs, a tracing. The linear and angular measuring tool in some software programs should be used to provide measures of specific angles or lines. The images used to illustrate the frontal measures will have the lines, angles, and specific measures superimposed on the image, but not necessarily the tracing behind the landmarks.

Landmark Identification and Reliability

Landmarks used in 2D frontal cephalometry[11–13] are defined in Table 4-1 and illustrated in Fig 4-12a. Some landmarks are apparent on the external skull, but many are useful only on a frontal cephalogram (Fig 4-12b). Because so many overlying structures make landmark identification difficult, it is helpful to know skull anatomy in order to best trace and identify the landmarks on either a lateral or frontal cephalogram.

The definitions of various landmarks have varied among authors since the beginning of cephalometry, making it difficult to define particularly the frontal landmarks. For example, the definition of menton is that it is the lowest point on the symphysis of the mandible and is used for lateral cephalograms. Many of the atlases reporting measurements from frontal cephalograms do not use this landmark probably because of the variation in the contour of the anterior portion of the chin.

Both median and bilateral landmarks are used, and some have the same name as used for lateral cephalometry. However, differences in image shape and distortion occur between lateral and frontal cephalograms[14] that affect reliability and even the definition of a landmark. For example, the definition of constructed gonion in 2D lateral cephalometry is dependent on bisecting the angle formed by a tangent to the posterior border of the ramus and the inferior border of the mandible. The gonion on a frontal cephalogram is the inferolateral point of the ramal outline at the mandibular angle.

Table 4-1 Frontal landmarks with abbreviation and definition

Landmark	Abbreviation	Definition	# labeled in Fig 4-12a
Crista galli	Nc	The most constricted point of the perpendicular plate of the ethmoid bone almost at the level of planum[11]	1
Anterior nasal spine	ANS		2
Upper central incisors	A1	The maxillary central incisor edge[12]	3
Lower central incisors	B1	The mandibular central incisor edge[12]	3
Lateral nasal	Ln	The most lateral point of the nasal aperture measured at the front of the face[11]	4
	NC (R & L)	The nasal cavity at its widest point (right and left)[12]	
Lateral orbit	Lo	The intersection of the lateral wall of the orbit with the greater wing of the sphenoid[11]	5
Zygomaticofrontal suture	Zt	The medial margin of the zygomaticofrontal suture[13]	6
	Zf (R & L)	The medial aspect of the zygomaticofrontal suture (right and left)[12]	
Condylion	Cd	The most superior point of the head of the condyle, centered mediolaterally[11]	7
Zygoma	Zyg	The most laterally positioned point on the zygomatic arches[11]	8
	Z (Za, aZ)	The center of the cross section of the zygomatic arch[13]	
Orbitale	Or (R & L)	The lowest point of the contour of the bony orbit (right and left)[11]	9
Maxillare	Mx (R & L)	The deepest point of the concavity formed by the lateral wall of the maxilla and the inferior border of the zygomatic process of the maxilla (located medial to the key ridge) (right and left)[11]	10
Jugal process	Ju	The midpoint of the most lateral point of the jugal process of the zygoma	10
	J (or Mx)	A point on the curve of the jugal process at the crossing of the outline of the tuberosity	
Upper molars	UM (R & L)	The most prominent lateral point on the buccal surface of the maxillary first molar (right and left)[12]	11
Lower molars	LM (R & L)	The most prominent lateral point on the buccal surface of the mandibular first molar (right and left)[12]	12
Mastoid process		The lowest point on the outline of the mastoid processes	13
Gonion	Go (R & L)	The point on the lateral aspect of the angle of the mandible at the junction of the corpus and ramus (right and left)[11]	14
Antegonion	Ag	The point at the lower border of the trihedral eminence or the antegonial tubercle	15
	Ag (R & L)	Antegonial notch (right and left)[12]	
Menton	Me	The point of the inferior border of the symphysis directly inferior to mental protuberance and inferior to the center of trigonium mentali[12]	16
Midsagittal plane	H	A perpendicular plane drawn from the neck of crista galli (Nc) to the Frankfort horizontal plane	NM
Frankfort horizontal plane	V	The connection between the lowest point of the contours of the bilateral bony orbits (Or)	NM

NM, not marked in figure.

The posterior border of the ramus cannot be seen on a frontal cephalogram, only the lateral border. If gonion is transferred from a lateral cephalogram to a frontal cephalogram, the range of landmark identification could be as much as 3 cm compared with a gold standard. The variability depends on the examiner and the cephalogram. Legrell et al[14] reported magnification of the image in a 2D lateral cephalogram to be so problematic that gonion could not be identified as right or left by experienced radiologists unless metal markers differentiated the two sides.

Antegonion, another landmark used for frontal cephalometry, is reported to be highly variable.[15,16] The variability is so great that Legrell et al[14] suggests that antegonion is invalid as a landmark for facial height and that differences up to 3 cm in the right- and left-side measures of gonion are probably identification error.

Some studies report that the reliability of landmark identification on 2D frontal cephalograms is lower than that on sagittal lateral cephalograms. Both El-Mangoury et al[15] and Major et al[16] report a considerable range of reliability for numerous landmarks on frontal cephalograms of patients. Major et al[16] analyzed cephalograms of multiple skulls versus actual patients with good facial symmetry in both the x-axis and the y-axis. Intraexaminer variability was considerable but was significant

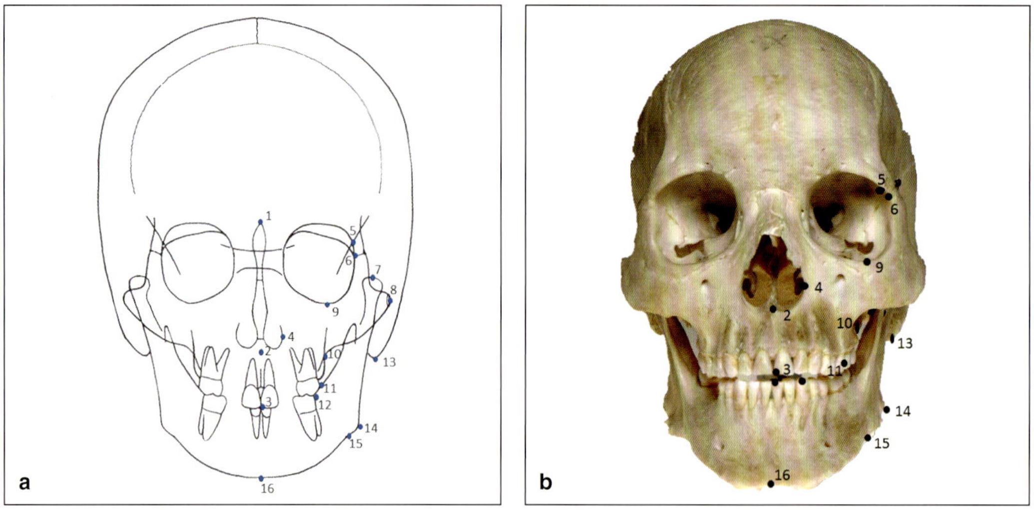

Fig 4-12 Frontal landmarks on a frontal radiograph *(a)* and on a dry skull (only external landmarks can be marked) *(b)*.

in both the axes for only three bilateral measures, only two of which (ie, the zygomaticofrontal suture and the cusp tips of the maxillary canines) might be considered clinically relevant. However, intraexaminer variability was significantly greater in the y-axis than in the x-axis for such medial measures as the center of crista galli and the midpoint on the nasal septum. Depending on the landmark, interexaminer variability was significantly larger than intraexaminer variability for multiple landmarks in both axes. Variability was also significant in the identification of certain landmarks on patient cephalograms as compared to skull cephalograms. The differences between skull and patient landmark identification could be caused by overlying soft tissue and bone or patient orientation. In some cases, the problem can be attributed to the definition of the landmark. For example, the definition of zygomaticofrontal suture does not indicate where on the wide suture the point should be made for the landmark.

Major et al[16] suggests that landmarks should be selected based on the magnitude of the x and y variability. For example, landmarks with a large x variability should not be used for width measures. They suggest avoiding landmarks with variabilities exceeding 1.5 mm and not using landmarks with a variability exceeding 2.5 mm.

Kim et al[17] tested methods of orienting and regenerating a frontal cephalogram from a CBCT. When the CBCT was oriented similar to a PA cephalogram using various cephalometric software, almost all the measures had no significant differences as compared with the 2D PA cephalogram using one software. The measures with significant differences included the landmark basion, which is difficult to find on a frontal cephalogram.

The intrainvestigator reliability of landmark identification using conventional 2D frontal cephalograms and 3D spiral CTs of the same patients by Bajaj et al[12] showed that numerous landmarks could be identified more reliably on a spiral CT, but not always the same landmark bilaterally.

van Vlijmen et al[18] indicated that 3D tracings are not suitable for longitudinal studies in which only 2D records were available originally because of the clinically relevant differences between 2D lines and 3D planes. They predicted that 3D growth norms would not become available.

Solem et al[19] determined the changes in mandibular structures with age by superimposing 3D CBCTs of growing children. They employed edge-finding algorithms used to detect condylar and mandibular boundaries to segment mandibles from 3D CBCTs. Following voxel-based registration at the mandibular symphysis in 3D, they hemisected the sides of the mandibles. More than 2,000 points were used on each mandibular half to compare changes over time. They suggested that metal implants similar to those used by Bjork, rather than anatomical landmarks, are the best reference for studying growth because no surface or structure on the mandible is stable over time.

2D Measures

Symmetry

Symmetry is evaluated easily as either vertical symmetry or horizontal symmetry. In both methods, following standardization of head position, a median line is drawn from crista galli through ANS and then through the middle of the chin (ie, menton) (Fig 4-13). In a patient with reasonable median symmetry, the line should be straight and perpendicular to the bottom edge of the radiograph. In addition, the midlines of both the maxillary and the mandibular teeth should be on the line. If the median line does not pass through the midlines of the two dentitions and the chin, the reason should be determined. For example, the asymmetry can be caused by crowding of the mandibular anterior teeth that resulted in the primary canine on one side being exfoliated early and the mandibular midline shifting in that direction when the permanent incisors erupted. Trauma, caries, or periodontal disease can cause loss of an incisor, resulting in asymmetry. Dental agenesis in either arch

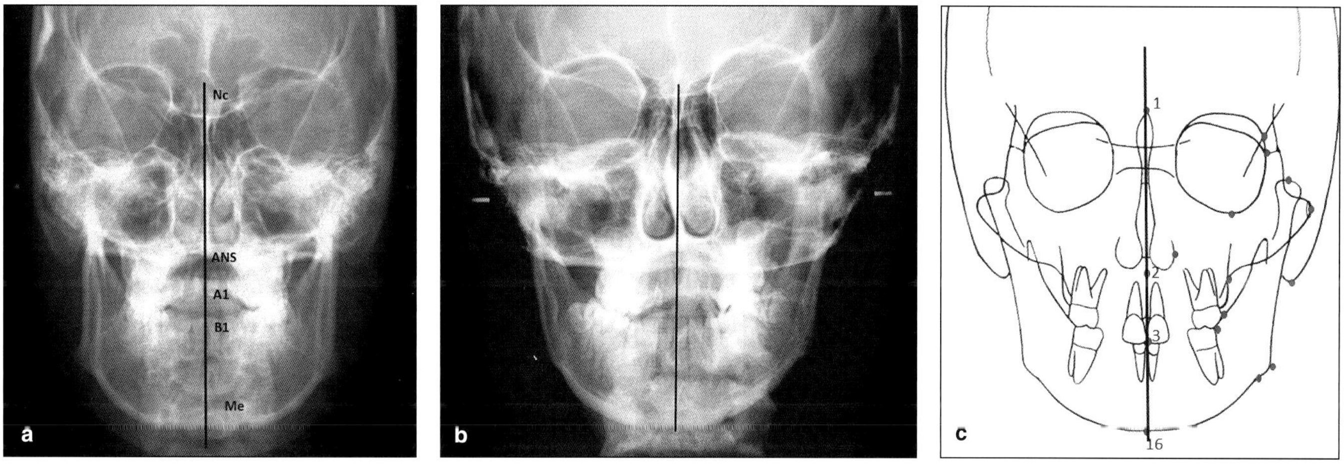

Fig 4-13 The midsagittal plane drawn from the neck of crista galli (Nc) through ANS on a frontal cephalogram of patients with different degrees of asymmetry as well as on a tracing. *(a)* In a patient with slight asymmetry, the line intersects both maxillary and mandibular midlines (A1 and B1) and the chin (menton [Me]). *(b)* In a patient with greater asymmetry, the line reveals nasal asymmetry, mandibular midline deviation, an asymmetric chin, and apparent differences in right and left gonial angles. *(c)* Line drawn on a conventional tracing.

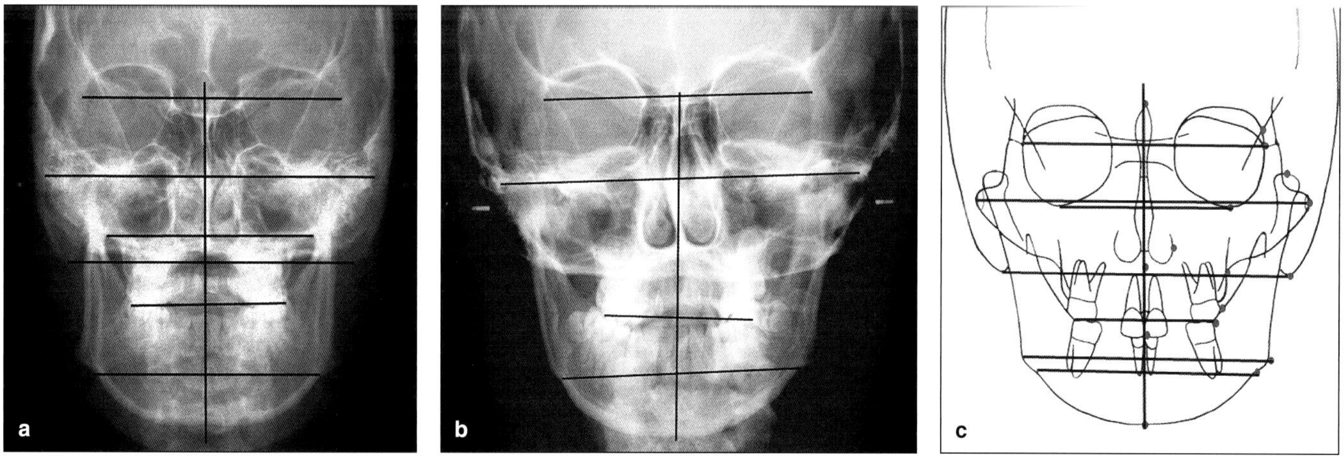

Fig 4-14 Frontal cephalograms with horizontal planes drawn connecting various bilateral landmarks. Even distances between most of the ends of the lines show nearly vertical symmetry *(a)*, whereas uneven distances show definitive asymmetry *(b)*. *(c)* Planes drawn on a conventional tracing showing relative symmetry.

can also cause dental asymmetry. If there is no sign of skeletal asymmetry, this case is a dental problem and could be relatively easy to correct, particularly in a young patient, depending on the existence of other problems.

In contrast, if the mandibular midline is asymmetric and the distances of the right and left occlusal line and the gonial line are unequal, the patient might have a dental interference causing a mandibular shift. Another cause of a mandibular shift could be a skeletal discrepancy between the widths of the maxilla and the mandible. In either case, correction should be performed as soon as possible in a young child to minimize significant and permanent asymmetry and muscle imbalance.

A thorough frontal analysis can aid intraoral examination. However, asymmetric glenoid fossae can cause the midline of the chin to swing to one side. This situation is best observed with an initial CBCT, which will minimize the number of radiographs taken. Thus, when asymmetry is noted on initial examination, a CBCT should be ordered rather than a series of 2D radiographs (eg, lateral cephalogram and panoramic radiograph, then a frontal cephalogram, then a submental vertex radiograph). These additional radiographs can be more costly and expose the patient to more radiation than one 3D CBCT.

Vertical symmetry

To determine vertical symmetry, draw a series of horizontal lines connecting bilateral landmarks such as the right and left frontonasal sutures at the intersection of the orbits, the bottom of the right and left orbits, the middle of the right and left jugal processes, and the bottom of the right and left mastoid processes (Fig 4-14). Then draw a horizontal line connecting the occlusal contacts between the maxillary and mandibular right first molars and left first molars. This line will tell you whether there is an occlusal cant affecting the occlusion. Draw another line connecting the right antegonial notch (or gonial angle) and the left antegonial notch (or gonial angle). This line will help to identify mandibular asymmetry.

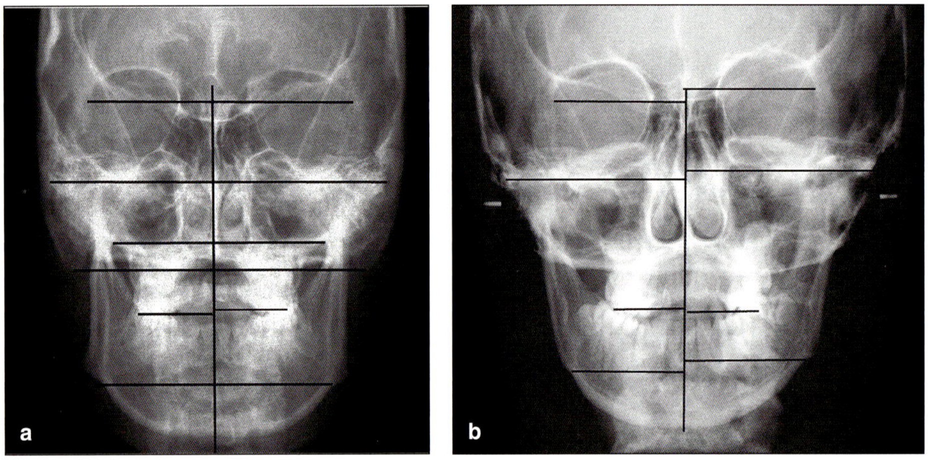

Fig 4-15 *(a)* Vertical symmetry shown on a frontal cephalogram with perpendicular lines from most bilateral landmarks touching the midsagittal plane at the same points but slight asymmetry at the occlusal plane. *(b)* In vertical asymmetry, the perpendicular lines do not touch at the same point. The distances between the perpendiculars from bilateral landmarks can be measured. Horizontal symmetry is determined by measuring the length of each line from the bilateral landmarks to the midsagittal plane.

All horizontal lines in a symmetric face should be perpendicular to the median line. Another way of saying it is that both right and left ends of each line should be equidistant from the line above and below it. Visual inspection is often adequate to determine symmetry, but in cases requiring surgery, measures will be necessary to determine the amount of bony corrections. In that case, construct a line perpendicular from each of the bilateral landmarks to the median line and measure the difference between the bilateral landmarks and the median line to quantify the asymmetry (Fig 4-15). Another way of measuring asymmetry is to make vertical lines from each of the landmarks to a reference plane (eg, zygomaticofrontal suture [Zf] or V plane [Frankfort horizontal plane]), similar to the measure for occlusal plane tilt described later in the chapter. However, the reference plane can also be asymmetric.

Slight differences, particularly in a nongrowing patient, are usually acceptable, whereas asymmetry in a young growing patient can become much worse with growth and should be evaluated and treated as soon as possible. Distinct differences among lines can point to the problem area, but when there are unequal distances between lines in the area of the skull, this usually means that the asymmetries seen in the face probably have their root in skull formation. Orthodontics alone might not be able to correct facial asymmetry. In fact, improper use of mechanics can exaggerate the asymmetry.

Horizontal symmetry

Evaluate horizontal symmetry by measuring the length of the lines extending from the median line to each set of bilateral landmarks (see Fig 4-15). Perfect symmetry means that the right side of each line should equal the left side at all points, but perfect symmetry is rare in an individual.[1,2] Acceptable symmetry is best considered the average measures of a population.

Discussion

The evaluation of horizontal symmetry can assist the orthodontist in evaluating facial asymmetry and its relation with the malocclusion. Asymmetry at the mandibular angle can indicate posterior crossbite or unilateral transverse discrepancies. Similar to vertical asymmetries, horizontal asymmetries starting in the area of the skull are difficult to manage by orthodontics alone.

Slight asymmetries are common. Symmetry is proposed to be one of the four main visual cues for determining facial attractiveness,[20] although it appears that other morphologic components overshadow the relative importance of asymmetry in assessing attractiveness.[21] The cant of the lips at the commissures and asymmetry of the floor of the nose appear to be the major factors of asymmetry affecting attractiveness ratings.[21] Both factors can be associated with malocclusion.

Basyouni and Nanda[11] reviewed the literature concerning frontal asymmetries and transverse discrepancies. The lack of standards for frontal cephalograms prompted them to produce an atlas containing numerous transverse measures of growing children based on the frontal cephalograms contained in the Denver Growth collection.

The Bolton-Brush Study[22] provided serial frontal templates based on the growth of children with ideal facial proportions. Frontal and lateral cephalograms were taken simultaneously. Because radiographic machines are not made so that both cephalograms can be taken simultaneously, mathematical methods of deriving 3D measurements were developed, but they were still not accurate.[23] The frontal cephalograms of growing children were duplicated, and each side was matched with itself and traced as a separate cephalogram. Then the tracings of the duplicated right and the duplicated left images were averaged. Although this method provided a reference for ideal growth, it masked the true asymmetries of the children.

Additional measurements

There are multiple measures of symmetry using frontal cephalometric landmarks. Ricketts and Grummons[13] suggested an extensive means of evaluating symmetry and predicting transverse discrepancies. Some of the measures are similar to each other but provide a somewhat different way of evaluating symmetry.

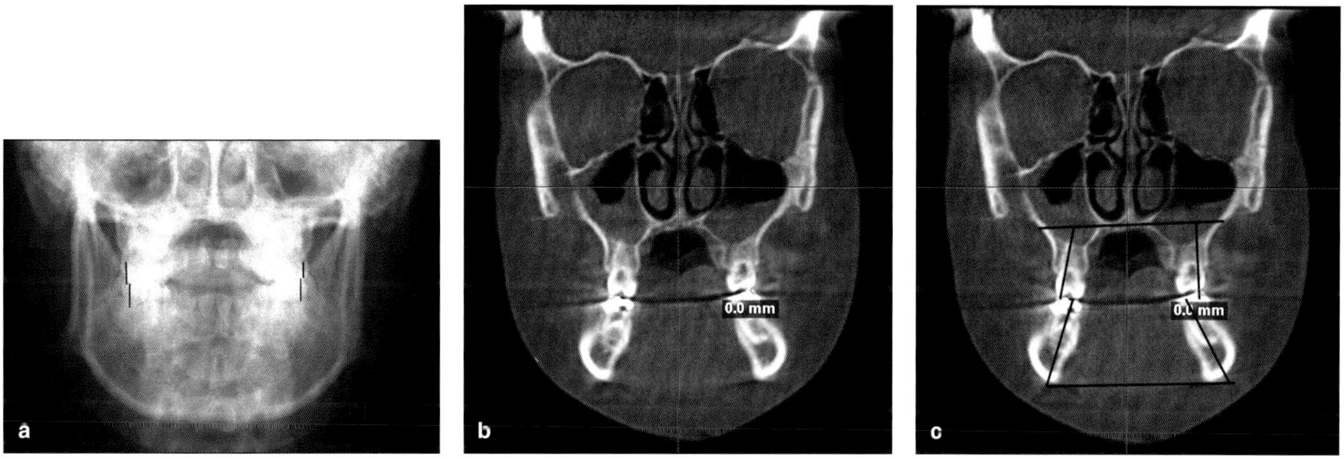

Fig 4-16 Molar relationships measured on a conventional frontal cephalogram *(a)* and on a CBCT *(b)*. 3D CBCTs also allow the inclination of teeth within each arch to be measured relative to a reference plane as well as the distance of the root from the buccal and lingual cortical plates *(c)*.

A few measures that are considered more helpful are measured more easily on 3D CBCTs rather than frontal cephalometric images because of the lack of interference by overlapping structures, particularly in the dental areas. Some measures were discussed previously and will not be reviewed. Some measures have not been applied commonly to 3D CBCTs.

Molar relation. The molar relation or overjet is the distance between the buccal surfaces of the maxillary and mandibular first molars measured along the occlusal plane (Fig 4-16a). These landmarks can be difficult to identify in 2D when the second molars and especially the third molars are erupted. In 2D, only the most buccal surfaces of the molars can be identified, not the cusp tips. The norm for each side is 1.5 mm, with buccal surfaces of the maxillary molars hanging buccal to the surface of the mandibular molars. Numbers larger than 3 mm are interpreted as a buccal crossbite with the maxillary teeth buccal to the mandibular teeth. Numbers that are negative indicate a lingual crossbite with the maxillary teeth lingual to the mandibular teeth. The size of the teeth also influences the amount of the overlap between the molars.

In 3D, slice the image to remove overlying structures and to more clearly see the molars on both sides (Fig 4-16b). Even cusp tips can be identified, allowing a more exacting measure of arch width. In addition, the buccolingual discrepancy or overlap of posterior teeth can be seen anywhere along the arches, including anywhere along the buccal surface of the molars. Standardization of position is necessary for accurate interpretation, particularly because some biomechanics (eg, molar rotation using a toe-in bend) can produce a distal end-to-end situation or even a crossbite of the maxillary and mandibular molars. The inclination of the root and the distance of the root from the buccal and lingual cortical plates can be measured (Fig 4-16c). These measures can be used either for initial decisions of treatment or posttreatment assessment of outcome.

Intermolar width. The intermolar width in 2D is the distance between the buccal surfaces of the mandibular first molars measured along the occlusal plane (Fig 4-17a). According to Ricketts and Grummons,[13] the norm is 55 mm for boys and 54 mm for girls, boys having slightly wider mandibles. The clinical deviation of this measure is 2 mm. Similar to molar relation, the overlap of other structures can make accurate landmark identification difficult in 2D.

In 3D, a little more care must be taken to specifically define the landmarks because the intermolar width can be measured anywhere along the buccal surfaces of the first molars using coronal slices of the arch (Fig 4-17b).

Intercanine width. The intercanine width is the distance between the tips of the mandibular canines (Fig 4-18a). By age 13 years, the distance between erupted mandibular canines is expected to be 27.5 mm, with a clinical deviation of 2 mm. This measure can indicate early width problems of the mandibular arch and potential crowding of the mandibular incisors. Overlying structures in 2D radiographs make identification of canine cusp tips difficult.

Similar to the molars in CBCT, 3D images allow sectioning of the arches to measure the intercanine width (Fig 4-18b). Coronal slicing of the arches removes overlying structures. Asymmetric canines are difficult to measure on one slice, but a sagittal slice in which the mandibular arch is segmented can allow an occlusal view of the teeth to facilitate measurement.

Maxillomandibular width. The maxillomandibular width, a bilateral measure, is the distance between the maxilla (jugal

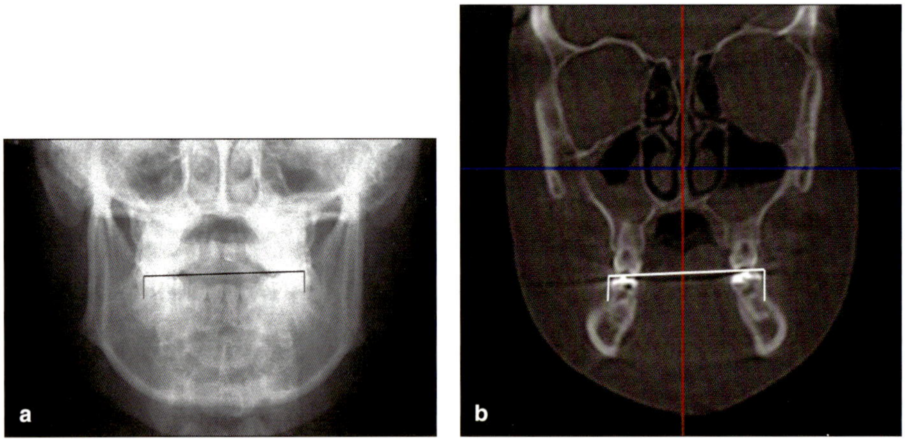

Fig 4-17 Intermolar width measured on a conventional frontal cephalogram *(a)* and on a CBCT *(b)*.

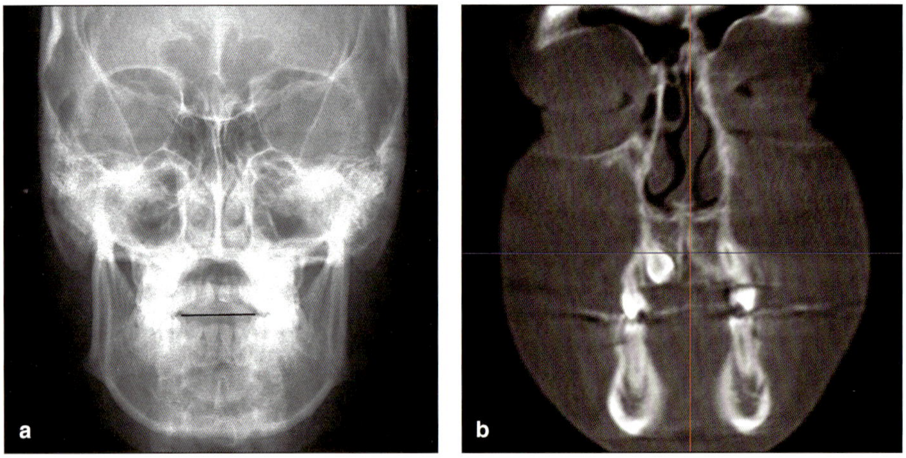

Fig 4-18 Intercanine width measured in the mandibular arch on a conventional frontal cephalogram *(a)* and on a CBCT *(b)*.

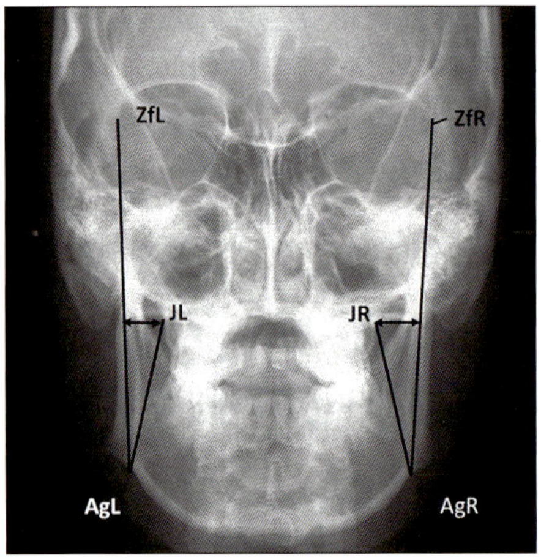

Fig 4-19 Maxillomandibular width shown on a conventional frontal cephalogram. J, jugal process; Ag, antegonion; L, left; R, right.

process) and the frontal facial plane on both the right and left sides (Fig 4-19). The norm is 10 mm for an average-size child at 8.5 years of age. The measure will be smaller for slighter patients and larger for robust patients. The clinical deviation is 1.5 mm. When a crossbite is present, this measure helps to determine if it is a skeletal or dental problem. Large values indicate a skeletal lingual crossbite, whereas small values indicate skeletal buccal crossbites. Small values also indicate that it will be difficult to expand the maxillary arch without interference from the mandible. These numbers can also show asymmetry caused by either skeletal discrepancies or a mandibular lateral slide.

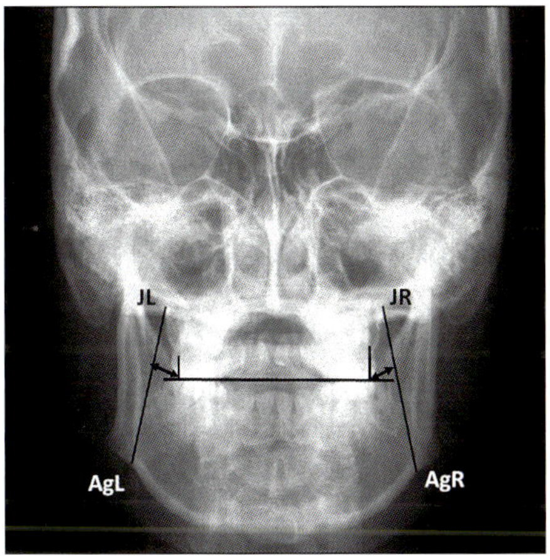

Fig 4-20 Molar to jaws measurement shown on a conventional frontal cephalogram.

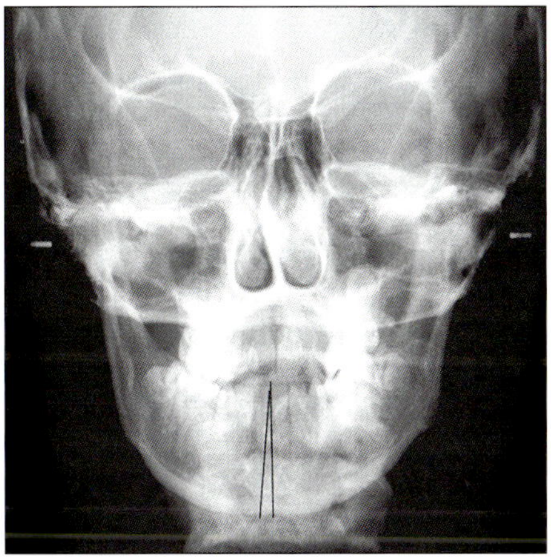

Fig 4-21 Dental to jaw midline measurement shown on a conventional frontal cephalogram.

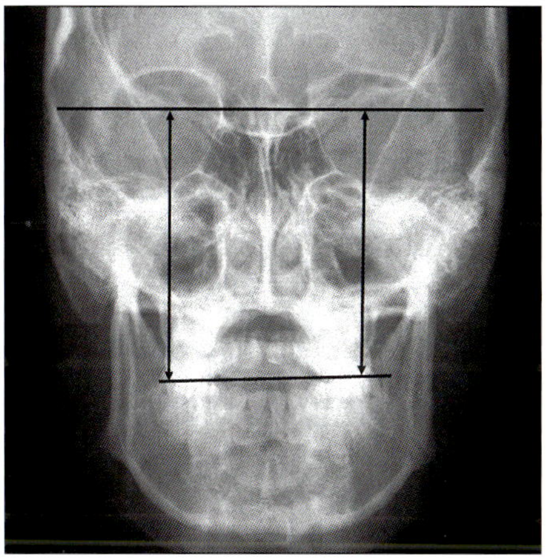

Fig 4-22 Occlusal plane tilt measurement shown on a conventional frontal cephalogram.

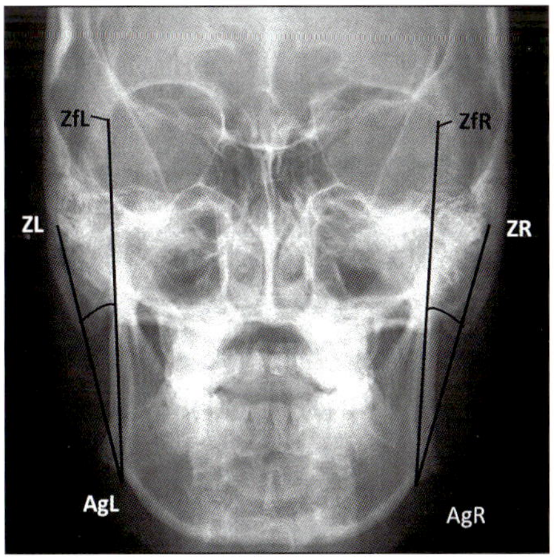

Fig 4-23 Postural symmetry measurement shown on a conventional frontal cephalogram. Z, zygoma.

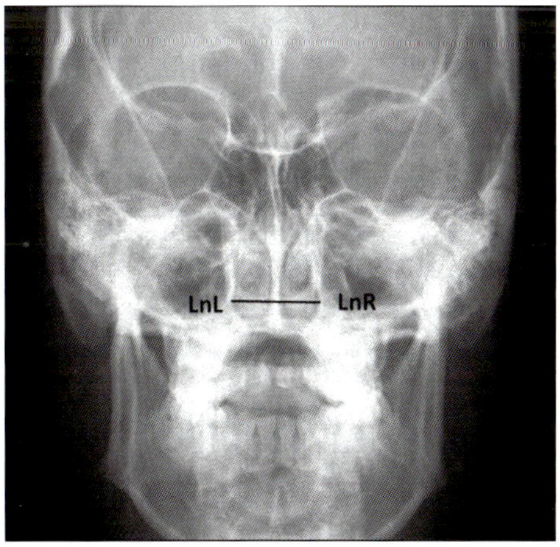

Fig 4-24 Nasal width measurement shown on a conventional frontal cephalogram. Ln, lateral nasal.

Molar to jaws. This measure is the distance between the buccal surface of the maxillary molar and the frontal jaw plane (Fig 4-20). The norm provided is 6.3 mm for an average-size child at 8.5 years of age but can vary depending on the size of the child. The clinical deviation is 1.7 mm. A large distance between the molar and the plane means that there might be room for buccal expansion of the maxilla, whereas a small distance indicates no room for buccal expansion.

Dental to jaw midline. This measure is the distance between the midline of the mandibular incisors and the jaw midline (Fig 4-21). The two midlines should be continuous with each other. Therefore, the norm is 0 degrees, with a clinical deviation of 1.5 mm. This measure is supposed to indicate the difference between a skeletal and a dental shift.

Occlusal plane tilt. This measure is the difference between the height of the occlusal plane at the right and left molars to the zygomaticofrontal suture line (Fig 4-22). This measures the occlusal cant.

Postural symmetry. This measure is the difference between the left and right angles formed by the zygomaticofrontal suture, the antegonial protuberances, and the zygomatic arches (Fig 4-23). The two angles should equal each other. This measure indicates jaw position in centric occlusion.

Nasal width. This measure is the widest aspect of the nasal cavity (Fig 4-24). The nasal opening is measured, and the widest diameter is identified.

Transverse discrepancies

Although various indices (eg, Pont's index, Schwarz and Gratzinger analysis, McNamara's rule of thumb, Korkhaus index, Howe's index), dental cast measurements, PA cephalograms, and CBCTs have been used to predict arch widths, a

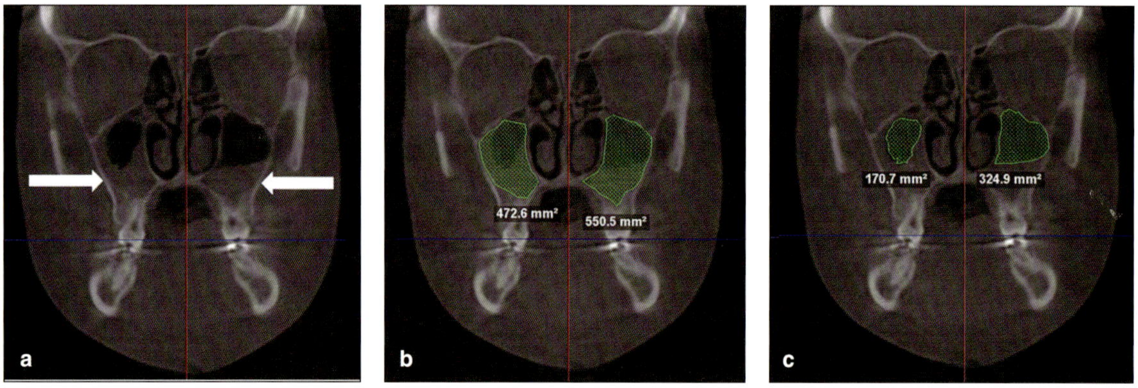

Fig 4-25 3D CBCT coronal slices through the sinuses. *(a) Arrows* pointing to the right and the left maxillary sinuses outlined by radiopaque bone. The right sinus shows a dark radiolucency representing air but almost surrounded by gray, which is probably inflamed soft tissue. The left sinus shows almost a flat line with gray below and black above. The gray is probably fluid because it is flat, and the black is air. *(b)* Following demarcation of the bony outline of the sinuses, the area tool was used to measure the area of both sinuses. *(c)* Area measures of both the right and left sinuses following demarcation of only the black area (air).

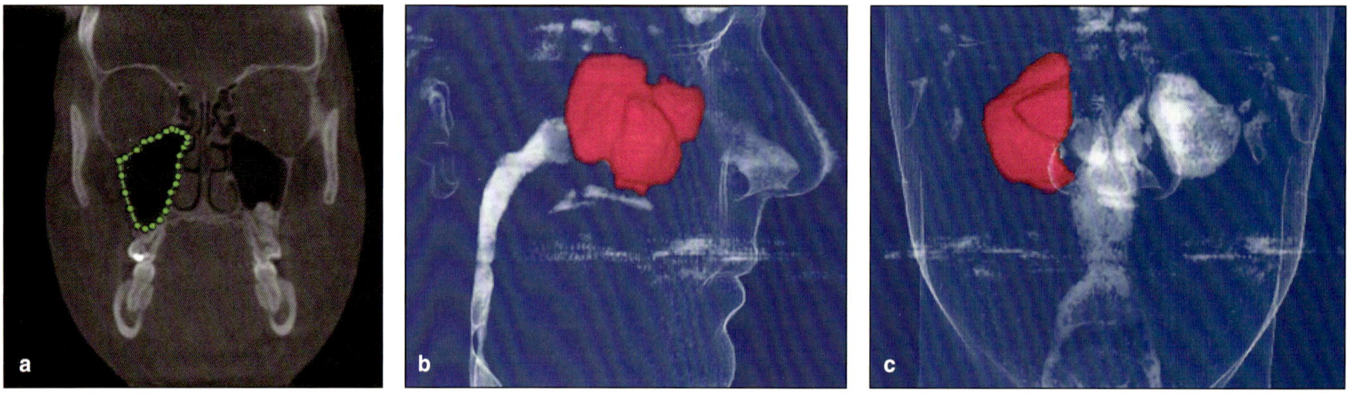

Fig 4-26 Measuring volume using a CBCT. *(a)* A slice through the maxillary sinuses is shown on a CBCT. *(b)* Segmentation of the sinus from the sagittal view. *(c)* Segmentation of the sinus from the frontal view.

recent systematic review of the literature[24] suggests that dental cast studies alone are inaccurate; a combination of dental cast measurements and frontal cephalogram landmarks are more accurate. Studies that compared CBCT and frontal cephalogram measurements to dry skull measurements show that CBCT images more accurately and reliably assessed maxillomandibular transverse discrepancies. The methods suggested for using CBCTs to analyze transverse discrepancies[25,26] are reliable and reproducible but need to be validated clinically.[24] Miner et al[25] suggested using CBCT measures comparing intermolar arch widths as well as molar inclinations that are not obtainable using frontal cephalograms.

3D CBCT Evaluation

Essentially all the measures taken on a 2D cephalogram can be made on a 3D CBCT, although the definition of some landmarks will need to add the y-axis. Overlying structures do not present the same problems seen in 2D cephalometry, although the position of the 3D CBCT image should be standardized to Frankfort horizontal plane and then to the midsagittal plane prior to measurement. This minimizes potential soft tissue and airway differences caused by position and will allow better comparison for growth and treatment among patients. The beauty of 3D CBCT is that the image can be reconstructed to view it similar to a skull (see Fig 4-5a) or that slices can be made through the skull to compare the right and left sides at any point. Selection of specific areas that need to be evaluated is performed by manipulating the colored axis indicators on the screen to a particular area on the skull.

Measures of area can be made using the software by outlining the structure (eg, maxillary sinus) and then selecting area measures in the software[27] (Fig 4-25). Volumetric measures can also be taken either by segmenting the entire structure (Fig 4-26) or by selecting volume measures.[28] However, the gray values (sensitivity settings) need to be adjusted to determine total volume, not just air volume. Alternatively, volume can be calculated by measuring the area and thickness of all the slices involved in a structure, but this is more time-consuming.

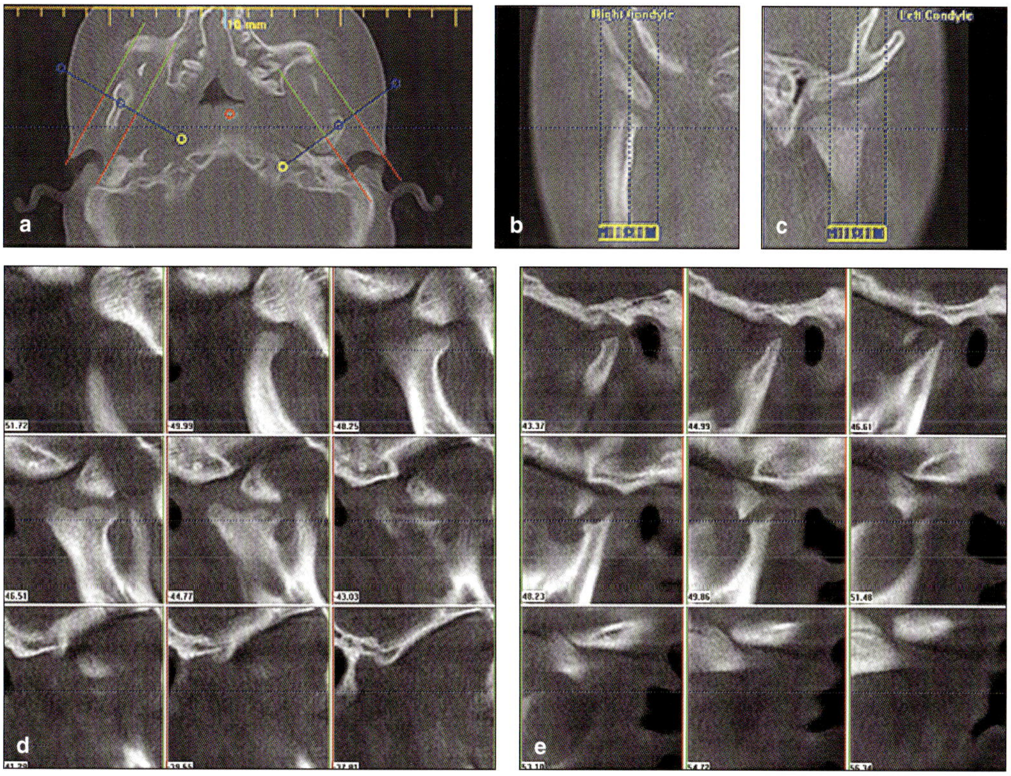

Fig 4-27 3D CBCT showing a submental vertex view *(a)*, coronal slices through the right and left condyles *(b and c)*, and sagittal slices through the right and left condyles *(d and e)*.

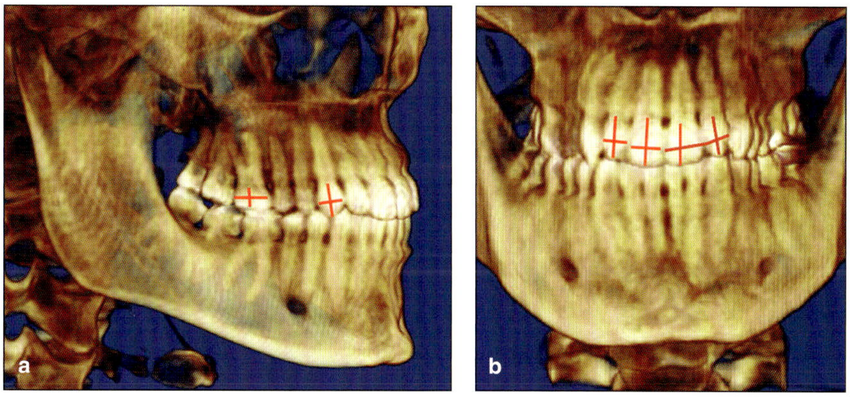

Fig 4-28 Crown height and width measured in sagittal *(a)* and frontal *(b)* views of a reconstructed CBCT.

A 3D CBCT will allow temporomandibular joint evaluations using a submental vertex view (Fig 4-27a) as well as individual coronal sections of both condyles (Figs 4-27b and 4-27c) and a sagittal section of the right and left condyles (Figs 4-27d and 4-27e). Depending on the FOV of the CBCT, various bones and sutures in the cranium can be evaluated for symmetry and early closure. However, suture evaluation is limited by the resolution of the CBCT.

Depending on crowding, the height and width of each tooth crown can also be measured using sagittal and frontal reconstruction[29] (Fig 4-28). Using segmentation, axial slices of the same CBCT allow an occlusal analysis of each arch to be made as well as measurements of individual teeth and Little's Irregularity Index (Fig 4-29).

Note that while CBCTs allow a 3D evaluation of the head and neck area, cephalometry still uses primarily 2D measures.

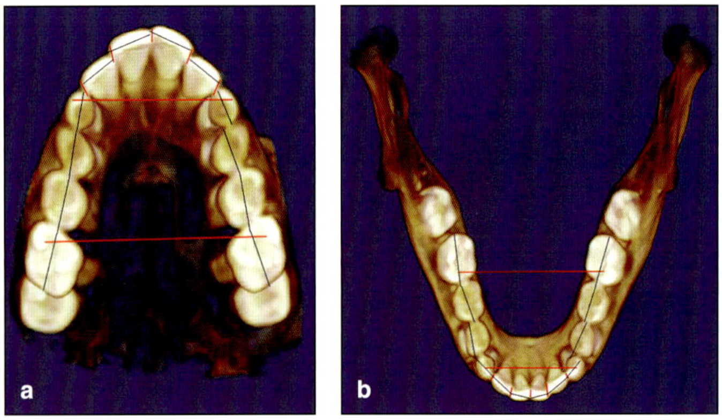

Fig 4-29 *(a and b)* Occlusal views of maxillary and mandibular arches segmented from a 3D CBCT showing tooth width measures in *black*. *Red lines* between the mandibular incisor contact points indicate Little's Irregularity Index, a measure of crowding. The intercanine and intermolar widths are also shown in *red*.

Conclusion

A 2D frontal analysis provides significant information concerning asymmetry that is necessary for diagnosis and treatment considerations, but the visibility of many structures is poor because of overlying structures. In contrast, following image orientation, a 3D analysis allows removal of overlying structures and provides considerably greater diagnostic information than a 2D analysis.

References

1. Lundström A. Some asymmetries of the dental arches, jaws, and skull, and their etiological significance. Am J Orthod 1961;47:81–106.
2. Farkas LG. Anthropometry of the Head and Face, ed 2. New York: Raven, 1994.
3. Smith RJ, Bailit HL. Prevalence and etiology of asymmetries in occlusion. Angle Orthod 1979:49:199–204.
4. Huang M, Hu Y, Yu J, Sun J, Ming Y, Zheng L. Cone-beam computed tomographic evaluation of the temporomandibular joint and dental characteristics of patients with Class II subdivision malocclusion and asymmetry. Korean J Orthod 2017;47:277–288.
5. Lundström F, Lundström A. Natural head position as a basis for cephalometric analysis. Am J Orthod Dentofacial Orthop 1992;101:244–247.
6. Moorrees CFA, Kean MR. Natural head position, a basic consideration in the interpretation of cephalometric radiographs. Am J Phys Anthropol 1958;16:213–234.
7. Kumar V, Ludlow J. Effect of cone beam CT study orientation on synthesized 2D radiographs from Dolphin 3D software. Paper presented at the American Association of Oral and Maxillofacial Radiology 57th Annual Meeting, Kansas City, MO, 16 Nov 2006.
8. Berco M, Rigali PH Jr, Miner RM, DeLuca S, Anderson NK, Will LA. Accuracy and reliability of linear cephalometric measurements from cone-beam computed tomography scans of a dry human skull. Am J Orthod Dentofacial Orthop 2009;136:17.e1–17.e9.
9. Cevidanes L, Oliveira AE, Motta A, Phillips C, Burke B, Tyndall D. Head orientation in CBCT-generated cephalograms. Angle Orthod 2009;79:971–977.
10. Gupta A, Kharbanda OP, Balachandran R, et al. Precision of manual landmark identification between as-received and oriented volume-rendered cone-beam computed tomography images. Am J Orthod Dentofacial Orthop 2017;151:118–131.
11. Basyouni AA, Nanda SK. An Atlas of the Transverse Dimensions of the Face, monograph 37, Craniofacial Growth Series. Ann Arbor: University of Michigan, 2000:235.
12. Bajaj K, Rathee P, Jain P, Panwar VR. Comparison of the reliability of anatomic landmarks based on PA cephalometric radiographs and 3D CT scans in patients with facial asymmetry. Int J Clin Pediatr Dent 2011;4:213–223.
13. Ricketts RM, Grummons D. Frontal cephalometrics: Practical applications, Part I. World J Orthod 2003;4:297–316.
14. Legrell PE, Nyquist H, Isberg A. Validity of identification of gonion and antegonion in frontal cephalograms. Angle Orthod 2000;70:157–164.
15. El-Mangoury NH, Shaheen SI, Mostafa YA. Landmark identification in computerized posteroanterior cephalometrics. Am J Orthod Dentofacial Orthop 1987;91:57–61.
16. Major PW, Johnson DE, Hesse KL, Glover KE. Landmark identification error in posterior anterior cephalometrics. Angle Orthod 1994;64:447–454.
17. Kim SJ, Park SB, Kim YI, Cho BH, Hwang DS. The reliability of cone-beam computed tomography (CBCT)—Generated frontal cephalograms. J Craniomaxillofac Surg 2012;40:e331–e336.
18. van Vlijmen OJ, Maal T, Bergé SJ, Bronkhorst EM, Katsaros C, Kuijpers-Jagtman AM. A comparison between 2D and 3D cephalometry on CBCT scans of human skulls. Int J Oral Maxillofac Surg 2010;39:156–160.
19. Solem RC, Ruellas A, Miller A, Kelly K, Ricks-Oddie JL, Cevidanes L. Congenital and acquired mandibular asymmetry: Mapping growth and remodeling in 3 dimensions. Am J Orthod Dentofacial Orthop 2016;150:238–251.
20. Bashour M. History and current concepts in the analysis of facial attractiveness. Plast Reconstr Surg 2006;118:741–756.
21. Hatch CD, Wehby GL, Nidey NL, Moreno Uribe LM. Effects of objective 3-dimensional measures of facial shape and symmetry on perceptions of facial attractiveness. J Oral Maxillofac Surg 2017;75:1958–1970.
22. Broadbent BH Sr, Broadbent BH Jr, Golden WH. Bolton Standards of Dentofacial Developmental Growth. St Louis: Mosby, 1975.
23. Hans MG, Palomo JM, Valiathan M. History of imaging in orthodontics from Broadbent to cone-beam computed tomography. Am J Orthod Dentofacial Orthop 2015;148:914–921.
24. Sawchuk D, Currie K, Vich ML, Palomo JM, Flores-Mir C. Diagnostic methods for assessing maxillary skeletal and dental transverse deficiencies: A systematic review. Korean J Orthod 2016;46:331–342.
25. Miner RM, Al Qabandi S, Rigali PH, Will LA. Cone-beam computed tomography transverse analysis. Part I: Normative data. Am J Orthod Dentofacial Orthop 2012;142:300–307.
26. Podesser B, Williams S, Bantleon HP, Imhof H. Quantitation of transverse maxillary dimensions using computed tomography: A methodological and reproducibility study. Eur J Orthod 2004;26:209–215.
27. Kula K, Hale LN, Ghoneima A, Tholpady S, Starbuck JM. Cone-beam computed tomography analysis of mucosal thickening in unilateral cleft lip and palate maxillary sinuses. Cleft Palate Craniofac J 2016;53:640–648.
28. Smith T, Ghoneima A, Stewart K, et al. Three-dimensional computed tomography analysis of airway volume changes after rapid maxillary expansion. Am J Orthod Dentofacial Orthop 2012;141:618–626.
29. Kula K, Cilingir HZ, Eckert G, Dagg J, Ghoneima A. The association of malocclusion and trumpet performance. Angle Orthod 2016;86:108–114.

5

Soft Tissue Analysis

Ahmed Ghoneima, BDS, PhD, MSD
Eman Allam, BDS, PhD, MPH
Katherine Kula, MS, DMD, MS

Throughout history, anthropologists, artists, and philosophers have tried to describe beauty and attractiveness. Envisioning that beauty could be measured, scientists have attempted to quantify the ideal proportions of the face.

As early as ancient Egypt, facial beauty was detailed in art using a proportional grid system for creating drawings and facial masks with ideal proportions as a hallmark of beauty and royalty. The Greek culture continued to idealize and define facial esthetics as symmetry and mutual harmony of all parts. Through his drawings, Leonardo da Vinci attempted to formulate facial esthetics and divided the profile into equal thirds. A German printmaker, Albrecht Dürer, used his finger as a measurement unit to create a proportional system for the human body and divided the facial profile into four equal parts. David Hume, the 18th-century Scottish philosopher, pointed out the fact that beauty is in the mind of the beholder and that each mind perceives a different beauty, indicating that individual history and cultural backgrounds influence perception of beauty. Thus, beauty can be an evolving perception. Research has shown that popular actresses and models considered beautiful do not necessarily meet "ideal" soft tissue norms that were established decades ago. However, it is generally agreed that facial beauty is directly related to the balanced proportions of the face.[1–5]

Orthodontists use multiple measures to evaluate soft tissue balance and harmony of the facial features and how treatment will affect the soft tissue. In some cases, the soft tissue of the face suggests the ideal orthodontic or surgical treatment, although the ideal might not be reached for various reasons that the orthodontist or surgeon cannot control. The purpose of this chapter is to describe the measurements of facial soft tissue that can be made using two-dimensional (2D) and three-dimensional (3D) imaging and to provide some norms for those measures.

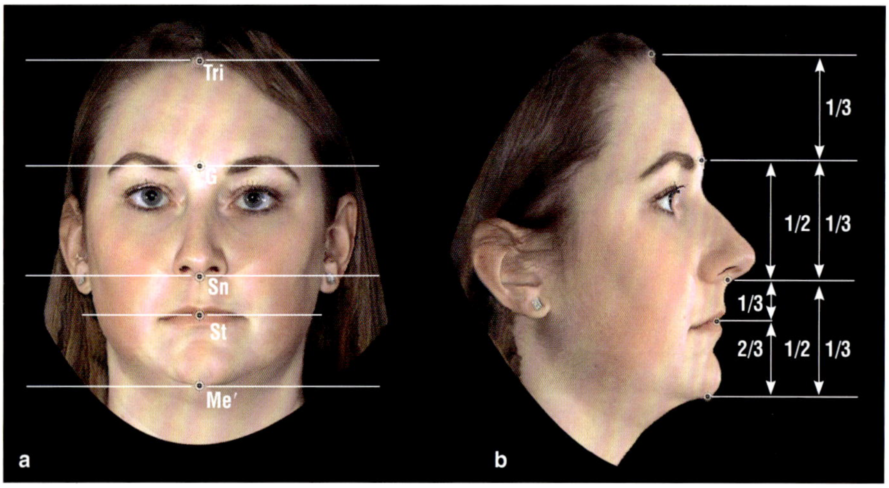

Fig 5-1 Frontal *(a)* and profile *(b)* views showing measures of facial proportions. St, stomion.

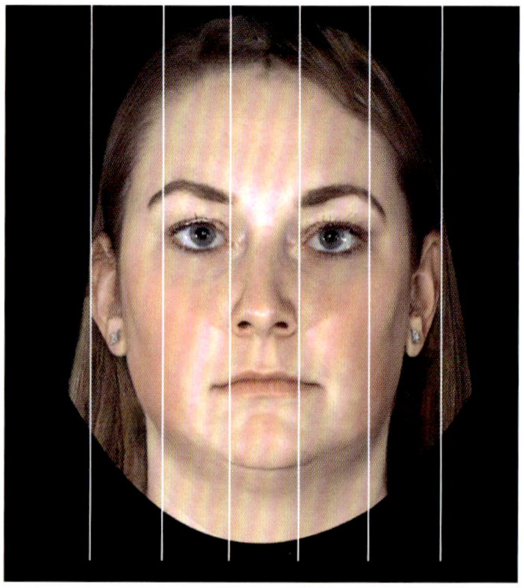

Fig 5-2 Frontal view showing proportions using vertical fifths.

Facial Proportions

To assess facial proportions using anatomical landmarks, an ideal face is divided into equal thirds defined by horizontal lines representing the hairline or trichion (Tri), glabella (G), subnasale (Sn), and soft tissue menton (Me′) (Fig 5-1). In the profile view, the head position is established prior to the image being taken in either the natural head position or with the Frankfort horizontal (FH) plane parallel with the floor. The lips should be relaxed. The upper third should extend from the hairline to glabella, the middle third from glabella to subnasale, and the lower third from subnasale to soft tissue menton. In an ideal lower third, subnasale to stomion (St; or the bottom of the upper lip) comprises the upper third, while menton to stomion (or the top of the lower lip) make up the lower two-thirds.

Lips not touching could indicate lip incompetence, although some researchers consider a slightly open mouth with somewhat protrusive lips to be normal. If the lips are together, one line (St) defining the meeting of the lips can be used as the bottom of the upper lip and the top of the lower lip. The space between the upper lip and the lower lip is called the *interlabial gap*. Ideally, the chin should not show puckering when the lips are together. The puckering usually indicates that the lips are being stretched to touch.[5–7]

Another method of determining facial proportions is to divide the frontal soft tissue of the face vertically into sections (Fig 5-2). The face is divided into five parts from helix to helix of the outer ears. Ideally, the sections should be equal. Vertical lines are dropped through the inner and outer canthus of each eye and then through the helix of each ear. Each eye usually measures one-fifth of the width of the face. The middle fifth is defined by the inner canthus of the eyes. Lines passing through the outer canthus should coincide with the gonial angles of the mandible and provide a frame for the lateral one-fifth on each side. In individuals with broad faces or masseter muscle hypertrophy, the face appears square, and the gonial angles fall outside the canthus line. Unequal proportions suggest hard tissue asymmetry and possible dental asymmetry, but they can also be just soft tissue asymmetry. Contralateral sections that do not match their bilateral counterpart indicate lack of proportionality.[5–7]

Facial Symmetry

Facial symmetry has been proposed as a standard of beauty. In the literature, *symmetry* is defined as the balance and equilibrium in size, form, and arrangement of facial parts on opposite sides of a constructed midsagittal plane. Midline landmarks should coincide with the midsagittal plane, and measurements to landmarks on both sides should be equal (Fig 5-3). Symmetry is rarely perfect because no face is completely symmetric (Fig 5-4). However, the lack of any outstanding asymmetry is essential for good facial esthetics and is considered a sign of attractiveness and good health. Soft tissue asymmetry can also be a clue for skeletal or dental asymmetry and should be evaluated prior to intraoral examination. Facial symmetry is an ultimate goal in plastic and orthognathic surgical corrections of the face.[1–3,8]

Deviation in the midsagittal plane can indicate a shift of the jaw into a crossbite upon closing or a true skeletal asymmetry. The cause of facial asymmetry in a child should be determined and corrected as soon as possible, because it usually increases with growth if untreated. Dental interferences can cause unilateral functional crossbites evident as facial asymmetry. Severe condylar trauma and fracture can also cause facial asymmetry. Recognition of soft tissue asymmetry should be followed by a thorough intraoral and radiographic examination. Currently, a 3D cone beam computed tomography (CBCT) scan would be more appropriate than a 2D radiograph to most efficiently identify the problem.[6,7]

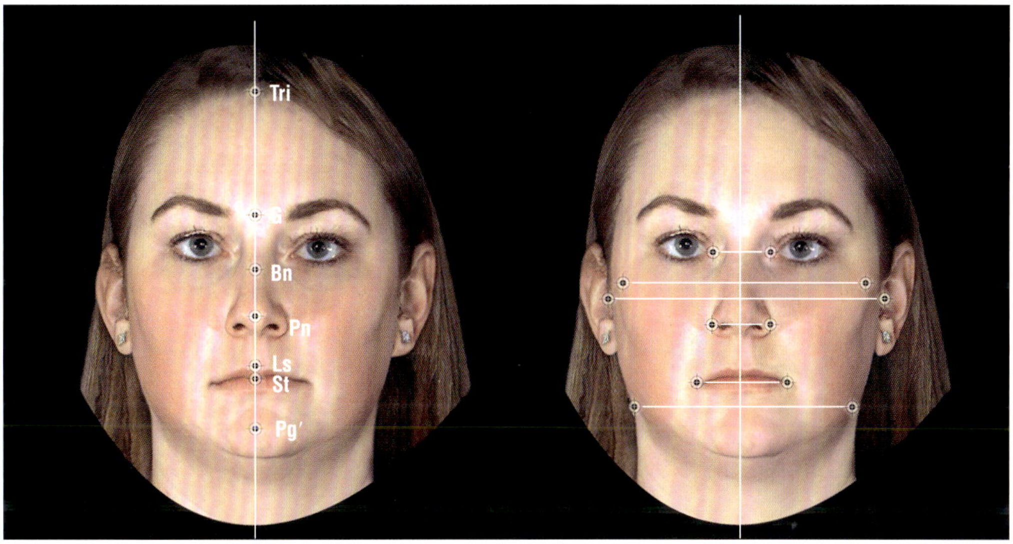

Fig 5-3 The symmetry of the face is defined by identical left and right sides of the midsagittal plane. Bn, bridge of nose; Pn, pronasale; Ls, labrale superius; Pg', soft tissue pogonion.

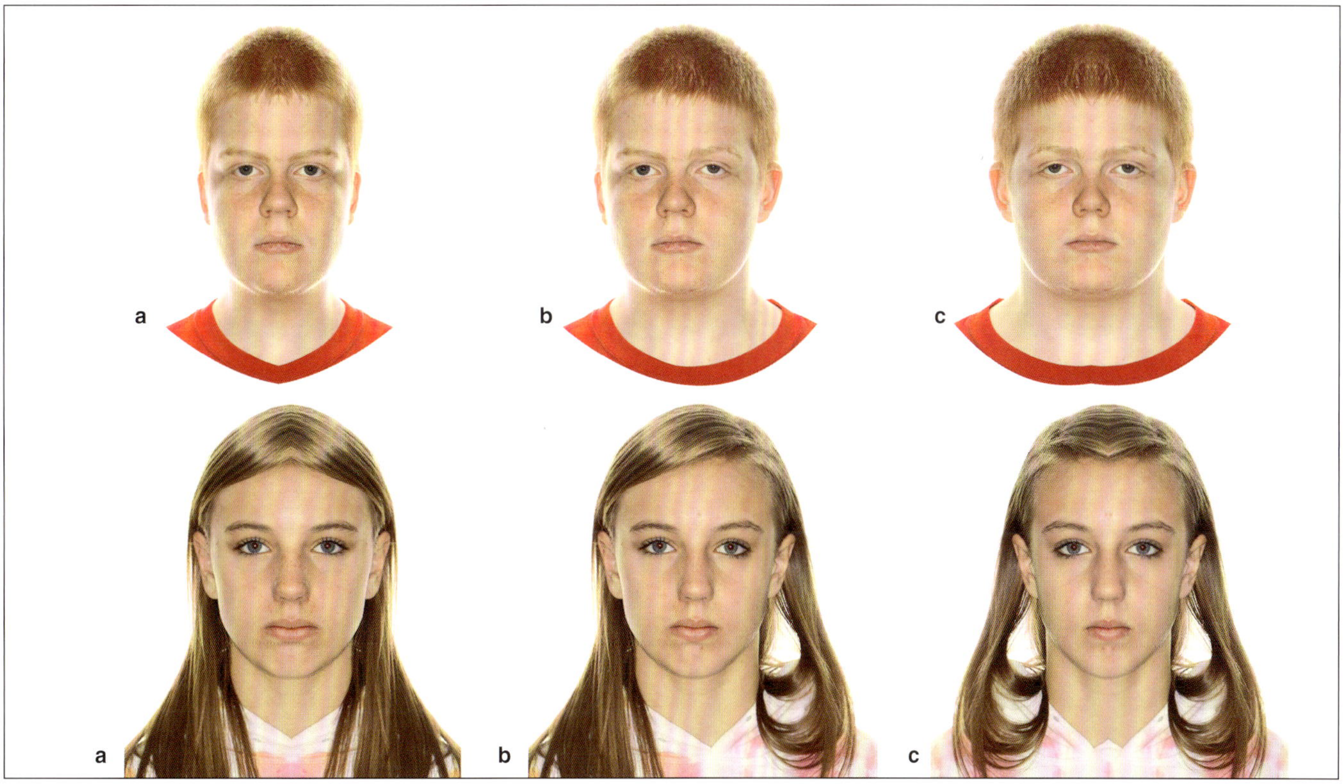

Fig 5-4 Symmetry is rarely perfect, as shown by these photographs that duplicate half the face. *(a)* Image constructed by reflecting the left half of the face onto the right half. *(b)* Original image of the face. *(c)* Image constructed by reflecting the right half of the face onto the left half. None of the constructed images is the same as the original face from which the halves were taken. Asymmetry can be remarkable *(top)*, where the right image produces a much thinner face and the left image produces a broader face, or mild *(bottom)*, where the demarcation between normal and abnormal bilateral facial asymmetry is not as noticeable.

Table 5-1 Soft tissue landmarks with abbreviation and definition

Landmark	Abbreviation	Definition	Midline or bilateral landmark
Trichion	Tri	The point of the hairline in the midline of the forehead	Midline
Glabella	G	The most prominent midline point in the midsagittal plane between the eyebrows	Midline
Soft tissue nasion	N′	The point of greatest concavity in the midline between the forehead and the nose	Midline
Bridge of nose	Bn	Midpoint on the midsagittal plane over the tip of the nasal bone	Midline
Endocanthion	En	The point at the inner commissure of the eye fissure	Bilateral
Exocanthion	Ex	The point at the outer commissure of the eye fissure	Bilateral
Orbitale	Or	The most inferior point of the orbital floor below the center of the eye	Bilateral
Zygomatic prominence	Zp	The most protrusive anterior point on the zygomatic arch	Bilateral
Zygion	Zy	The most lateral point of each zygomatic arch	Bilateral
Tragion	T	The point located at the upper margin of each tragus	Bilateral
Pronasale	Pn	The most prominent midline point on the tip of the nose	Midline
Alare	Al	The most lateral point on each alar contour	Bilateral
Subnasale	Sn	The point at which the columella (nasal septum) merges with the upper lip in the midsagittal plane	Midline
Superior labial sulcus	Sls	The point of greatest concavity in the midsagittal plane of the upper lip between Sn and labrale superius	Midline
Labrale superius	Ls	A point indicating the mucocutaneous border of the upper lip (usually the most anterior point of the upper lip)	Midline
Stomion	St	The contact point between the upper and lower lip at the mouth slit	Midline
Cheilion	C	The most lateral point located at each labial commissure	Bilateral
Labrale inferior	Li	The most anterior aspect of the lower vermilion border of the lower lip in the centerline	Midline
Inferior labial sulcus	Ils	The point of greatest concavity in the midsagittal plane of the lower lip between Li and soft tissue pogonion (also known as *labiomental sulcus*)	Midline
Soft tissue pogonion	Pg′	The most anterior point on the chin in the midsagittal plane	Midline
Soft tissue gnathion	Gn′	The most anterior and inferior point on the soft tissue chin in the midsagittal plane	Midline
Soft tissue menton	Me′	The most inferior point on the soft tissue chin	Midline
Tragus	Trg	The most lateral and posterior point of the right tragus of the ear	Bilateral

Soft Tissue Cephalometric Landmarks

Cephalometry is a standard tool for describing the short- and long-term changes of growth and treatment on the skeletal, dental, and soft tissues. Soft tissue analysis is essential to determine facial esthetics before and after orthodontic treatment. On a 2D lateral cephalogram, soft tissue analysis can be performed on either the facial profile or frontal view, while a 3D image will allow soft tissue evaluation to be performed in multiple planes and different dimensions. Table 5-1 outlines the 2D and 3D facial landmarks commonly used by most orthodontic clinicians for cephalometric soft tissue analysis[9–13] (Fig 5-5).

Soft Tissue Analysis and Orthodontic Applications

Orthodontic treatment has historically been based on the hypothesis that achieving ideal occlusion allows facial beauty to follow. It was assumed that the soft tissue profile configuration was principally related to the underlying skeletal structures and that a linear relationship exists between them. This basic philosophy of orthodontic diagnosis was based on the idea that the dentoskeletal structures acted as the scaffold onto which soft tissue drapes, so treatment planning basically depended on moving the dentoskeletal structures.

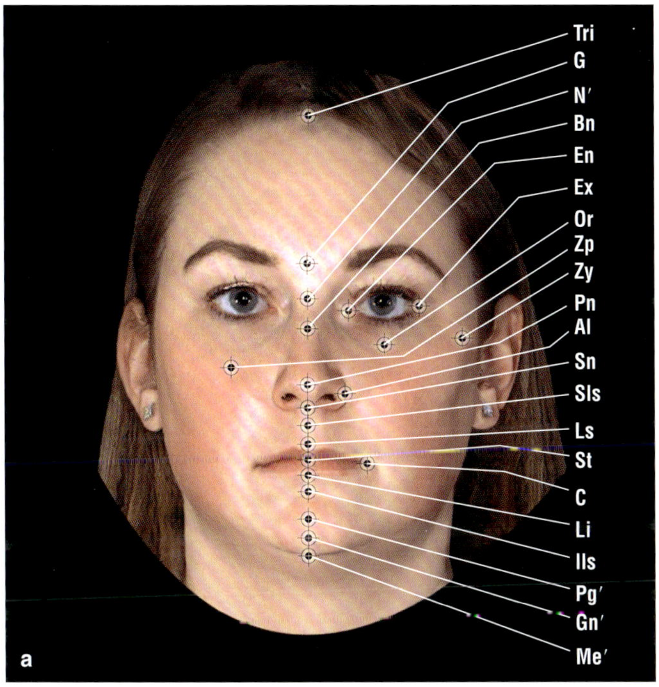

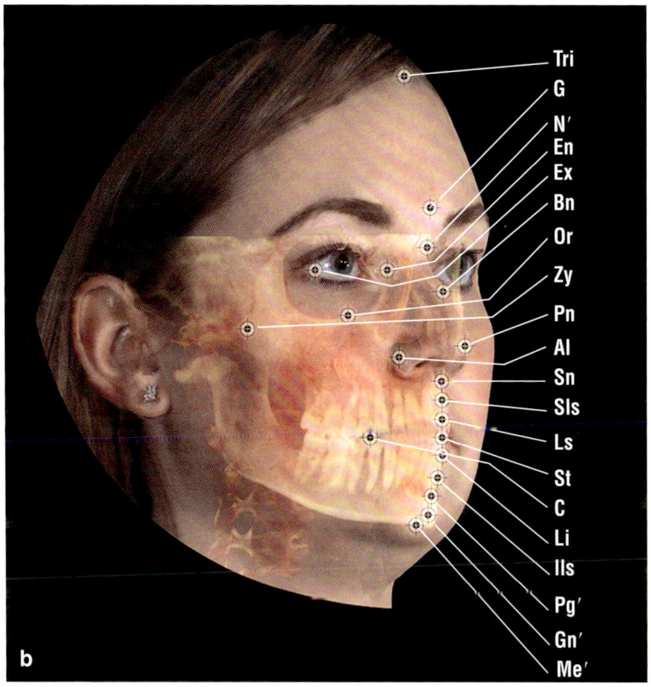

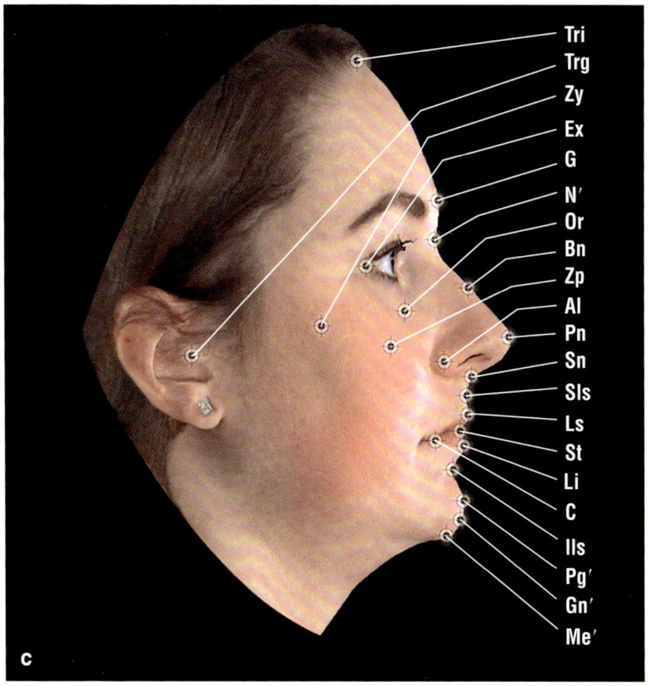

Fig 5-5 Soft tissue landmarks. *(a)* Frontal view. *(b)* Lateral oblique view. *(c)* Lateral or profile view.

Assessment of the soft tissue on its own merit and developing soft tissue profile objectives was a paradigm shift led by the introduction and promulgation of cephalometric soft tissue analysis. A change in treatment philosophy stressed harmonious facial characteristics compatible with sound functionality as the main goal in orthodontic treatment.[14,15] This change in treatment philosophy indicated that more emphasis should be placed on the soft tissue and the external facial profile evaluation and that clinicians should consider mainly treatment plans that fit within the patient's limits of soft tissue adaptation and facial contours.

Orthodontists should also recognize that facial cephalometric measurements and standard values are variable, especially when different ethnic populations are involved. Studies measuring human faces from various ethnic populations indicate that ethnic variations in soft tissue are greater than skeletal and dental variations.[16–18]

Soft tissue cephalometrics is considered a reliable guide for measuring and quantifying positions and relationships of facial parts. Diagnosis and treatment planning of an orthodontics patient involves the clinical analysis of dental components combined with a thorough soft tissue examination and quantitative assessment of facial morphology. Assessment of facial convexity, the patient's nose along with the lip positions, soft tissue chin prominence, and profile soft tissue thickness are of considerable importance in successful diagnosis and treatment planning. This section describes the parameters that could be used for such assessment. The colored and textured images shown in profile will be used to demonstrate 2D cephalometric measures.

Facial convexity

There are a number of measures for facial convexity, many of which sound the same. However, there is a distinction between *skeletal profile convexity*, *soft tissue profile convexity*, and *total profile convexity*. Skeletal profile convexity is represented by soft tissue nasion–A-point–soft tissue pogonion (N′APg′), with a mean value of 175 to 177.5 degrees. Skeletal convexity decreases with age. Soft tissue profile convexity is represent-

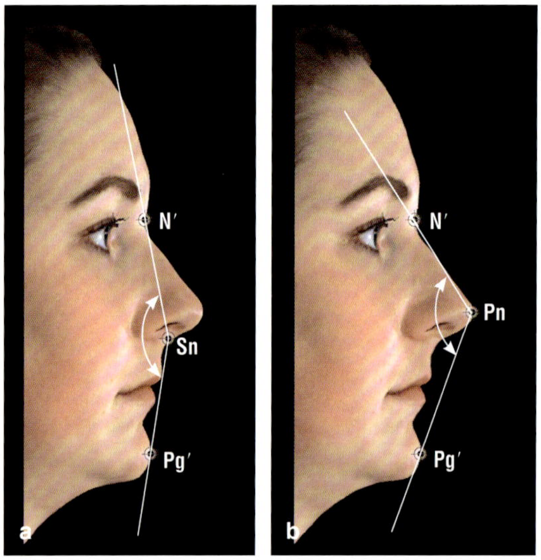

Fig 5-6 *(a)* Soft tissue profile convexity. *(b)* Total profile convexity.

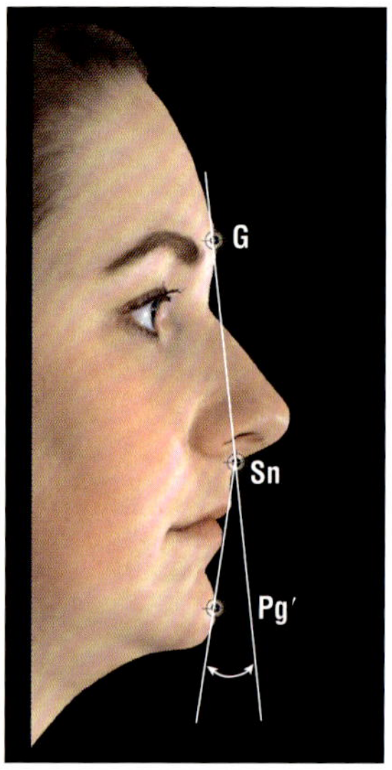

Fig 5-7 Angle of facial convexity.

ed by the intersection of the soft tissue nasion–subnasale line (N′Sn) and the subnasale–soft tissue pogonion line (SnPg′) (Fig 5-6a). The mean value is 161 degrees, and this is generally considered stable and does not change with age. Total profile convexity includes the nose and is represented by the intersection of the soft tissue nasion–pronasale line (N′Pn) and the soft tissue pogonion–pronasale line (Pg′Pn) (Fig 5-6b). The mean value is 137 degrees for males and 133 degrees for females. This convexity increases with age. The age-dependent changes in total profile convexity make it evident that soft tissue changes are not parallel to skeletal profile changes. The increase in total profile convexity is suggested to be due to the forward growth of the nose.[9,19–21]

The angle of facial convexity (Fig 5-7) is measured as the angle formed between the glabella-subnasale line (GSn) intersecting with the SnPg′ line, with an estimated mean value of 12 ± 4 degrees. In females, a more convex profile is considered esthetically pleasing, whereas straighter profiles are generally preferred for males. Values range from 11 ± 4 degrees for males and 13 ± 4 degrees for females.[9,19–21]

Nose

The nose, the most prominent feature in the face, is considered by orthodontists as a keystone of facial esthetics. An ideal nose should be in complete harmony with the other features of the face and in balance with the profile convexity. Nasal characteristics directly relate to the individual's race, sex, and other facial features. Evidence indicates that the nose grows in a downward and anterior direction, with an average length increase of 1.0 to 1.5 mm annually until early adulthood. An excessively large or small nose significantly affects the facial harmony as well as orthodontic treatment results.

In evaluating treatment results, orthodontists must assess the positional balance and harmony between the lips, chin, and nose. The tip of the nose (pronasale) grows more than any other part of the soft tissue profile. While nose growth in males is about 1.5 to 2 times that in females, the vertical growth in males tends to compensate for the horizontal nasal growth, keeping the convexity in males from being significantly more prominent than in females.[7,19,22]

The nasal angle is measured as the angle formed between a line drawn tangent to the lower border of the nose and the vertical line passing through Sn (SnV). The nasolabial angle is the angle formed between a line tangent to the lower border of the nose and the line connecting Sn with Pg′. The nasofacial angle is determined by the intersection of the glabella–soft tissue pogonion line (GPg′) with a line drawn tangent to the bridge of the nose[9] (Fig 5-8).The measurement of the nasolabial angle ranges from 90 to 110 degrees, with no great difference between the sexes. This angle is important in assessing the upper lip position, and it greatly depends on anteroposterior (AP) position or the inclination of the maxillary anterior teeth and is also influenced by the inclination of the lower border of the nose. It is critical for evaluating the AP position of the maxilla and for extraction decisions. The nasolabial angle is more obtuse in Class III patients and more acute in Class II patients. An acute angle suggests the need for maxillary incisor retraction or a maxillary setback, while an obtuse angle suggests the need for maxillary advancement, advancement of the maxillary incisors, or both.[9,21,23] The nasolabial angle is also closely related to the thickness of the upper lip. The upper lip is typically thick and everted in black individuals and flat in white individuals. The sulcular depth of the upper lip increases with prominent lips and decreases with flat lips.[24,25]

Profile

Variations in soft tissue facial profile are generally perceived in the discrepancies of skeletal convexity, soft tissue thickness, protrusion of the lips, and position of the mandibular incisors. Although evidence indicates that growth and maturation con-

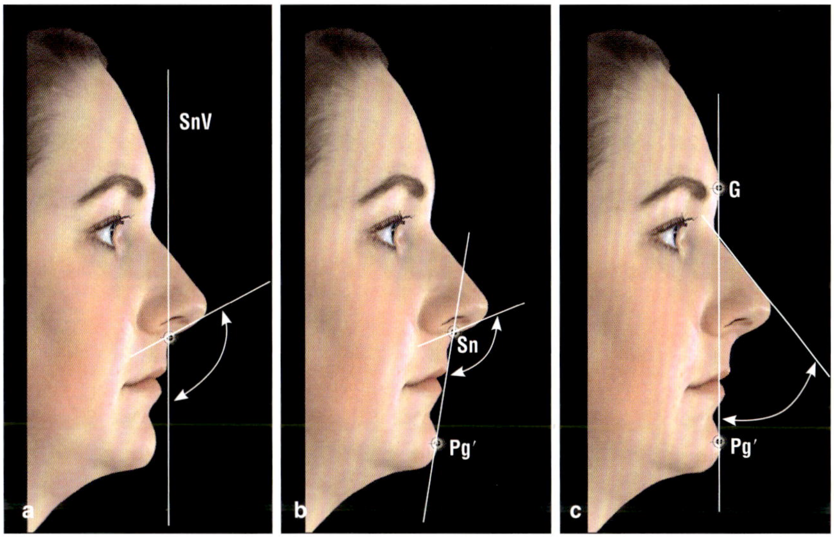

Fig 5-8 *(a)* Nasal angle. *(b)* Nasolabial angle. *(c)* Nasofacial angle.

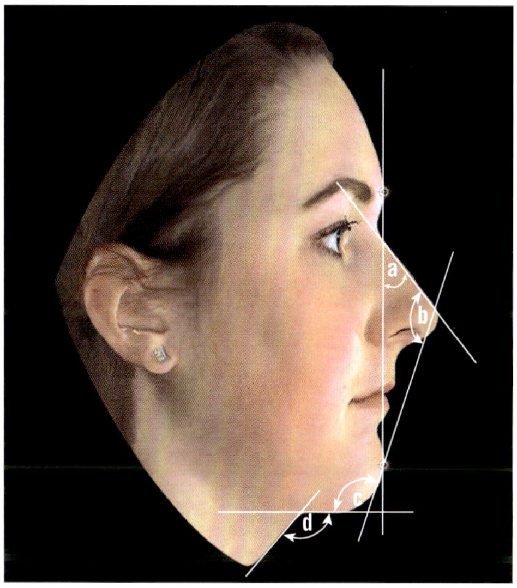

Fig 5-9 *(a)* Nasofacial angle. *(b)* Nasomental angle. *(c)* Mentocervical angle. *(d)* Submental-neck angle.

tinue throughout life, most facial profile changes occur before early adulthood, and changes are more evident in males than in females. With continuous growth, the facial profile becomes more concave. Principally, as the nose and the chin grow, the lips become more retruded.

Many angles can be used for profile analysis, such as the nasofacial angle, nasomental angle, mentocervical angle, submental-neck angle, and mentolabial sulcus (Fig 5-9). In white individuals, ideal ranges for these angles are as follows: nasofacial angle, 30 to 35 degrees; nasomental angle, 120 to 132 degrees; mentocervical angle, 110 to 120 degrees; and submental-neck angle, 126 degrees in males and 121 degrees in females.[6,26,27]

Mentolabial depth is measured as the angle of intersection between two tangent lines of the lower lip and the upper part of the chin (Fig 5-10a). The average value is 130 degrees. It can also be measured as the linear distance between the deepest point on the mentolabial sulcus to the lower lip–soft tissue pogonion line (LiPg′) (Fig 5-10b). The average value is 4 ± 2 mm. The depth of the mentolabial sulcus is affected by various factors such as flared mandibular incisors, a flaccid lower lip, extruded maxillary incisors causing rolling of the lower lip, and a prominent chin. The presence of excessively uprighted incisors usually results in a deficient mentolabial sulcus, giving the lower facial third a flat appearance. A short lower face height is usually associated with an excessive mentolabial sulcus. A more pronounced mentolabial angle can be seen in Class II patients and patients with vertical maxillary deficiency. Uprighting of the mandibular incisors tends to enlarge the angle, whereas proclination of the mandibular incisors decreases the angle.[11,12,28]

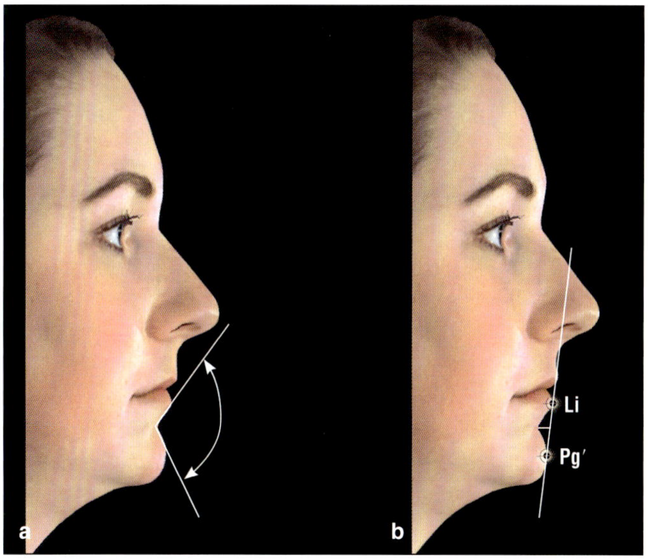

Fig 5-10 *(a and b)* Measurements for mentolabial depth.

Lips

Lip measurements, postural position, the interlabial gap, and relative proportionality with other facial features are important components in the clinical analysis of the orthodontic patient. The length of the upper lip is measured from subnasale to stomion (SnSt) and is about 22 ± 2 mm for males and 20 ± 2 mm for females at age 12 years. In most adults, the upper lip increases in length with age, especially in males. A slight increase in length between 6 and 12 years of age is expected in Class II patients (1.9 mm) and Class III patients (0.9 mm). The upper lip length also increases during the course of orthodontic treatment as a result of both growth changes and opening of the bite.[9,11,29] A shorter upper lip usually results in more tooth exposure at rest.

The length of the lower lip is measured from gnathion to stomion (Gn′St). The mean value is 49 ± 2 mm in males and 46.5 ± 2 mm in females. The lower lip gradually increases in length

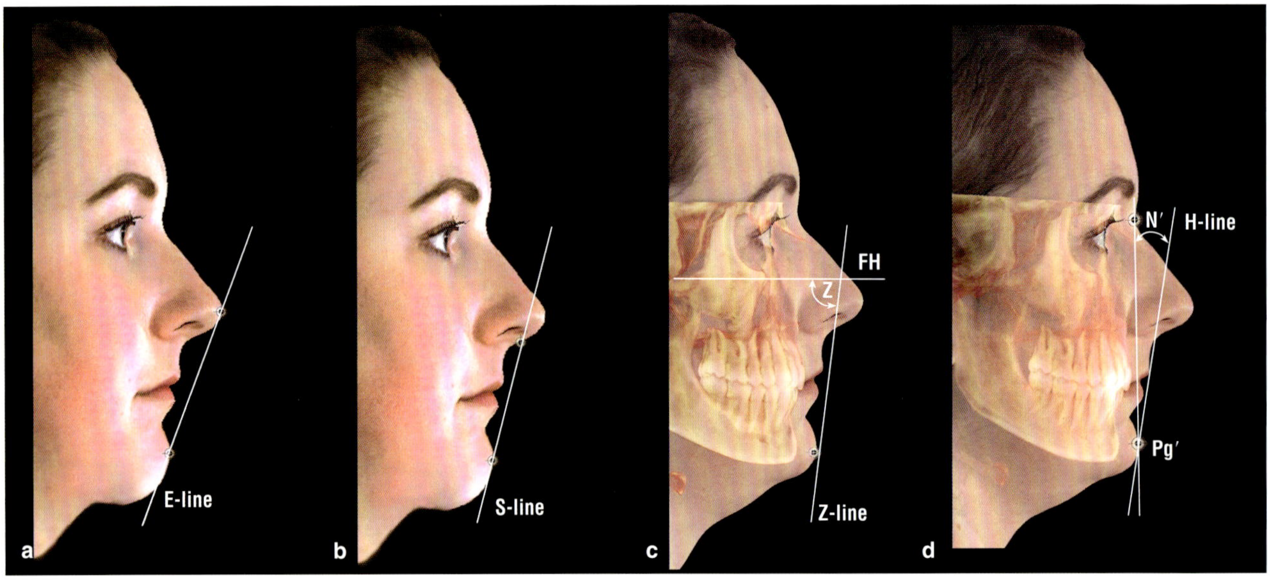

Fig 5-11 *(a to d)* E-line, S-line, Z-angle, and H-angle.

with age, slightly more in patients with Class III malocclusion (1.9 mm) than in those with Class II (1.5 mm) malocclusion. During treatment, the lower lip shows a greater increase in length in Class III patients than in Class II patients. The changes are principally connected with growth in AP and vertical directions.[9,11,29] The upper and lower lip length measurements are relatively larger in black individuals than in white individuals.[25]

The interlabial gap is the distance between the inferior border of the upper lip and the upper border of the lower lip. The acceptable average values are 2 ± 2 mm in normal occlusion or at the end of treatment. A little amount of lip incompetence is still considered normal. An increase in the interlabial gap is related to several factors, including tooth position, lip length and posture, vertical maxillary excess, and facial patterns.[9,11,29]

Reference planes for lip profile analysis

There are several measures for evaluating lip profile, with some minor differences between them (see Fig 5-11). The lips are supported primarily by the teeth, but the reference lines are based usually on chin and nose position. All of these measures are therefore influenced by nasal and chin growth, but some are influenced less by nasal growth than the others. These measurement tools along with clinical examination of tooth position and gingival support and cephalometric evaluation of the bone around the incisors help to determine whether extractions or surgery is indicated.

Studies on small groups of patients indicated significant ethnic variations in lip position. Upper and lower lips were positioned more anteriorly with a greater degree of lip protrusion in Asian populations than in white populations. Black individuals had fuller, more prominent lips and greater protrusion of both upper and lower lips as related to the facial plane when compared with white individuals.[16,17,29–31]

Ricketts E-line

The Ricketts E-line (esthetic plane) is drawn from the tip of the nose (Pn) to Pg′ (Fig 5-11a). Ideally, the upper lip (Ls) is about 4 mm behind this reference line, while the lower lip (Li) lies about 2 mm behind it. Upper and lower lips become more retruded to the E-line between 5 and 25 years of age, with an average of 5.6 mm in males and 5.0 mm in females for the upper lip and about 4.1 mm in males and 2.6 mm in females for the lower lip. However, tooth positions and dental support for the upper and lower lips as well as the chin position can significantly affect these values.[32,33]

Steiner lip analysis (S-line)

The upper reference point for Steiner analysis is at the center of the S-shaped curve between the tip of the nose and Sn. Pg′ represents the lower point (Fig 5-11b). Lips lying behind the line connecting these two points are too flat, and those lying anterior to it are too prominent. Ideally, the most prominent point in the upper and lower lips should touch this line.[34]

Merrifield profile line (Z-angle)

The Merrifield Z-angle is formed by the intersection of FH and a line connecting Pg′ and the most protrusive lip point (either upper or lower lip) (Fig 5-11c). It generally reflects the relationship of the lips to the chin. The average value is 80 ± 9 degrees.[35]

Holdaway lip analysis

The Holdaway H-angle (Fig 5-11d) describes the degree of soft tissue protrusion of the maxilla relative to the mandible and is ideally about 10 degrees. This angle, similar to other lip anal-

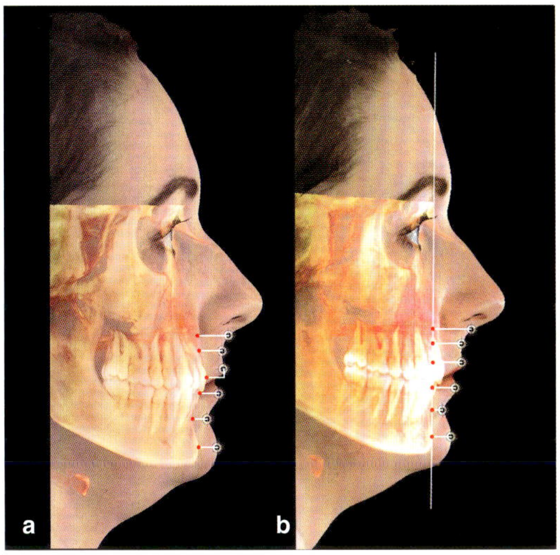

Fig 5-12 Thickness of soft tissue profile according to Burstone analysis *(a)* and Bowker and Meredith analysis *(b)*.

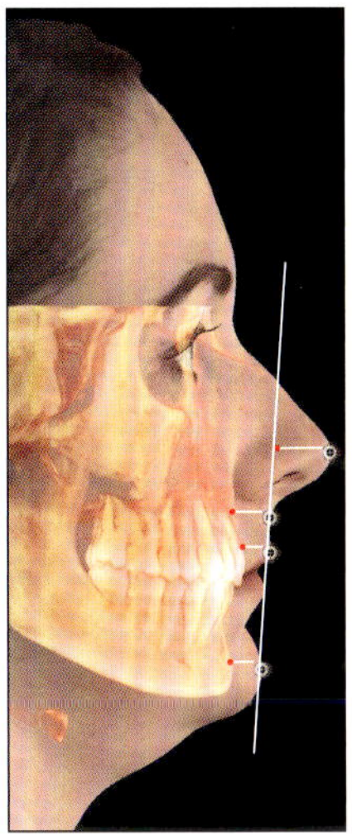

Fig 5-13 Soft tissue thickness of the nose, upper lip, and chin.

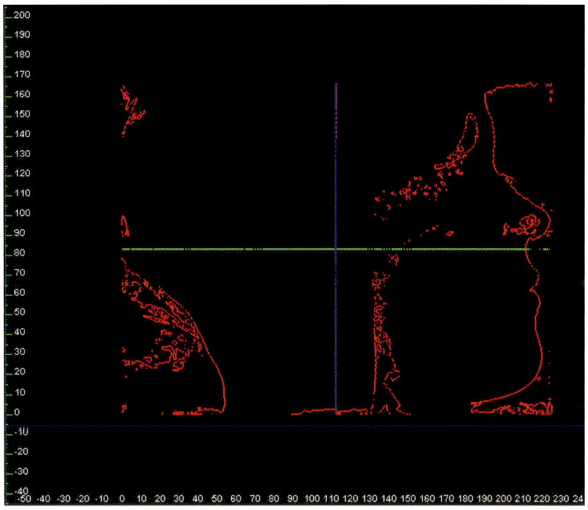

Fig 5-14 Screenshot of CBCT soft tissue segmentation showing the 2D outline of skin.

ysis measures, can be manipulated by orthodontics. According to Holdaway, a perfect profile should have an A-point–soft tissue nasion–B-point (ANB) of 2 degrees, an H-angle of 7 to 15 degrees, a lower lip touching the H-line, an H-line bisecting the S-shaped curve between Pn and Sn, the tip of the nose at 9 mm anterior to the H-line, and no lip tension on closure. Both the lips and the chin should align near the H-line.[36]

Soft tissue thickness

Soft tissue thickness is measured at the following points: Sn, soft tissue A-point, the upper lip (Ls), the lower lip (Li), soft tissue B-point, and Pg′ on a straight line to the underlying skeletal and dental tissues (Fig 5-12a). It also can be measured at the same aforementioned soft tissue landmarks to the facial plane (N′Pg′) (Fig 5-12b). A greater increase in maxillary soft tissue thickness than mandibular soft tissue thickness occurs with age and would explain the tendency for the soft tissue convexity to increase with age despite the tendency of the skeletal profile to straighten.[37,38]

Upper lip thickness is measured from labrale superius (Ls) to the labial surface of the maxillary central incisor and from a point on the outer alveolar plate to the outer border of the upper lip. The ideal upper lip thickness is about 15 mm. Soft tissue–chin thickness is measured as the distance between the bony and soft tissue facial planes (Pg to Pg′). An ideal average value for chin thickness is 10 to 12 mm. In individuals with prominent chins, the mandibular incisors may be allowed to remain in a more prominent position as an important facial harmony consideration. Nose thickness is also critical for facial and labial balance and harmony. The distance from Pn to H-line should not exceed 12 mm in individuals 14 years of age and older[9,12] (Fig 5-13).

Capturing Soft Tissue Images

2D cephalometry limits soft tissue analysis to the patient's profile. This limitation requires that additional records (traditional 2D facial photographs) be taken to evaluate the intricate details of a patient's facial anatomy. These 2D facial photographs consequently reveal limitations in describing the 3D structures of a patient's face.

Advanced imaging techniques such as CBCT and 3D stereophotogrammetry allow the human face to be explored in three dimensions with multiple useful applications that range from measuring all the esthetic facial parameters to orthodontic diagnosis and evaluation of the craniofacial growth and development. They also allow superimposition of craniofacial structures to show the position of each.

Soft tissue segmentation of the CBCT data can be created by adjusting the threshold and Hounsfield units manually to the closest soft tissue segmentation level or by using the software default value of skin segmentation (Fig 5-14). Depending on the protocol for taking CBCTs, the image might be recorded with the eyes closed rather than open as used in orthodontic records (Fig 5-15). The CBCT soft tissue image shows a nonsmiling patient, thereby requiring an additional photograph to capture the smile for orthodontic records. The soft tissue segmentation can be viewed from multiple angles but lacks color and texture.

Stereophotogrammetry can be considered a valid method of capturing a patient's face in 3D by means of one or more stereo pairs of photographs being taken simultaneously.[39] The 3D photo camera is used to capture the soft tissue surface of the face with correct geometry, color, and texture information. The technique is based on the triangulation and fringe projection method. Image fusion (ie, registration of a 3D photograph upon a CBCT) results in a reliable and photorealistic digital 3D data set of a patient's face[39] (Fig 5-16). It is quick (requiring

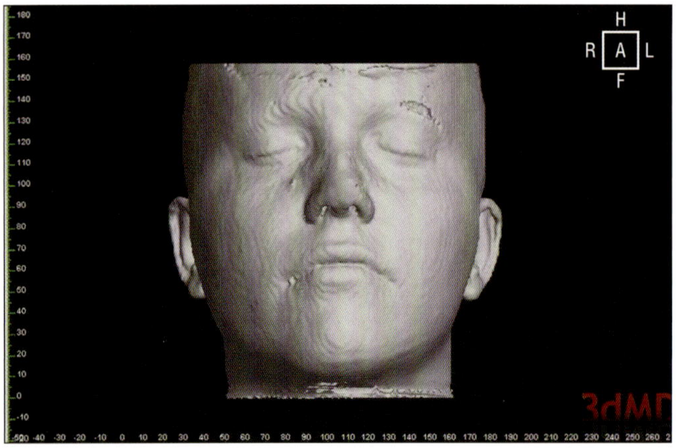

Fig 5-15 Screenshot of CBCT soft tissue segmentation showing the 3D reconstruction of skin outlines.

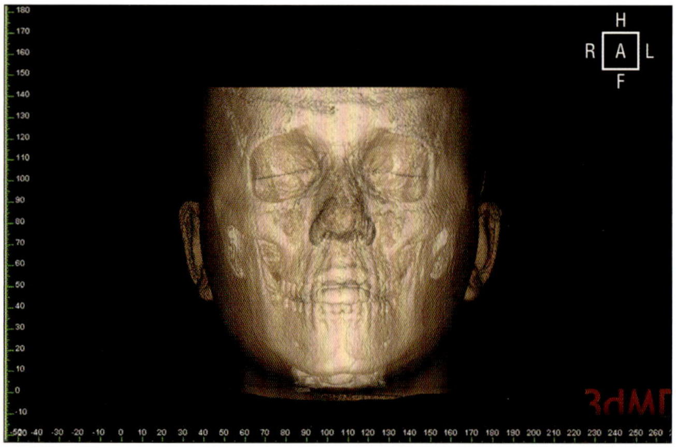

Fig 5-16 Superimposition of CBCT soft tissue segmentation over hard tissue.

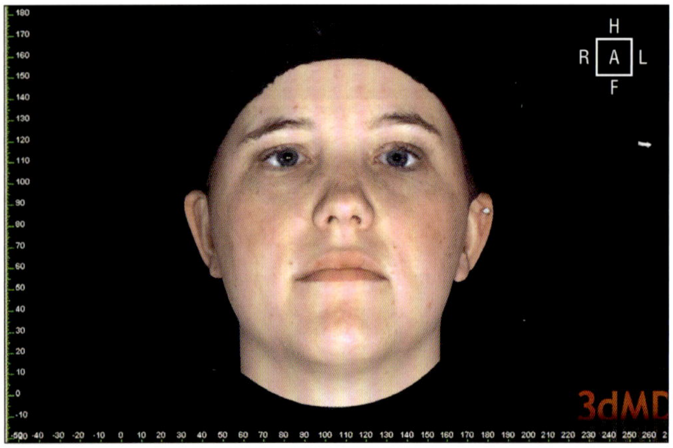

Fig 5-17 Stereogrammatic image of the same patient shown in Figs 5-14 to 5-16.

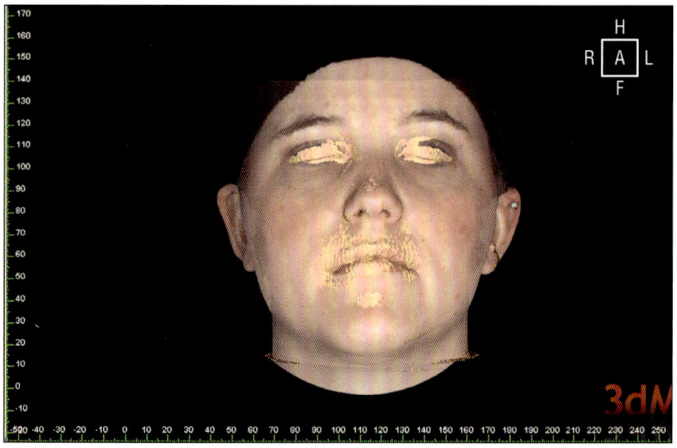

Fig 5-18 Superimposition of a stereogrammatic image over the CBCT soft tissue reconstruction showing nonalignment in the area of the eyes because of eye closure in the CBCT image versus open eyes in the stereogrammatic image. The lips were held slightly differently in the two images, resulting in nonalignment there as well.

only milliseconds), reliable, and does not expose the patient to radiation. Using various software, stereogrammatic soft tissue images can be superimposed with surface registration onto the reconstructed 3D CBCT soft tissue images of the same patient for better color and surface texture (Fig 5-17) or onto the 3D hard tissue images shown previously in this chapter.

Various commercial products allow 180- or 360-degree photographs of the patient. One disadvantage of this method is the reduced reliability at the edge of the field of view due to the inability to capture the ears or chin on some patients. Hair and whiskers can also make landmark identification difficult.[39] Finally, if differences exist in the way the images were taken (eg, eyes open versus closed in CBCT and stereogrammatic images), superimposition can result in nonalignment of landmarks (Fig 5-18).

Conclusion

Esthetics is most commonly the reason patients seek orthodontic treatment. A beautiful dentition and pleasant smile together with symmetric and balanced facial proportions identify perfect esthetics. Assessment of the soft tissues during orthodontic examination and an understanding of the changes associated with growth and treatment are essential. Quantitative analysis of the human face and identification of facial asymmetry is thus considered a major focus for orthodontic diagnosis. The clinical observation of abnormal facial features may indicate the presence of a particular trait or possible skeletal or occlusal discrepancy. Facial analysis, as a key component in orthodontic treatment planning, entails the use of several 2D and 3D linear and angular measurements to allow the clinician to analyze and develop a comprehensive plan tailored to each specific patient's needs and esthetic expectations. One key to remember is that the soft tissue can hide skeletal relationships.

References

1. Peck H, Peck S. A concept of facial esthetics. Angle Orthod 1970;40:284–317.
2. Peck S, Peck L. Selected aspects of the art and science of facial esthetics. Semin Orthod 1995;1:105–126.
3. Rhodes G, Proffitt F, Grady JM, Sumich A. Facial symmetry and the perception of beauty. Psychonom Bull Rev 1998;5:659–669.
4. Elam K. Facial Proportions. In: Elam K. Geometry of Design: Studies in Proportion and Composition. New York: Princeton Architectural Press, 2001:18–19.
5. Zimbler MS, Ham J. Aesthetic facial analysis. In: Cummings CW (ed). Otolaryngology: Head and Neck Surgery, ed 4. Philadelphia: Mosby, 2005:513–528.
6. Sarver D, Jacobson RS. The aesthetic dentofacial analysis. Clin Plastic Surg 2007;34:369–394.
7. Morris W. An orthodontic view of dentofacial esthetics. Compendium 1994;15:378–382.
8. Naini FB, Moss JP, Gill DS. The enigma of facial beauty: Esthetics, proportions, deformity, and controversy. Am J Orthod Dentofacial Orthop 2006;130:277–282.
9. Rakosi T. Soft tissue analysis. In: An Atlas and Manual of Cephalometric Radiography. London: Wolfe, 1982.
10. Scheideman GB, Bell WH, Legan, HL, Finn RA, Reisch JS. Cephalometric analysis of dentofacial normals. Am J Orthod 1980;78:404–420.
11. Bergman RT. Cephalometric soft tissue facial analysis. Am J Orthod Dentofacial Orthop 1999;116:373–389.
12. Jacobson A, Vlachos C. Soft tissue evaluation. In: Jacobson A, Jacobson RL (eds). Radiographic Cephalometry: From Basics to 3D Imaging, ed 2. Chicago: Quintessence, 2006:205–218.
13. Ferrario VF, Sforza C, Serrao G, Ciusa V, Dellavia C. Growth and aging of facial soft tissues: A computerized three-dimensional mesh diagram analysis. Clin Anat 2003;16:420–433.
14. Ackerman JL, Proffit WR, Sarver DM. The emerging soft tissue paradigm in orthodontic diagnosis and treatment planning. Clin Orthod Res 1999;2:49–52.
15. Turley PK. Evolution of esthetic considerations in orthodontics. Am J Orthod Dentofacial Orthop 2015;148:374–379.
16. Arnett GW, Bergman RT. Facial keys to orthodontic diagnosis and treatment planning. Part I. Am J Orthod Dentofacial Orthop 1993;103:299–312.
17. Hwang HS, Kim WS, McNamara JA Jr. Ethnic differences in the soft tissue profile of Korean and European-American adults with normal occlusions and well-balanced faces. Angle Orthod 2002;72:72–80.
18. Farkas LG, Katic MJ, Forrest CR, et al. International anthropometric study of facial morphology in various ethnic groups/races. J Craniofac Surg 2005;16:615–646.
19. Subtelny JD. A longitudinal study of soft tissue facial structures and their profile characteristics, defined in relation to underlying skeletal structures. Am J Orthod 1959;45:481–507.
20. Bishara SE, Hession TJ, Peterson LC. Longitudinal soft-tissue profile changes: A study of three analyses. Am J Orthod 1985;88:209–223.
21. Reyneke JP. Systematic patient evaluation. In: Essentials of Orthognathic Surgery, ed 2. Chicago: Quintessence, 2010:11–56.
22. Chaconas SJ, Bartroff JD. Prediction of normal soft tissue facial changes. Angle Orthod 1975;45:12–25.
23. Rifkin R. Facial analysis: A comprehensive approach to treatment planning in aesthetic dentistry. Pract Periodontics Aesthet Dent 2000;12:865–871.
24. Flynn TR, Ambrogio RI, Zeichner SJ. Cephalometric norms for orthognathic surgery in black American adults. J Oral Maxillofac Surg 1989;47:30–39.
25. Sutter RE Jr, Turley PK. Soft tissue evaluation of contemporary Caucasian and African American female facial profiles. Angle Orthod 1998;68:487–496.
26. Prendergast PM. Facial proportions. In: Erian A, Shiffman MA (eds). Advanced Surgical Facial Rejuvenation: Art and Clinical Practice. Berlin: Springer-Verlag, 2012:15–22.
27. Fernández-Riveiro P, Suárez-Quintanilla D, Smyth-Chamosa E, Suárez-Cunqueiro M. Linear photogrammetric analysis of the soft tissue facial profile. Am J Orthod Dentofacial Orthop 2002;122:59–66.
28. Anić-Milosević S, Lapter-Varga M, Slaj M. Analysis of the soft tissue facial profile by means of angular measurements. Eur J Orthod 2008;30:135–140.
29. Burstone CJ. Lip posture and its significance in treatment planning. Am J Orthod 1967;53:262–284.
30. Connor AM, Moshiri F. Orthognathic surgery norms for American black patients. Am J Orthod 1985;87:119–134.
31. Fonseca RJ, Klein WD. A cephalometric evaluation of American Negro women. Am J Orthod 1978;73:152–160.
32. Ricketts RM. Esthetics, environment, and the law of lip relation. Am J Orthod 1968;54:272–89.
33. Bishara SE, Jakobsen JR, Hession TJ, Treder JE. Soft tissue profile changes from 5 to 45 years of age. Am J Orthod Dentofacial Orthop 1998;114:698–706.
34. Steiner CC. The use of cephalometrics as an aid to planning and assessing orthodontic treatment. Am J Orthod 1960;46:721–735.
35. Merrifield LL. The profile line as an aid in critically evaluating facial esthetics. Am J Orthod 1966;52:804–822.
36. Holdaway RA. A soft-tissue cephalometric analysis and its use in orthodontic treatment planning. Part I. Am J Orthod 1983;84:1–28.
37. Burstone CJ. The integumental profile. Am J Orthod 1958;44:1–25.
38. Bowker WD, Meredith HV. A metric analysis of the facial profile. Angle Orthod 1959;29:149–160.
39. Metzger TE, Kula KS, Eckert GJ, Ghoneima AA. Orthodontic soft-tissue parameters: A comparison of cone-beam computed tomography and the 3dMD imaging system. Am J Orthod Dentofacial Orthop 2013;144:672–681.

6

A Perspective on Norms and Standards

Katherine Kula, MS, DMD, MS
Ahmed Ghoneima, BDS, PhD, MSD

Forensic scientists can determine age, sex, and ethnicity of skeletal remains based on differences in various bones and teeth. Orthodontists use some of these same characteristics to assist in determining the potential for growth and development in their patients as well as the potential interaction of orthodontic treatment with growth and development.

Many cephalometric studies have been published measuring the position or size of the craniofacial bones and teeth. Several studies have even published norms or standards based on age, sex, or ethnicity. In most individual cases, cephalometric norms or standards should be used along with other data (eg, extraoral and intraoral examination; cast evaluation; medical, dental, and behavioral history) to predict and to compare treatment effects because variation can be considerable and still allow normal occlusion.[1]

To best use and understand norms or standards, the terms *norm* and *standard* should be defined. This is particularly true if the use of norms affects treatment decisions. A *norm* is defined as a fixed or ideal standard, whereas *normal* simply means it agrees with the regular and established type.[2] A *standard* is defined as something established as a measure or model to which other similar things should conform. A problem with using norms to determine orthodontic treatment is that many individuals will not be able to be treated to those ideal norms for various reasons. However, their orthodontic treatment will be considered successful if treatment greatly improves their function and esthetics. Treating to ideal numbers is not always cost-effective or practical for many reasons: medical or financial inability, lack of desire to undergo orthognathic surgery, little change for the cost of the procedure, poor oral hygiene, poor patient cooperation, esthetic perceptions, as well as many other reasons. The issue of some cephalometric parameters not meeting the norms can also be related to the influence of other cephalometric parameters for a given patient—eg, the desired incisor mandibular plane angle (IMPA) can be influenced by the mandibular plane to Frankfort horizontal.

The esthetic perceptions of the patient and his or her family as well as the culture within which a clinician operates frequently influence orthodontic treatment. For example, a patient's profile is influenced by bone structure and position as well as dental position, and the soft tissue drape is a characteristic that varies ethnically and with age and sex. The influence of orthodontic treatment on the profile has been contentious for decades and is the subject of considerable cephalometric research and commentary.[3-6] However, cephalometric software programs frequently provide comparisons of an individual patient's cephalometric values to the same norm (average and standard deviation) despite differences in sex, age, and ethnic group.

In order to better understand the influence of norms of dental and skeletal relations, one should study potential changes in the facial structure. Within the United States, many studies have been performed to determine the growth patterns of Americans of Caucasian, African, and other ethnic descent. Although studies concerning ethnic and racial groups in other countries have been published, the purpose of this chapter is to provide and discuss two-dimensional (2D) cephalometric norms using examples developed from American ethnic groups, how they were established, and their limitations and uses. Understanding these norms and their limitations should help orthodontists in all countries understand and use their norms appropriately. Discussion of changes in norms relative to age and sex should also explain their limitations.

Clinical cephalometric studies can be divided into longitudinal studies, in which data are collected from the same individuals over time, and cross-sectional studies, in which the data are gathered from a population or multiple individuals at a limited point in time (eg, a certain age). Each type of study can provide valuable information, but each has its limitations in describing growth and development of the face.

Longitudinal Studies

Our understanding of the changes in the craniofacial complex that occur with growth are the result of ambitious and laborious long-term studies over decades involving thousands of children in various areas of the United States and Canada. The collection, retrieval, and interpretation of records and data often involved generations of researchers, considerable organization, and transition of data analysis and storage using various technologies. These studies required considerable financial support to collect, maintain, and analyze the records. The results of several of these studies were published as atlases of norms or standards of growth, and others were published as journal articles answering particular questions. The addition of the publications from these studies was a tremendous asset to the understanding of the growth of the craniofacial complex.

Currently, there are 11 known collections of craniofacial records/radiographs of various magnitudes known in the United States and Canada. Understanding the potential for degradation of the records, cost of upkeep, and difficulty in accessing records, the American Association of Orthodontists Foundation (AAOF) Legacy Collection established a website[7] containing samples of lateral and frontal radiographs, primarily of orthodontically untreated Caucasian children, from nine of these collections. However, the site does not contain all the records from each study. The choice of records was based first on the criteria that the AAOF established. The records available on this website are categorized by Angle's molar classification, sex, age, and the availability of such longitudinal records as lateral cephalogram, frontal cephalogram, hand-wrist films, dental casts, and photographic images, as well as whether cephalometric landmarks were added. The rationale for the caretakers of individual collections to choose the specific records that fit the AAOF criteria is unknown. Indeed, these records might not represent the entire collection but only individuals for whom all or most of the requested records were available.

The following sections highlight studies that published norms for various cephalometric measures and provide a short review of some of the other studies. Investigators did not always produce data for the same measures as in other studies (see Table 6-2). In some publications such as the atlases, the norms of multiple parameters are produced for each year in a 10+-year span in the growth and development of children. The reproduction of all these norms would be too unwieldy to handle within a chapter. Not all cephalometric parameters will be compared because many are used just for research and do not affect clinical decisions. Therefore, the authors have selected norms based on clinical usefulness.

Norms are usually based on a bell-shaped curve and provide the mean or average for the ideal as well as one standard deviation (SD) from that average measure. Values within one standard deviation on either side of the mean generally are considered acceptable. Understanding the selection process of a particular study will help determine whether the cephalometric values produced are actually norms or normals or just average values of the group selected. However, the entire research design should be considered and not just the conclusions of the study.

Each cephalometric parameter should be interpreted in context with other parameters (eg, mandibular incisor to mandibular plane angle or to nasion–B-point [NB]). In some cases, parameters support the indications of another parameter, but in other cases they contradict each other. Thus, several parameters might need to be reviewed to best explain the skeletal or dental position. This chapter reviews the established growth studies and discusses the problems and relevance of published norms developed from these studies.

Caucasian American Children

Broadbent-Bolton Study

With the support of the Bolton family, serial cephalograms were taken of 5,000 children in the Cleveland, Ohio area for 30 years (1928 until the 1960s), after which time the organizers of the study decided to emphasize the analysis of more than 22,000 radiographs rather than acquiring more data.[8] The lateral standards were developed for children ages 1 to 18 years, whereas the frontal standards were developed for ages 3 to 18 years.

Transparent templates of composite cephalometric tracings of selected male and female faces were produced at 3-year intervals. The inclusionary criteria for the tracings included

Table 6-1 **Comparison of normal (Michigan) versus ideal (Bolton) norms for three skeletal measures (mean ± SD) by age of Caucasian American children**

	SNB (degrees)				SNA (degrees)				ANB (degrees)			
	Michigan[a]		Bolton[b]		Michigan		Bolton		Michigan		Bolton	
Age (y)	Female	Male	Female	Male	Female	Male	Female	Male	Female	Male	Female	Male
6	76.0 ± 3.5	76.5 ± 2.6	79.1 ± 2.2	77.6 ± 3.4	80.7 ± 3.0	81.9 ± 3.3	83.2 ± 2.4	81.4 ± 3.8	4.7 ± 2.2	5.3 ± 2.2	4.1 ± 1.1	3.9 ± 1.9
7	76.3 ± 3.1	75.7 ± 2.8	79.4 ± 1.9	76.7 ± 3.1	81.9 ± 3.0	80.7 ± 3.0	83.6 ± 1.9	80.4 ± 3.7	5.7 ± 2.7	5.0 ± 2.3	4.2 ± 1.4	3.7 ± 2.0
8	76.7 ± 3.3	76.3 ± 2.8	79.4 ± 1.7	77.7 ± 3.1	81.2 ± 3.3	81.0 ± 3.1	83.1 ± 2.3	81.0 ± 3.6	4.6 ± 2.4	4.8 ± 2.2	3.7 ± 1.4	3.3 ± 1.7
9	76.5 ± 3.4	76.4 ± 2.5	79.4 ± 1.7	78.2 ± 3.1	80.6 ± 3.2	80.6 ± 3.0	82.5 ± 2.4	81.8 ± 3.4	4.0 ± 2.6	4.2 ± 1.9	3.1 ± 1.2	3.6 ± 1.8
10	76.7 ± 3.5	76.5 ± 2.5	80.2 ± 1.6	78.3 ± 3.1	80.7 ± 3.7	80.8 ± 3.1	83.3 ± 2.2	81.7 ± 3.6	4.0 ± 2.7	4.3 ± 2.0	3.1 ± 1.1	3.5 ± 1.8
11	77.3 ± 3.9	76.5 ± 2.6	80.5 ± 1.8	78.5 ± 3.1	81.1 ± 3.8	80.8 ± 3.0	83.7 ± 2.1	81.9 ± 3.6	3.8 ± 2.2	4.3 ± 1.9	3.2 ± 1.4	3.4 ± 2.0
12	77.7 ± 3.4	77.3 ± 2.7	80.0 ± 1.7	78.4 ± 3.2	81.4 ± 3.6	81.2 ± 3.3	82.5 ± 1.7	82.0 ± 3.4	3.7 ± 2.4	3.9 ± 2.1	2.5 ± 1.3	3.6 ± 1.9
13	77.5 ± 3.9	77.5 ± 3.0	81.2 ± 2.3	79.1 ± 2.7	81.0 ± 3.8	81.2 ± 3.4	84.0 ± 2.4	83.0 ± 2.9	3.5 ± 2.4	3.7 ± 2.0	2.8 ± 2.0	3.9 ± 1.9
14	77.9 ± 3.8	77.3 ± 3.1	81.9 ± 2.1	79.7 ± 2.9	81.3 ± 3.5	80.7 ± 3.4	84.5 ± 2.7	83.2 ± 2.9	3.4 ± 2.5	3.4 ± 2.0	2.6 ± 1.8	3.5 ± 1.8
15	78.9 ± 3.9	77.6 ± 3.0	81.2 ± 1.9	80.3 ± 2.9	81.8 ± 3.5	80.9 ± 3.2	83.2 ± 2.2	83.1 ± 3.1	2.9 ± 2.7	3.3 ± 2.1	2.0 ± 1.7	2.8 ± 1.5
16	79.2 ± 2.3	78.2 ± 3.9	81.9 ± 2.1	79.9 ± 3.0	81.8 ± 3.7	81.4 ± 4.4	84.3 ± 2.4	83.1 ± 2.9	2.6 ± 2.4	3.2 ± 2.3	2.3 ± 1.6	3.2 ± 1.7

SNB, sella-nasion–B-point; SNA, sella-nasion–A-point; ANB, A-point–nasion–B-point.
[a] Data derived from Riolo et al.[9]
[b] Data derived from Broadbent et al.[8]

excellent health history, very good dentition with normally developing or "excellence of static" occlusion that had not undergone orthodontics, longitudinal radiographic records from ages 1 to 18 years, and favorable comparison to an "optimum" face. These tracings consisted of "optimal" or "aesthetically favorable" faces as determined by the investigators, not "normal" faces. In actuality, only 16 males and 16 females were selected from this large group of subjects for the composite tracings of both lateral and frontal cephalograms. As described in the *Bolton Standards of Dentofacial Developmental Growth*, "rather than there being a statistical mean drawn at random from the population, they are instead a representation of the 'optimum.'"[8] In some cases, the cephalograms of other individuals of similar size and morphology were used to replace missing records of the original subjects.

The composite tracings for both male and female lateral standards were made by averaging the hand tracings of pairs of males or females and then continually averaging two of the remaining averages to form another composite until the final two composites were averaged. Mathematically, this method of averaging can produce a different number than the method of lumping all the numbers together for a particular value and dividing by the total number of data points. Broadbent et al[8] recognized that the continual averaging of the image tracings with each other also masked the variability of growth spurts of the individuals.

Although the magnification factor (5.9%) is provided for the older children, the cephalograms of children during the first 2 years of life were taken with the baby's head lying against the film. However, the distance of the film to the center of the target was not mentioned nor was the exact positioning of the head. Thus, neither total magnification for younger children nor the amount of distortion is known.

The objective of the Bolton frontal standards was to show how an ideal face grew transversely and vertically. The tracing of the frontal cephalogram of a child was averaged with a cephalometric tracing that was then reversed over itself and retraced. The average of the double-lefts and double-rights was traced again. This minimized the difference between the right-side versus left-side magnification and asymmetries. Problems that existed with vertical standardization of the frontal cephalograms were corrected using an orientator, a device used to reference the lateral and the frontal cephalograms to each other when tipping of the head occurred.

To compare a patient with the standards, transparent templates based on age were developed. A template is laid over the tracing of an orthodontic patient of the same age, and the differences are visually compared.

In 1975, the purpose, methodology, and longitudinal norms of numerous cephalometric linear and angular measures for these boys and girls with esthetically pleasing faces were published in *Bolton Standards of Dentofacial Developmental Growth*.[8] Data provided from these "ideal" faces is presented in Table 6-1 to compare against "normal" faces.

Michigan Study

In the 1930s, the University of Michigan under the tutelage of Dean Willard Olson and Professor Byron Hughes began a longitudinal, multidisciplinary growth study of children from the time they enrolled in the University School around the age of 3 years until the children graduated from the 12th grade (about 18 years of age).[9] Originally, lateral jaw and occlusal plane films were included in the various data collected but were discontinued in 1953 when lateral cephalograms were substituted.

The sample reported in *An Atlas of Craniofacial Growth*[9] included 47 males and 36 females who were primarily of Northern European descent. The children continually attended the University School from their 6th to 16th birthdays. These children were orthodontically untreated prior to or during the time of data collection. Annual records were taken on birthdays when the birthdays fell within the school year. When birthdays were not within the school year, annual records were taken 6 months before a birth month through 5 months after a birth month, adding some variability in age. However, the published data also showed inconsistent numbers of subjects at various ages.

Four tracings with landmark identifications were made of each cephalogram, and the first three were discarded. A second investigator reviewed the tracing, and landmarks were identified numerically. A third reviewer checked the series of landmarks prior to digitization and storage.

Computerization evolved from analysis of the linear and angular manual measures taken either directly from the radiographs or from the tracings to depicting shapes and areas as a series of x,y coordinates to scanning the cephalometric tracings by an automatic computer-controlled line that produced x,y coordinates for storage on magnetic or paper tape. Various landmarks and lines were flagged, and linear and angular measurements were computed using the x,y coordinates. Magnification of all linear measures reported in the atlas was 12.97%. The distance from the x-ray target to the midsagittal plane of the subject's head was 5 feet, and the distance from the midsagittal plane of the head to the film was 7.75 inches.

The resulting data for 104 linear and 74 angular cephalometric measures were presented in the atlas for both males and females from 6 years of age to 16 years of age. A tracing identifying the involved landmarks was included for each parameter. Each parameter was accompanied with a data table and a line graph plotting the value by age for each sex. More than 60 papers and 8 books and chapters used this data.

Data from this study is presented in Table 6-1 to allow comparison for three skeletal norms of normal faces and occlusions with norms for ideal faces and occlusions.

University of Toronto Burlington Growth Study

The Burlington Growth Centre at the University of Toronto was initiated by Robert Moyers in 1952 and continued to develop under the direction of Frank Popovich from 1961 to 1989.[10,11] At the initiation of the study, the ethnicity of the original subjects who composed 90% of the children in the age groups in the town of Burlington was primarily Anglo-Saxon Caucasian. The economic status was above average. Initially, multiple orthodontic and health records were collected on 1,258 subjects aged 3, 6, 8, 10, and 12 years. Records were collected annually as the 3-year-olds continued in the study, but data were collected on the other original groups at 8, 10, 12, and 20 years, when possible. In addition, records were collected on 111 various-aged siblings and 312 parents, when possible. Approximately 20% of the children in the serial experimental group dropped out of the study by age 12 years. More than 60% were treated orthodontically. In the control group, 20% of the children were treated orthodontically. Comparisons made at early ages between the groups that dropped out and those that remained showed no differences. Collection was essentially completed in 1971 when the remaining subjects reached 20 years of age. Cephalograms and dental casts were duplicated for study purposes, and the originals were stored. Cephalograms and dental casts were digitized using a Gradicon 100 digitizer that derived the x,y coordinates of each point. These coordinates were used to derive measurements using an IBM 1130 computer and an IBM 370-165 computer. Growth analyses were corrected for distortion and magnification error and stored in a data bank.

Norms in the form of The Burlington Craniofacial Growth Templates were constructed to show growth from ages 4 to 20 years. More than 400 studies including such topics as diastema closure, the effects of digit sucking, increase of Class II malocclusion with age, and dental agenesis were published based on this data.[12]

University of Oklahoma Denver Growth Study

Multiple longitudinal records were collected from 1927 to 1967 on children of European Caucasian descent living in the Colorado area.[13] Lateral cephalometric radiographs were collected on 292 children. Cephalograms of 57 males and 56 females with a minimum of four films per person between the ages of 8 years and 16–18 years were supplied for the AAOF website. Some of the subjects have cephalograms collected from the age of 4 years 9 months to over 21 years of age.

Fels Longitudinal Study

The Fels Longitudinal Study was started in 1929 in southwest Ohio to study human growth and composition changes with age.[14] The Fels Longitudinal Study is still actively recruiting new subjects and collecting data from the original participants who mostly live in Ohio, Indiana, Kentucky, and West Virginia. It is the world's oldest and largest human growth study. The data on newborns and young children have been used by the National Center for Health Statistics for national growth charts.

Examinations are scheduled at 1, 3, 6, 9, and 12 months of age and then at 6-month intervals until age 18 years. Thereafter, participants have biennial examinations. More than 200 nuclear and extended generational families continue lifelong examinations in the study. In all, more than 1,200 longitudinal subjects and their family members participated. This study could be classified as a study of normal variation because subjects were not selected for any particular craniofacial feature (eg, Class II, orthodontically untreated, pleasant features).

Lateral radiographs were taken from 1931 to 1982 when the study moved to Wright State University under Dr Roche and currently resides in the Department of Population and Public Health Sciences. Although most subjects had radiographs up to the age of 18 years, some have more than 30 lateral cephalograms spanning 45 years.

Forsyth Institute Twin Sample

Coenraad Moorrees collected longitudinal radiographic and other data on more than 500 Boston-area families who contained a set of twins or triplets.[15] This prospective, longitudinal study involved 148 males and 128 females and their parents who were observed annually. Landmarks located within a rectilinear coordinate system were used to analyze proportionate changes in the craniofacial complex from ages 8 to 16 years. Although analysis of data primarily focused on tooth formation and eruption, Moorrees used this database to develop a mesh diagram for analysis of facial growth. The database was also used to confirm the Tanner-Whitehouse system of analyzing bone development and to study tooth eruption.

Iowa Facial Growth Study

From 1946 to 1960, Drs Howard V. Meredith and L. B. Higley directed the Facial Growth Study at the University of Iowa.[16] Multiple records included lateral and frontal cephalograms of 183 children of Northwest European descent. Dental casts, anterior and profile photographs, and full intraoral radiographs were secured semiannually, while posteroanterior and lateral cephalometric radiographs were taken at 3-month intervals until age 5 and twice yearly after the children reached their 5th birthday. After age 12, records were made annually until 1960, when many of the subjects were 18 years of age.

Krogman Philadelphia Growth Study

The original study was started by Dr Wilton Krogman, an anthropologist, and continued by Dr Sol Katz.[17] Lateral, posteroanterior, and hand-wrist films were gathered on a sample of 600 Caucasian and 150 African American children aged 12 to 18 years. In addition, data was collected from 410 sets of twins as well as some children with cleft palate and orthodontically treated children.

UOP Mathews Growth Study

From 1967 to about 1977, Dr J. Rodney Mathews surgically inserted Bjork-type implants into 36 children aged 4 to 7 years who were selected from the University of California at San Francisco Dental Clinic.[18] These children were primarily of Northern European descent, and some received orthodontic treatment. Various cephalograms (lateral, posteroanterior, and oblique) were taken annually midway between successive birthdays, although not all subjects were imaged at all time points. This group of longitudinal records appears to be the only ones available worldwide with Bjork-type implants. Studies of these records[19,20] led Matthews and Perera[20] to state that the reliability of identifying metallic implants in growing children was highly variable. The interrater variability for each landmark resulted in a wide range of values for any measure that used that landmark, for example as much as a 3-degree range for sella-nasion–A-point (SNA), a 9-degree range for sella-nasion–B-point (SNB), and a 6-degree range for A-point–nasion–B-point (ANB). They suggested that potential remodeling resorption in young patients—that is, palatal implantation—could cause displacement of the implant into a sinus, or that the pin could have been placed improperly. They also suggested that some landmarks, such as B-point, were really not points but fields or areas.

Hixon Oregon Growth Study

From the 1950s to the 1970s, extensive longitudinal records including lateral cephalograms were collected at the Child Study Clinic on orthodontically untreated Caucasian children either annually or semiannually.[21] The records include 357 children from ages 3 to 18 years and 206 from the ages of 10 to 18 years. Twenty pairs of twins are included.

Caucasian American Adults

An extension of the Broadbent-Bolton Study[22] allowed a better understanding of the changes that occur to both male and female faces after the age of 18 years. Technically, the 153 subjects were not a subset of the Bolton Standards, a small group with faces judged to be ideal by the investigators. Although some (117) were participants in the original study who had records taken at 16 years of age or older, other subjects (36) included in the aging study were people working on the project. All subjects were in good health, could undergo another examination and cephalogram, and did not have more than three missing posterior teeth. Most had orthodontic needs, but they did not have comprehensive orthodontic treatment. However, some who received limited orthodontics were included as another group if their treatment was completed at least 2 years prior to the study. Many of the measures reported in the atlas were the same as the Broadbent-Bolton Study, but not all. The magnification factor was adjusted to 6%.

Table 6-2 Characteristics of cross-sectional cephalometric studies of various ethnic groups in the United States

Study (year)	Subject source	Selection criteria
African American		
Cotton et al[30] (1951)	San Francisco Bay Area	No real malocclusion; three different ethnic populations measured by different orthodontists
Altemus[31] (1960)	Washington, DC high schools	Normal occlusion; complete permanent dentition except for third molars
Drummond[32] (1968)	Baylor University College of Dentistry, Dallas, Texas	Clinically acceptable occlusion with Angle Class I molar relationship; face not deformed in any way; seeking dental care
Alexander and Hitchcock[33] (1978)	Grades 3 to 8 from schools in Jefferson County, Alabama	Never had any orthodontic appliance; exemplified best occlusions of 560 children examined (Class I molar with acceptable anterior tooth relationships and acceptable profile)
Richardson[34] (1980)	Meharry Medical College, Nashville, Tennessee	Participants in growth study; random sampling; acceptable occlusion
Anderson et al[35] (2000)	Altemus's sample from Washington, DC	Normal occlusion; complete permanent dentition except for third molars
Faustini et al[36] (1997)	Montefiore Medical Center, Bronx, New York	Seeking orthodontic treatment, but no history of prior orthodontics; late mixed or permanent dentition; Class I occlusion; minimal crowding (≤4 mm); esthetically pleasing face (determined by panel of four diverse individuals)
Bailey and Taylor[37] (1998)	Private practices in two Alabama cities and University of Alabama School of Dentistry	Normal skeletal (Class I) relationship; Class I molar relationship; no severe vertical, transverse, or anteroposterior discrepancies; balanced facial profile (consensus of three-fourths of examiners); no history of orthodontics
Huang et al[38]	University of Alabama at Birmingham pedodontic clinic, pediatric dentistry faculty practice, two orthodontic practices	Acceptable profile; Class I occlusion without stainless steel crowns; missing teeth or premature loss of secondary primary molars (unknown as to how many were seeking orthodontic treatment)
Caucasian American		
Alexander and Hitchcock[39] (1966)	School smile contest, Birmingham, Alabama	Winners of contest; normal occlusion; untreated orthodontically; pleasing or at least acceptable facial development; families of predominantly Southern extraction for two generations
Japanese American (Nisei)		
Cotton et al[30] (1951)	Seattle, Washington	
Chinese American		
Cotton et al[30] (1951)	San Francisco, California	Born in United States; normal arch relationships; good facial pattern
Chinese versus Caucasian American		
Gu et al[40] (2011)	Peking, China	Chinese: Not from Guangdong or Fujian provinces
	Ann Arbor, Michigan	Normal occlusion with no or minimal crowding; spacing less than 1 mm; midline discrepancy <1 mm; well-balanced profile determined by Chinese orthodontists and laypeople; nongrowers

M, male; F, female; NR, measurement not reported.

Other investigators also extended the data of child growth studies at the University of Iowa,[23,24] the University of Oklahoma,[25] and the University of Michigan[26,27] into adulthood by recalling some of the original participants. Investigators[28] at The Fels Longitudinal Study at Wright State University also published various studies on changes in the maturing craniofacial skeleton. These studies confirmed that some cephalometric values continue to change through adulthood. Recently, the University of Toronto's Burlington Growth Study extended the age of their sample to 40 years for the original 3-year-old sample and to 70 years for the original parent sample.[29]

No. of subjects	Ages (y)	Method of reporting	Reliability tests	% magnification
20 (10 M:10 F)	1–34	Numerical values of lines and angles	NR	NR
80 (40 M:40 F)	12–16	Numerical values of lines and angles	NR	NR
40	8–23	Numerical values of lines and angles	NR	NR
50	8–14(?)	Numerical values of lines and angles	Measures made by two orthodontic students (if differences <1 mm or degree, then values averaged; if >1 mm or degree, then values remeasured)	NR
40 (20 M:20 F)	13–16	Numerical values of lines and angles	NR	NR
80 (40 M:40 F)	12–16	Numerical values of lines and angles	Repeat measures of 20 randomly selected cephalograms	7%, not corrected
43 (18 M:25 F)	F mean 13.8 M mean 15.0	Mesh diagram	10 randomly selected tracings measured twice on different days	NR
71 (42 M:29 F)	8–20 divided into four groups: 8–12 (M and F) and 13–20 (M and F)	Mesh diagram and numerical values of lines and angles	Three tracings per subject to determine "accuracy" of landmark identification; all linear and angular measures for adolescent female group measured twice; intraclass correlation coefficients and coefficient of variation not provided	NR
136 Caucasian American: 32 M:35 F; African American: 39 M:30 F	6–18 (6–11, 12–18)	Numerical values of angles	All cephalograms measured twice by the same investigator at least 1 week apart; if measures exceeded accepted standards, a third measure was made and the two closest measurements averaged	8%, not corrected
40 (17 M:23 F)	8–15	Numerical values of lines and angles	Measures made by two orthodontic students (if differences <1 mm or degree, then values averaged; if >1 mm or degree, then values remeasured)	NR
20 (10 M:10 F)	Adult (mean 21)	Numerical values of lines and angles	NR	NR
20 (10 M:10 F)	11–16	Numerical values of lines and angles	NR	NR
Chinese: 65 (25 M:40 F) Caucasian: 90 (30 M:60 F)	Chinese: M 19.3 ± 3.0 F 20.3 ± 3.4 Caucasian: M 24.1 ± 5.7 F 22.9 ± 5.2	Lines and angles	60 randomly chosen cephalograms measured twice by same examiner	Standardized to 8%

African American Children

Meharry Growth Study

Although several cross-sectional studies[30–38] (Table 6-2) reported cephalometric standards for African American children, only one study[41] was performed in a longitudinal design. This longitudinal study used a modified random sampling technique without replacement and with socioeconomic stratification.

Originally, 150 children aged 3, 4, and 5 years were selected randomly from lists of Americans of African descent who lived in the metropolitan area of Nashville, Tennessee. The only

Table 6-3 Cephalometric norms for ethnicity and sex from two separate studies of normal individuals at 16 years of age

	Caucasian[a]		African American[b]	
	Female	Male	Female	Male
Skeletal parameters (units)				
SNA (degrees)	81.8 ± 3.7	81.4 ± 4.4	84.2 ± 3.5	84.4 ± 4.0
SNB (degrees)	79.2 ± 2.3	78.2 ± 3.9	80.6 ± 3.7	80.5 ± 5.1
ANB (degrees)	2.6 ± 2.4	3.2 ± 2.3	4.8 ± 2.4	3.7 ± 1.8
SNPg (degrees)	80.2 ± 2.5	79.3 ± 3.5	80.7 ± 3.6	80.4 ± 5.1
SNGoGn (degrees)	31.3 ± 3.1	32.6 ± 5.2	30.8 ± 4.4	32.4 ± 8.9
SN-MP (MeGoI) (degrees)	31.2 ± 3.0	32.9 ± 5.2	30.8 ± 4.4	32.4 ± 8.9
MP-FH (degrees)	25.8 ± 3.0	28.7 ± 5.2	22.4 ± 4.9	24.7 ± 7.2
OP(Downs)-FH (degrees)	8.3 ± 1.5	9.7 ± 3.5	6.2 ± 3.9	7.6 ± 3.6
SN/ANS-PNS (degrees)	8.0 ± 2.2	7.0 ± 3.0	5.1 ± 3.0	5.3 ± 3.6
ANS-PNS/MP(MeGoI) (degrees)	23.2 ± 3.7	25.9 ± 5.1	25.7 ± 4.8	27.2 ± 6.9
NAPg (degrees)	3.2 ± 5.6	4.4 ± 6.0	7.0 ± 5.7	10.0 ± 6.5
NMe (mm)	123.2 ± 5.1	136.8 ± 7.9	126.9 ± 7.2	134.8 ± 10.3
N-ANS (mm)	50.7 ± 2.4	55.8 ± 2.3	74.2 ± 6.6	80.4 ± 7.8
ANS-Me (mm)	69.3 ± 5.2	79.5 ± 6.2	74.2 ± 6.6	80.4 ± 7.8
PgNB (mm)	2.1 ± 1.6	2.4 ± 2.5	1.5 ± 1.3	1.4 ± 1.4
SGo (mm)	79.1 ± 4.3	88.2 ± 5.9	82.0 ± 5.2	86.3 ± 6.4
ArGo (mm)	49.6 ± 3.9	54.3 ± 4.1	50.3 ± 4.1	52.4 ± 4.7
Dental relations				
U1-NA (mm)	3.8 ± 2.7	5.5 ± 2.7	NR	NR
U1-NA (degrees)	21.4 ± 6.9	23.1 ± 6.1	NR	NR
L1-NB (mm)	3.4 ± 3.6	6.1 ± 2.9	NR	NR
L1-NB (degrees)	22.4 ± 9.6	26.4 ± 7.3	35.0 ± 6.9	34.8 ± 5.8
U1-1 (degrees)	133.6 ± 13.0	126.0 ± 10.0	NR	NR
U1-MP (degrees)	92.1 ± 9.0	95.3 ± 6.6	103.1 ± 6.4	102.1 ± 7.3
U1-OP (Downs) (degrees)	71.1 ± 10.1	64.7 ± 6.8	61.3 ± 5.7	60.3 ± 7.6
U1-SN (degrees)	103.1 ± 6.5	105.2 ± 6.4	108.6 ± 6.8	108.3 ± 6.2
U1-APg (degrees)	0.8 ± 2.8	2.8 ± 2.9	D	D

[a] Data derived from Riolo et al.[9]
[b] Data derived from Richardson.[41]
MP, mandibular plane; FH, Frankfort horizontal; OP, occlusal plane; U1, maxillary incisor; L1, mandibular incisor; NR, measurement not reported; D, criteria for measurement different from most studies. For landmark abbreviations and definitions, see Table 3-1.

selection criteria for the growth study were based on economic stratification (lower, middle, and upper middle groups), volunteerism, and age. These lists contained children from multiple socioeconomic backgrounds including public housing projects, blue-collar worker neighborhoods, and professional families. Occlusion and facial esthetics were not included in the selection criteria; therefore, the sample could be considered representative of a normal population.

The children were assigned numbers, and 50 from each of the socioeconomic groups were randomly selected. Younger and older siblings were also accepted into the study to comprise a group of 180 participants, although records were taken on only 160 children. Longitudinal records (lateral, posteroanterior, and oblique cephalograms; alginate impressions; and medical history) were taken semiannually to the age of 14 years and then annually until age 16 years. Records were taken year round on or near the child's birthday. Ultimately, records of 82 children (41 boys, 41 girls) were analyzed for the atlas. Lateral cephalograms were taken from 1965 to 1981, and the magnification factor was reported as 9.2%. Each child was followed to the age of 16 years, and none were orthodontically treated during record collection.

All lateral radiographs were traced manually on acetate tracing paper by two different individuals and compared. If a landmark varied by less than 1 mm, the midpoint between the two was used. The tracings were digitized with Cartesian coordinates. The data were published in the *Atlas of Craniofacial Growth in Americans of African Descent*[41] and can be used for comparison with data from studies performed on Caucasian children (Table 6-3).

One-third of the lateral radiographs were randomly selected to test for systematic and random tracing and measurement error. The coordinates were analyzed using an IBM PC-AT. Several cephalometric values used in other longitudinal studies were not reported (see Table 6-3).

The longitudinal study of African Americans from ages 6 to 16 years showed changes in various cephalometric measures that probably continued beyond the age of 16 years, suggesting that the potential for change with age needed additional study.

Cross-Sectional Studies of Children

The United States is composed of multiple ethnic groups who migrated across the country's borders from all directions. Immigration patterns to the United States show large groups of the same ethnicity settling in certain geographical areas; for example, the South has a predominance of people with Scottish, Irish, and English heritage, while Iowa has a predominance of Germans, with certain areas settled by Norwegians and Czechs.

Realizing that an astute eye could identify some differences between these groups within the United States, some orthodontists[28] were stimulated to study their particular group of patients because of their concern that cephalometric standards developed for research would not help with their diagnoses. Numerous cross-sectional studies reported the craniofacial characteristics of the African American child[30–38] (see Table 6-2). Few actually compared one ethnic group to another using data gathered within the study, whereas others compared published studies to their own sample.[34]

Current Relevance of Published Norms

Prior to cephalometrics, our understanding of craniofacial growth was based primarily on soft tissue measurements with their inherent limitations, particularly repeatability, and the bones of deceased children that prevented longitudinal studies. Cephalometric radiographs allowed serial records of bony structures to be documented and records maintained for decades. The lateral cephalograms and sometimes frontal cephalograms taken on children either annually or semiannually for many years provided longitudinal and cross-sectional data for many studies. The longitudinal records of children in some studies were enhanced by records collected when they became adults.[22–24] 2D lateral and frontal cephalometric parameters in the form of angles and linear measures provided the best knowledge of longitudinal growth and development of the living human face at that time. However, understanding these studies and their limitations is important when using or citing these studies so that the norms can be used appropriately.

Many of these cross-sectional studies were published decades ago and, understandably, have quite a few problems with research design. In fact, many studies providing data for various cephalometric analyses for adults have similar problems and should be reviewed with the following points in mind. Indeed, the current relevance of longitudinal studies published decades ago could be questioned for numerous reasons.

Research design problems

In some studies (see Table 6-2), the number of subjects was low, the age range was wide, the selection criteria were not randomized, and criteria such as an "acceptable" or "pleasing" profile or occlusion were not well defined or were subjective and possibly did not represent the population from which they were drawn. In some cases, the sample did not differentiate between potential growers and nongrowers and simply averaged their cephalometric values. With a few exceptions,[34] many papers did not mention reliability studies.

The report by Cotton et al[30] is actually a compilation of three separate populations, each measured by a different person and only published when a commentator compiled the data and wrote the discussion. No mention is made of the magnification factor of the three different radiographic machines used for measurement. In general, most studies represent the cephalometric values of subjects with minimal dental or skeletal malocclusion, whereas other studies are based on individuals seeking orthodontic treatment for unknown reasons.

Magnification differences

Nonuniform magnification was a problem with early cephalometers. Most studies did not report magnification or whether they corrected for magnification. The film placed close to the head was another source of uncontrolled magnification with early cephalograms. Eventually, placement of a standardized ruler or chain was used to calculate magnification and allow correction of linear distances.

Magnification of cephalometric images

Differences in magnification possibly occurred within studies. For example, the distance from the anode tube to the center of the patient's head was fixed in the Bolton-Brush cephalometer, providing uniform magnification to the radiographs. However, the distance between the anode and the center of the head was increased to account for the largest-size head, and this increased distance probably contributed to variations in magnification because the heads were of different sizes. Because other early cephalograms did not use a standardized distance between the anode tube and the center of the patient's head, radiographs taken with other machines could not be compared to each other or to those taken with the Bolton-Brush cephalometer. In the Broadbent-Bolton Study, the right and left sides of bilateral structures were both traced and then averaged, possibly producing a small amount of investigator error but definitely masking magnification differences of the right versus left side and any natural asymmetry. Tracings were not performed randomly but were made progressively from the youngest age of the child to the oldest or started at the oldest age of the child and worked backward.

Differences in magnification also occurred between studies. The Broadbent-Bolton Study reported a magnification of 5.9% for children over the age of 3 years, whereas the Michigan Study reported a magnification of 12.9% for all linear measures reported in *An Atlas of Craniofacial Growth* when they fixed the midsagittal plane of the head to the film surface at 7.75 inches. It is not clear whether the differences seen in various cephalometric parameters (see Table 6-1) are due to actual physical differences or lack of correction for magnification.

Dibbets and Notte[42] showed that radiographic magnification played a major role in interpreting differences among studies, especially in interpreting the differences between ethnic groups. They arithmetically corrected the magnification of various linear parameters selected from published cephalometric atlases (the Bolton, Michigan, Meharry, and Philadelphia growth studies). When the means of the linear parameters were compared by age, several parameters showed little difference among the groups, whereas others showed great differences. Some parameters were not compared because they were not reported in all studies. Thus, magnification differences or the lack of information concerning magnification made it difficult to compare ethnic groups.

However, one cross-sectional study (Huang et al[38]) that compared cephalometric data from Caucasian Americans with African Americans gathered from four separate clinics or practices did report that all cephalometric machines were set to the same magnification (see Table 6-2). Although the published data were not corrected for magnification, they showed that adolescent African Americans had significantly larger maxillae (SNA), mandibles (SNB), and maxillomandibular differences (ANB) as well as greater hyperdivergency (upward-tilted palates and downward-tilted functional planes) than Caucasian Americans. The measures comparing the maxilla, the mandible, and the maxillomandibular differential were angles, not the linear measures that Dibbets and Notte[42] used, suggesting that multiple cephalometric parameters used to analyze growth and development are needed to really make cephalometrics useful. In other words, patient diagnosis might depend on the selection of parameters.

Nonetheless, even the cephalometric values provided by Huang et al[38] cannot be used to compare individual patients by age because of their method of lumping age groups together. In general, clinicians should be careful when using absolute values from most of these studies to help determine treatment for their patients unless they know that the magnification of their machine is the same.

Changes in ethnic population

With time, migrations of various ethnic groups occurred within the United States from multiple ports of entry to other areas in the United States. Although large communities of similar ethnic groups tended to settle in specific areas, the population of these areas changed with time as new ethnic groups arrived and the previous groups moved or became a smaller percentage of the population. Admixtures of genetic pools occurred.[43] For example, some admixtures of African Americans occurred from approximately 1910 to 1970 with European Americans, Asian Americans, and Native Americans when economic opportunities drove many southern African Americans to migrate north and west. These admixtures might change the current cephalometric norms or phenotypes of these groups. In some cases though, strong cultural mores probably limited admixtures outside of a particular ethnic group, and various cephalometric characteristics could have minimal changes as had been proposed for the Alabama studies. More recent changes in economics and cultural mores appear to allow the possible blending of many superficial facial characteristics and, possibly, cephalometric characteristics. This makes it difficult to group or lump some individuals into simple categories such as African Americans or Chinese Americans.

Also, within each continent or country with a large landmass, differences in cephalometric values among ethnic groups are not always known. Although the origin of many African Americans is from West Africa and West Central Africa, some evidence of Southwest and Southeast African heritage is present within the African American genetic pool.[44] Chinese Americans also migrated from a large geographic landmass and might have local or ethnic differences among themselves.[40]

Changes in nutrition

The effects of time, socioeconomic status, and changes in nutrition on craniofacial measures are also unknown. The 2002 study[45] by the Centers for Disease Control and Prevention showed that the average height of 10-year-old American boys and girls increased by 0.5 to 0.9 inch and for 15-year-old adolescent boys by 0.9 inch since 1963.[45,46] The change in height is noted earlier in Philadelphia[47] as well as in other countries (eg, Germany,[48] China,[49] and Canada[50]). The effect that this height difference has on cephalometric values (linear and angular) is unknown, although one could hypothesize that linear measures might change, and if the linear changes in structures are not proportionate to each other, then angular changes might occur. Cephalometric values of children born in the United States during the 1930s could be different from those born during the 1980s or in 2000.

Effect of age

Some parameters change with age or with maturity (see Table 6-1). Therefore, parameters measured in a 10-year-old

Table 6-4 Comparison of SNB and SNPg (mean ± SD) in growing normal populations of Caucasian and African American children based on longitudinal studies

Age (y)	SNB (degrees)				SNPg (degrees)				PgNB (mm)			
	Caucasian[a] (Michigan)		African American[b] (Nashville, TN)		Caucasian (Michigan)		African American (Nashville, TN)		Caucasian (Michigan)		African American (Nashville, TN)	
	Female	Male	Female	Male	Female	Male	Female	Male	Female	Male	Female	Male
6	76.0±3.5	76.5±2.6	78.2±4.3	77.5±3.7	75.6±3.6	76.0±2.4	76.6±3.8	76.9±4.4	−0.7±1.5	−1.0±1.7	1.8±1.4	2.3±1.6
7	76.3±3.1	75.7±2.8	77.9±4.4	77.8±3.7	75.9±3.1	75.4±2.6	77.2±3.8	77.0±4.3	−0.6±1.3	−0.5±1.5	1.4±1.0	1.9±1.4
8	76.7±3.3	76.3±2.8	78.2±4.5	78.1±3.7	76.8±3.3	76.4±2.7	77.7±3.7	77.4±4.3	0.2±1.3	0.2±1.4	1.3±1.0	1.8±1.3
9	76.5±3.4	76.4±2.5	78.5±4.4	78.0±3.6	76.7±3.3	76.7±2.5	77.7±3.8	77.9±4.4	0.5±1.6	0.5±1.3	1.3±0.9	1.5±1.5
10	76.7±3.5	76.5±2.5	79.5±4.5	78.5±3.4	77.2±3.5	76.9±2.4	78.3±3.5	78.8±4.6	0.9±1.1	0.8±1.6	1.2±1.0	1.7±1.5
11	77.3±3.9	76.5±2.6	79.2±4.7	78.8±3.9	77.9±3.9	77.1±2.5	78.7±4.0	78.7±4.7	1.2±1.2	1.2±1.5	1.3±1.0	1.5±1.3
12	77.7±3.4	77.3±2.7	79.6±4.4	79.8±3.9	78.4±3.4	77.9±2.6	79.4±4.1	79.3±4.4	1.3±1.5	1.3±1.6	1.2±1.1	1.5±1.2
13	77.5±3.9	77.5±3.0	79.9±4.8	79.5±3.9	78.4±4.0	78.2±2.8	79.4±4.2	79.6±4.7	1.7±1.3	1.5±1.8	1.4±1.2	1.4±1.3
14	77.9±3.8	77.3±3.1	80.2±4.0	80.1±4.0	78.8±4.1	78.2±3.0	80.1±4.1	79.9±4.2	1.7±1.6	1.9±1.6	1.4±1.2	1.4±1.4
15	78.9±3.9	77.6±3.0	80.3±4.7	80.3±4.3	79.8±4.1	78.5±3.1	80.2±4.3	80.1±4.8	1.9±1.4	2.1±.8	1.3±1.3	1.6±1.3
16	79.2±2.3	78.2±3.9	80.5±5.1	80.6±3.7	80.2±2.5	79.3±3.5	80.7±3.6	80.4±5.1	2.1±1.6	2.4±2.5	1.5±1.3	1.4±1.4

[a] Data derived from Riolo et al.[9]
[b] Data derived from Richardson.[41]
Measures show that the average B-point (B) and chin point (Pg) both move forward with age, but the forward movement of Pg is usually not as great as that of SNB. Although the values provided for PgNB appear to be positive for both Caucasian and African Americans, the drawing in the *Atlas of Craniofacial Growth in Americans of African Descent* actually shows a reversal of the sign for Pg (in African Americans, Pg distal to NB is marked as positive; in Caucasians, Pg mesial to NB is marked as positive). By age 16 years, the chin point does not differentiate from average B-point in African Americans as compared to Caucasian Americans.

should not be compared to those of a young adult, much less an older adult.[22,25,27,41] Age-specific norms would be more representative for children and adolescents, although some children mature early and others much later than the chronologic age averages. The use of some adult norms assumes minimal or no change, although studies show that numerous cephalometric values change with age in adults.[22,24]

Sex differences

There are sex differences in numerous parameters,[8–10,22,40,41] although some of these differences are not obvious until puberty.

Differences in interpretation based on selection of cephalometric parameters

As previously discussed, comparison of studies of various ethnic groups is complicated for multiple reasons. It can be difficult to compare studies using the same-age subjects because not all studies report the same cephalometric parameters. For example, comparing the protrusion of B-point with pogonion in African Americans can be difficult because some studies[33] did not report measures including pogonion because of the unreliability of identifying pogonion as the most anterior point of the chin. In some cases, the author reversed the conventional sign used to express a cephalometric value. For example, one study[41] used a positive sign instead of a negative sign to record values for pogonion when pogonion was posterior to nasion–B-point (Table 6-4). Unless the methodology of the original study was read, the value provided for PgNB for African American children could be interpreted as a protrusive chin but is not. Pogonion was used to measure the Holdaway number, but skeletal A-point and soft tissue pogonion are used, not skeletal pogonion.[41]

Many studies comparing ethnic groups do not include more than one ethnic group in which they have controlled the variables or actually do the measures. Instead, they refer to previously published data. For example, Richardson[34] concluded that the difference in variability within ethnic or racial groups was often greater than the differences in the means of craniofacial parameters among or between the groups. Unfortunately, this comparison is difficult to interpret because the criteria for subject selection was not uniform among the papers (see Table 6-2) and the cephalometric magnifications were either not the same, not corrected, or not reported. Some of the studies reported only the mean and not the variation of data, and some did not report the same parameters.[34]

Differences in esthetic perception

The concept that biologic norms and esthetic values are different[35] can affect treatment and must be applied to the differences among ethnic and cultural groups. For example, the application of various cephalometric measures used to analyze esthetics in Caucasians has been attempted in other ethnic groups. The differences between measures such as ANB, upper incisor to NA, and lower incisor to NB were so great between African American and European American children that 75% of African American children would require either a genioplasty or eight premolars extractions to meet Steiner's criteria[51] to improve the profile.[35] The difficulty in using norms to treatment plan cases suggests that the esthetic values of the practitioner and the patient might better be used to treatment plan the patient than the attempts to meet cephalometric norms for ethnic groups.

Proclination and protrusion of the incisors appear to be the most frequent difference among ethnic groups. Almost all cephalometric studies of African Americans report significant inclination and protrusion of the incisors.[30,35] However, within a single country (eg, China), incisor protrusion can vary between ethnic groups.[40]

Superficial facial differences related to the skeleton appear to exist within a continent. Chinese people also have some significantly different skeletal measures when compared with Korean and Japanese peoples, although these comparisons were made to published data.[40] Thus, these differences should be considered when decisions are made relative to treatment.

The Downs analysis was used to compare four American-born ethnic groups, each with normal occlusion and good facial patterns: Negroes, Chinese, Japanese, and whites.[30] Although there are many problems with the study, it was apparent that the mean values of most of the skeletal parameters for Negro and Chinese groups were usually greater than standard for the white group, although the Japanese values were quite similar. Relative to dental standards of other ethnic groups, the dentition of the white group tended to be more retrusive and reclined.

Choice of cephalometric parameters

Interpretation of ethnic differences might also depend on the particular cephalometric measure reported. For example, compared with Caucasians, both male and female Chinese people have significantly more protrusive mandibular incisors when lower incisor to APg is measured, but not IMPA.[40] The relative size of the maxilla (condylion–A-point) is significantly greater in Caucasians, whereas SNA is not. In females only, the mandible is significantly retrusive when PgN is measured in Chinese people as compared with Caucasians, whereas SNB is not. The retrusive chin could also help explain the relatively retrusive mandibular incisors. Both male and female Chinese people have significantly steeper mandibular planes than Caucasians.

Population differences

The subject selection was not always random; the selection criteria varied with the study. Each study concentrated on a specific population in the United States or Canada. Immigrants from various countries tended to settle more so in some parts of the United States and form large communities. Thus, many studies were composed of individuals from similar or limited ethnic backgrounds. However, the ethnic structure of the communities under study changed over time so that "new" faces entered some studies and "old" faces gradually vanished for various reasons. Therefore, some longitudinal studies do not report data consistently from the same individuals. Through the decades, a great deal of "amalgamating" of ethnic groups has occurred, making it difficult to characterize those groups and use the norms as originally intended. African Americans, for example, have considerable DNA diversity.[30,41] Whereas these limitations do not affect the actual norm values, they could affect their current usefulness and application.

It cannot be assumed that all the adults in the extended studies were in the original study as a child.[22] Careful reading of materials and methods can show that various adults were added or subtracted throughout some studies.

Secular changes in height

Physical changes in the United States population and other countries have occurred over time. For example, US national growth data[46] as well as data from other countries such as Germany,[48] China,[49] and Canada[50] have shown changes in height and weight of children during the past 50 or more years.

Understanding these studies would help to make more discriminating use of the data. From 1946 to 1976, the Stuart/Meredith Growth charts were used extensively to compare height and weight data on children.[45] These data were drawn from small samples of Caucasian children living in two dramatically different geographic areas—near Iowa City, Iowa or in Boston, Massachusetts—from 1930 to 1945. In addition to the limited ethnic backgrounds and geographic areas, the Great Depression and World War II raged, possibly affecting nutrition and socioeconomic status of some study participants. In addition, statistical curve fitting was not applied to the data. Later these charts were replaced by the National Center for Health Statistics Growth Charts, which were compilations of several cross-sectional studies: the National Health Examination Survey (NHES) II, which was run from 1963 to 1965 and provided the data for ages 6 to 11 years; the NHES III from 1966 to 1970, which provided the data for ages 12 to 17 years, and the first National Health and Nutrition Examination Survey (NHANES) from 1971 to 1974, which provided the data for ages 1 to 17 years. The birth to 3-year-old data was drawn from a formula-fed, Caucasian, middle-class population studied longitudinally by the Fels Research Institute in Yellow Springs, Ohio. The growth curves were smoothed to fit the multiple sources of data.

In 1978, the US Centers for Disease Control (CDC) replaced these growth curves with normalized curves to better quantify growth at the extremes and to compare growth to a reference population. In 2000, these normalized growth curves were replaced. The reader is directed to the CDC publication to best understand the limitations of these curves.[45] The infant charts now include a mix of both breast-fed and formula-fed children.

Cross-sectional studies showed that the average height of males aged 20 to 74 years increased from 5'8" in 1960 to 5'9" in 2002 and that the average height of females of the same age increased from 5'3" in 1960 to 5'4" in 2002. The increase is frequently thought to be related to socioeconomic status and diet but could also be due to changes in ethnicity within the US population. The potential effect of this height increase on the outcomes of bony changes of the face is not known, although one might surmise that linear measures might change more than angular measures. However, disproportionate growth of parts could change angular measures also. Thus, the application of growth data from 60+ years ago might not be applicable to today's children and adolescents.

Conclusion

The relevance of the growth studies and the development of norms as applied to current patients are best based on an understanding of their limitations. These studies have provided significant understanding of 2D growth of the craniofacial complex of individuals living at the time the data was collected. Prior to citing any of the studies, one should read the original materials and methods to best understand the study. Comparisons of differences in outcomes among the studies should not be based just on data presented in tables of published studies but also on the understanding of the populations studied and the methodologies of each study. The best use of these norms is to detect trends repeated from study to study; the specific numbers themselves are not as relevant. In fact, all cross-sectional studies providing norms used to provide diagnosis and treatment outcome should be evaluated for limitations and relevance.

References

1. Casko JS, Shepherd WB. Dental and skeletal variation within the range of normal. Angle Orthod 1984;54:5–17.
2. Dorland's Illustrated Medical Dictionary, ed 27. Philadelphia: Saunders, 1988.
3. Iared W, Koga da Silva EMK, Iared W, Rufino Macedo CR. Esthetic perceptions of changes in fixed profile resulting from orthodontic treatment with extractions of premolars: A systematic review. J Am Dent Assoc 2017;148:9–16.
4. Dai ML, Xiao M, Yu Z, Liu DX. Effect of extraction and nonextraction treatment on frontal incisor esthetics: A meta analysis. Shanghai Kou Qiang Yi Xue 2015;24:499–504.
5. Meyer A, Woods MG, Manton DJ. Maxillary arch width and buccal corridor changes with orthodontic treatment. Part 2. Attractiveness of the frontal facial smile in extraction and non-extraction outcomes. Am J Orthod Dentofacial Orthop 2014;145:296–304.
6. Bowman SJ, Johnston LE. The esthetic impact of extractions and nonextration treatments on Caucasian patients. Angle Orthod 2000;70:3–10.
7. American Association of Orthodontists Foundation Legacy Collection website. http://www.aaoflegacycollection.org/aaofhome.html. Accessed 5 March 2018.
8. Broadbent BH Sr, Broadbent BH Jr, Golden WH. Bolton Standards of Dentofacial Developmental Growth. St Louis: Mosby, 1975.
9. Riolo ML, Moyers RE, McNamara JA, Hunter WS. An Atlas of Craniofacial Growth: Cephalometric Standards from the University School Growth Study, monograph 2, Craniofacial Growth Series. Ann Arbor: University of Michigan, 1974.
10. Burlington Growth Study. http://www.aaoflegacycollection.html?id=UTBurlington. Accessed 16 March 2018.
11. Thompson GW, Popovich F. A longitudinal evaluation of the Burlington Growth Centre Data. J Dent Res 1977;56(special issue C):C71–C78.
12. The University of Toronto Burlington Growth Study. http://www.aaoflegacycollection.org/aaof_collection.html?id=UTBurlington. Accessed 5 March 2018.
13. The University of Oklahoma Denver Growth Study. http://www.aaoflegacycollection.org/aaof_collection.html?id=UOKDenver. Accessed 5 March 2018.
14. Fels Longitudinal Study Collection. http://medicine.wright.edu/epidemiology-and-biostatistics/fels-longitudinal-study-collection. Accessed 5 March 2018.
15. The Forsyth Institute Twin Sample. http://www.aaoflegacycollection.org/aaof_collection.html?id=Forsyth. Accessed 5 March 2018.
16. The Iowa Facial Growth Study. http://www.aaoflegacycollection.org/aaof_collection.html?id=UIOWAGrowth. Accessed 5 March 2018.
17. http://www.aaoflegacycollection.html?id=Krogman(Philadelphia). Accessed 4 November 2017.
18. The UOP Mathews Growth Study. http://www.aaoflegacycollection.org/aaof_collection.html?id=UOPMathews. Accessed 5 March 2018.
19. Matthews JR, Ware WH. Longitudinal mandibular growth in children with tantalum implants. Am J Orthod 1978;74:633–655.
20. Matthews Jr, Perera PSG. Quantification of computerized lower incisor changes: A longitudinal implant study in man. Angle Orthod 1980;50:218–229.
21. The Oregon Growth Study. http://www.aaoflegacycollection.org/aaof_collection.html?id=UOGrowth. Accessed 5 March 2018.
22. Behrents RG. Growth in the Aging Craniofacial Skeleton. Ann Arbor: University of Michigan, 1985.
23. Bishara S. Jakobsen JR. Changes in overbite and face height from 5 to 45 years of age in normal subjects. Angle Orthod 1998;68:209–216.
24. Bishara S, Treder JE, Jakobsen JR. Facial and dental changes in adulthood. Am J Orthod Dentofacial Orthop 1994;106:175–186.
25. Formby WA, Nanda RS, Currier GF. Longitudinal changes in the adult facial profile. Am J Orthod Dentofacial Orthop 1994;105:464–476.
26. West KS, McNamara JA. Changes in the craniofacial complex from adolescence to midadulthood: A cephalometric study. Am J Orthod Dentofacial Orthop 1999;115:521–532.
27. Pecora NG, Baccetti T, McNamara JA. The aging craniofacial complex: A longitudinal cephalometric study from late adolescence to late adulthood. Am J Orthod Dentofacial Orthop 2008;134:496–505.
28. Lewis AB, Roche AF. Late growth changes in the craniofacial skeleton. Angle Orthod 1988;58:127–135.
29. Kulshrestha R, Trivedi H, Tandon R, et al. Growth and growth studies in orthodontics—A review. J Dent Oral Care 2016;2:1–5.
30. Cotton WN, Takano WW, Wong WW, Wylie WL. The Downs' Analysis applied to three other ethnic groups. Angle Orthod 1951;21:213–220.
31. Altemus LA. A comparison of cephalofacial relationships. Angle Orthod 1960;23:217–240.
32. Drummond RA. A determination of cephalometric norms for the Negro race. Am J Orthod 1980;50:301–311.
33. Alexander TL, Hitchcock HP. Cephalometric standards for American Negro children. Am J Orthod 1978;74:298–304.
34. Richardson ER. Racial differences in dimensional traits of the human face. Am J Orthod 1980;50:301–311.
35. Anderson AA, Anderson AC, Hornbuckle AC, Hornbuckle K. Biological derivation of a range of cephalometric norms for children of African American descent. Am J Orthod Dentofacial Orthop 2000;118:90–100.
36. Faustini MM, Hale C, Cisneros G. Mesh diagram analysis: Developing a norm for African American. Angle Orthod 1997;67:121–128.
37. Bailey KL, Taylor RW. Mesh diagram cephalometric norms for American of African descent. Am J Orthod 1998;114:218–223.

38. Huang WJ, Taylor RW, Dasanayake AP. Determining cephalometric norms for Caucasians and African Americans in Birmingham. Angle Orthod 1998;68:503–512.
39. Alexander TL, Hitchcock HP. Cephalometric standards for American Negro children. Am J Orthod 1978;74:298–304.
40. Gu Y, McNamara JA, Sigler LM, Baccetti T. Comparison of craniofacial characteristics of typical Chinese and Caucasian young adults. Eur J Orthod 2011;33:201–211.
41. Richardson ER. Atlas of Craniofacial Growth in Americans of African Descent, monograph 26, Craniofacial Growth Series. Ann Arbor: University of Michigan, 1991.
42. Dibbets JM, Notte K. Comparison of linear cephalometric dimensions in Americans of European descent (Ann Arbor, Cleveland, Philadelphia) and Americans of African descent (Nashville). Angle Orthod 2002;72:324–332.
43. Baharian S, Barakatt M, Gignoux CR, et al. The great migration and African-American genomic diversity. PLOS Genet 2016;12(5):e1006059.
44. Scheible M, Just R, Sturk-Andreaggi K, et al. The mitochondrial landscape of African Americans: An examination of more than 2500 control region haplotypes from 22 U.S. locations. Forensic Sci Int Genet 2016;22:139–148.
45. Kuczmarski RJ, Ogden CL, Guo SS, et al. 2000 CDC Growth Charts for the United States: Methods and Development: Data from the National Health Examination Surveys and the National Health and Nutrition Examination Surveys. Hyattsville, MD: Department of Health and Human Services, 2002.
46. Longley R. Americans getting taller, bigger, fatter, says CDC. http://usgovinfo.about.com/od/healthcare/a/tallbutfat.htm. Accessed 5 March 2018.
47. Eveleth PB, Bowers EJ, Schall JI. Secular change in growth of Philadelphia black adolescents. Hum Bio 1979;51:213–228.
48. Greil H, Schilitz A. Secular changes are different in distinct subgroups of the growing population. Anthropologischer Anzeiger 2005;63:45–61.
49. Morgan SL. Richer and taller: Stature and living standards in China, 1979–1995. China J 2000;44:1–39.
50. Binning G. Earlier physical and mental maturity among Saskatoon public school children. Can J Public Health 1958;49:9–17.
51. Steiner CC. Cephalometrics in clinical practice. Angle Orthod 1959;29:8–29.

The Transition from 2D to 3D Cephalometrics: Understanding the Problems of Landmarks and Measures

Manuel Lagravère, DDS, MSc, PhD
Connie P. Ling, DDS, MSc

The analysis of human craniofacial patterns was first initiated by anthropologists and anatomists who recorded various dimensions of ancient dry skulls. The first measurements obtained for craniofacial patterns were based on osteologic landmarks (craniometry). With time, measurements were made directly on living subjects using palpation or by pressing the supra-adjacent tissue. Finally, with the discovery of x-rays, measurements were made on cephalometric radiographs (cephalometry).[1,2]

Since the development of cephalometric radiology, numerous cephalometric analyses have been proposed. They have been useful in describing how individual patients vary from norms derived from other studies and also for establishing descriptive communication among clinicians.[2]

A cephalometric analysis is a two-dimensional (2D) type of diagnostic rendering from a three-dimensional (3D) structure, and cephalometric measurements on radiographic images are subject to projection, landmark identification, and measurement errors.[2,3] Furthermore, 2D radiographs produce magnification, distortion, and superimposition of adjacent structures. Magnification occurs because the x-ray beam originates from a point source that is not parallel to all the points of the object being examined. Distortion occurs because of different magnifications occurring between different planes. Even though many landmarks used in cephalometric analysis are located in the midsagittal plane, some landmarks and many bilateral structures that are useful for the description of craniofacial form are affected by distortion due to their location in different depth fields.[2,3]

Landmark identification errors are also considered a major source of cephalometric error. This type of error is influenced by many factors such as the quality of the radiographic image, the precision of landmark definition, the reproducibility of the landmark location, the operator, and the recording procedure.[2,3] Despite all of these potential errors, cephalometric radiographs are still widely used and in many cases are essential in the diagnosis and treatment of the orthodontic patient. Since the mid-1970s, 3D analyses and related procedures in orthodontics have been attempted through several different approaches. The first step in this broad area was the fabrication of 3D models that imitated oral structures.[4–6]

3D Imaging

3D craniofacial imaging requires the application of various techniques from disciplines such as applied mathematics, computer science, and statistics.[7] Although several computer 3D methods have been developed to assist orthodontic diagnosis[8,9] and others to predict the results of treatment,[10–13] the data obtained present potential problems in their analysis because few accepted standards or conventions for managing this computational data in human jaws exist.[14] Clinical use of this data involves transformation of the information from a 3D to a 2D format so that the practitioner can understand it better. Other shortcomings are lack of perspective, superimposition effects, imaging artifacts, information voids, and lack of motion.[15]

Advances in the use of 3D imaging software have permitted important changes in our perception of 3D craniofacial structures. For example, this software can be used to evaluate the temporomandibular joint under the influence of functional appliances.[16,17] Digital volume tomography is another technique used with machines like the i-CAT (Imaging Sciences), 3D Accuitomo (J. Morita), and CB MercuRay (Hitachi), among others.[18] Cone beam computed tomography (CBCT) produces a lower radiation dose than spiral CT and is comparable with a full-mouth series of periapical radiographs.[18] It also allows secondary reconstructions, such as sagittal, coronal, and para-axial cuts, and 3D reconstructions of different craniofacial structures due to its volumetric data.[19] For these reasons, there is a trend in the orthodontic profession to move from traditional 2D analog radiographs to 3D digital imaging systems. It is understood by researchers and clinicians that accurate patient information would allow the construction of patient-specific models that could be used for therapeutics, research, and education.[15]

Compared with traditional cephalometric radiographs, CBCT has been reported to produce images that are anatomically true (1 to 1 in size) 3D representations from which slices can be displayed from any angle in any part of the skull and provided digitally on paper or film. Presently, 3D volumetric imaging provides useful information for clinicians in identifying teeth and other structures for diagnostic and descriptive purposes.[20] CBCT provides the opportunity to visualize craniofacial structures not available from traditional 2D cephalometrics. In particular, cranial base structures including the various foramina can be visualized in detail.

Since this technology was introduced in North America around 2000, the current challenge for clinicians is to understand and interpret 3D imaging and also to decide on a particular imaging modality as a function of the information/diagnostic yield versus patient risk and cost-benefit analysis.[15] Currently, there is no specific way to analyze these types of 3D images, and interpretation limitations still exist. For this reason, new standards are required, and clinicians need special training when dealing with these types of images.

Landmark Reliability

Before establishing CBCT as a common orthodontic diagnostic approach, landmark reliability has to be assessed. This has been extensively done for traditional lateral cephalograms. However, landmark reliability assessment for CBCT is very limited, and additional research is required in this area.[21,22]

The error involved in landmark identification is considered an important issue in cephalometric analysis.[23] Chen et al[24] stated that it is impossible to estimate the landmark positions without error. Efforts should be made to minimize the effect of error in landmark identification on cephalometric measurements because they are the major source in producing tracing errors.[25,26] There are several factors that contribute to the reliability of landmark identification, such as the nature of cephalometric landmarks, the density and sharpness of the images, anatomical complexity and superimposition of hard and soft tissues, the definition of the landmark, and the training level or experience of the observers.[26–28] McWilliam and Welander added that landmark identification may be related to pattern recognition, which is more applicable for experienced observers.[27] Intra-observer landmark identification error has been stated to be generally less than interobserver landmark identification error.[25] Intra-observer differences may be due to the nature of the cephalometric landmark, the image quality, and blurring of the anatomical structures, while interobserver differences may be caused by variations in training and experience of the observer.[29,30]

The appearance of CBCT in dentistry has offered an imaging solution without the anticipated projection error associated with magnification and that avoids the superimposition problems associated with traditional cephalometric imaging and analysis.[31] Also, CBCT offers a wide range of tools such as 3D reconstructions and orthogonal slices in any direction that facilitate correct location of landmarks. Studies[32,33] have reported excellent accuracy on 3D CT using phantoms and metallic markers. This approach demonstrates the accuracy of the imaging but does not simulate the clinical situation where precision is influenced by difficulty identifying the landmark.[21]

Kragskov et al[21] indirectly compared landmark reliability through linear and angular measurements obtained from traditional cephalometric analysis in lateral and posteroanterior cephalometric radiographs with the same measurements obtained from 3D spiral CT. Their findings suggest that landmarks and measurements were less reliable in 3D CT image analysis. It was argued that the reason behind these findings was that distances calculated between landmarks on the 2D cephalograms present only x and y coordinates, whereas 3D CT images present x, y, and z coordinates, thus adding an extra deviation.[21] Hildebolt et al[34] have shown that 2D CT measurements are inferior to 3D CT measurements when landmarks were located on different CT slices,[34] while measurements made on the same slice have been reported to be accurate and reliable.[31,35,36] Another aspect to consider is locating points outside the scanner planes. For example, A-point lies outside the scan plane on a normal transverse CT scan, but it is easy to locate in 3D CT image reconstructions.[21]

The magnitude of the landmark identification error depends on the position of the landmark and is expected to be smaller in clear borders with high-density contrast and larger in blurred areas of the craniofacial structure.[20,28] Baumrind and Frantz stated that landmarks that are placed on anatomically formed edges or crests are easy to identify, while those placed on curves with wide radii show greater error of measurement.[29] Although these two statements were made with respect to 2D imaging, they are also applicable to 3D imaging. Some landmarks were more difficult to locate in CBCT than in lateral cephalograms. Gonion, condylion, and porion points are landmarks that are difficult to define in a 3D projection because of their location on three-dimensionally flat surfaces or widely curved bone structures. Curved and flat surfaces in traditional lateral cephalograms appear as a curved line, which would only involve location variations in 2D, whereas in CBCT a third dimension is added, increasing the variation of the respective landmarks.[21] Other points located in areas of low density are more difficult to identify in CBCT images than in 2D lateral cephalograms. Root apices also can be difficult to locate because a clear division between the end of the root apex and its surrounding cortical bone is not easily identified. Two proximate dense structures like this can create some error when trying to view just one in 3D reconstruction because software categorizes the densities of both structures as similar.

If a landmark is used to measure angles or distances similar to cephalometric analysis, only two dimensions would have an impact on the final values, while a third dimension would have no influence at all. Linear measurements will be influenced by all three dimensions. Furthermore, the tolerance for landmark identification differences will depend on how the craniofacial measurements will be used. Intra-examiner landmark identification reliability is very important in the research setting, whereas interexaminer landmark reliability is very important in clinical diagnosis and treatment planning. It is reasonable to assume that mean differences in landmark identification less than 1 mm are clinically acceptable. It is also reasonable to accept that mean differences between 1 and 2 mm will be useful in most analyses, while landmarks with mean differences greater than 2 mm should be used with caution.

Establishing New Landmarks with CBCT

Traditional landmarks used in lateral cephalometric analysis have been defined and used based on what can be visualized on 2D images. In 3D imaging using CBCT, these traditional landmarks may not necessarily represent useful anatomical structures. At the same time, important structures that could not be visualized in 2D imaging due to superimpositions are now available for analysis. For example, multiple maxillary and mandibular skeletal landmarks as well as multiple landmarks within the cranial base were typically overlapped by adjacent structures in traditional 2D cephalograms but can now be identified with accuracy and reliability (see "3D Landmarks Previously Not Visible on Cephalograms").

Therefore, with the transition from 2D to 3D cephalometrics, new landmarks should be defined and evaluated. These could be located on osseous and dental surfaces or inside the bone or teeth depending on the objective to be analyzed. These landmarks would give us new tools for diagnosis and measurement of growth and treatment changes and may overcome limitations found in 2D imaging. For example, dental pulp chambers can be used to assess 3D changes in tooth position. Ideal locations for landmarks in CBCT would be edges, foramina, apices, and other structures that are easily pinpointed using the tools available in 3D imaging. Landmarks that can be easily viewed using 3D reconstruction and can be verified with 2D slices should be preferred. Other good locations for landmarks would be locations between structures with different densities, thereby eliminating the possibility of being lost during thresholding or distinguishing the limits between anatomical structures. Furthermore, 3D landmarks within the cranial base would be relatively unaffected by growth and would allow superimposition of image sets taken over time independent of patient positioning.[25] This would allow 3D assessment of craniofacial growth and treatment effects. CBCT also provides new opportunities for soft tissue landmarks.

Landmarks used as superimposition references should be located in nongrowing structures and at a distance from the region being influenced by treatment to reduce the effect of individual landmark placement. Ideally, several reference landmarks would be chosen that are located a significant distance from each other and in different planes of space to obtain a 3D coordinate system. Constructed landmarks based on two distant, well-defined landmarks are especially useful. Landmarks also need to be identified in the "region of interest" that will be representative of the structure being evaluated. The landmarks should be easily identified at any stage of growth and treatment. Finally, the choice of landmarks should be customized based on the type of treatment or growth effects that are being assessed.

The use of CBCT overcomes limitations present in traditional 2D cephalometric analysis, where overlapping of structures produces landmark identification errors, which affect the determination of real changes present (eg, in maxillary expansion treatments).[37–39] Several studies[38–41] have analyzed 3D changes using CBCTs and CTs in maxillary expansion treatment. A common factor among all these studies is the use of only linear and angular measurements instead of a 3D coordinate system to verify changes.

In 2D analysis, landmarks have been used to represent structures given the limitations of that type of imaging. With the use of 3D imaging, one landmark may not necessarily represent how an entire anatomical structure would react to growth or treatment. For this reason, thought should be given to considering multiple landmarks within a single structure of interest. For example, landmarks located on various parts of a tooth will allow measurement of movement in all planes of space, including rotational movement.

Swennen et al[42] understood the need for a 3D-based measurement analysis when using a 3D Cartesian system. They selected commonly used 2D cephalometric landmarks to determine a standardized reference position to locate skull structures and then determined 3D position changes using different landmarks. The disadvantage of their approach was the use of landmarks located in skull structures prone to growth-based changes (landmarks forming Frankfort horizontal plane, sella, and nasion) that could occur concurrently with treatment changes, thus potentially skewing the results depending on the time of follow-up.

Tausche et al[43] used a similar 3D Cartesian system approach to determine changes after maxillary expansion treatments. The advantage of their approach was the use of landmarks present in the cranial base to standardize the skull position. However, the study did not reach its full potential of reporting changes in 3D but instead reported changes with respect to linear and angular measurements.

Published reliability values with respect to coordinates for landmarks used in lateral and posteroanterior cephalometrics are not very common. Some studies[3,27,44,45] did report reliability values for x and y coordinates for several points, and one meta-analysis presented an overall analysis on reliability values for some lateral cephalometric landmarks.[46] Points such as orbitale, piriform, and porion showed the largest errors in these studies.

Clinical significance of error in repeated landmark location is difficult to define and will depend on the purpose of analysis. For diagnostic purposes, population norms are compared with a specific patient; interexaminer reliability should be carefully considered, and variations higher than 1.5 mm could be considered clinically significant. When different time points are analyzed, the impact of cumulative landmark location errors should be considered. In situations where the effect of growth or treatment intervention is being evaluated with superimposition, intra-examiner reliability is of primordial importance. In this case, landmarks with variations higher than 1.0 mm would be of clinical significance. The size of the structure being investigated and the magnitude of change to be detected will also influence the clinical significance of landmark identification error. Landmark identification error may be different in x, y, and z coordinates, and some landmarks may be useful for detecting change in one axis but not in another. For example, piriform has low intra-examiner landmark identification error in the transverse dimension but high error in the vertical dimension. Piriform may be useful to assess changes in nasal width in cases of maxillary expansion but should not be used to assess vertical change.

Redefining 2D Landmarks

A major challenge during this transition from 2D to 3D cephalometrics is the redefining of historic 2D landmarks into the 3D space. For example, the anterior limit of the maxillary and mandibular apical jaw bases are identified as a single point on a 2D planar image. However, on a 3D hard tissue model, those points are in fact two surfaces and not a 3D point that can easily be defined. Furthermore, these two points are also subjected to bone remodeling during orthodontic tooth movement. With the growing interest in 3D anatomical quantification, more investigations are needed to formally transform historic 2D landmarks into the 3D space without potentially introducing new identification errors. The following requirements for selected landmarks must still be met: stable throughout treatment and continued growth, anatomically accurate, and easily reproducible. Additionally, these landmarks must be representative of skeletal and dental features that can be practically used for further studies.

Only a few studies[47,48] have looked at the accuracy and reliability of 3D skeletal and dental landmarks. To the authors' knowledge, there is still limited evidence to support the accuracy and reliability of 3D landmarks. Because every landmark can have non-uniform error for all three axes, there is a need to determine the most accurate landmark measurements for each axis after treatment. Traditional 2D landmarks should be reviewed to determine if new landmarks need to be added (Table 7-1) and whether some of the traditional landmarks should be deleted. The validity of skeletal and dental landmarks to represent the region of interest would have to be determined by comparing diagnostic measures from untreated normal populations with those of untreated abnormal populations. Large standard deviations or no differences in landmark location between these populations would suggest that it is not useful for diagnostic analysis.

For example, piriform landmarks are located in the outer portion of convexity of the nasal cavity. The bone in this area is thin and of low density, and thus visualization of this bone is very dependent on the threshold used in the software. Some teeth apices are difficult to visualize due to low-density contrast with the adjacent bone. The auditory canal is a cylinder-type structure, and in the x-axis dimension, the external auditory meatus could be placed in a variety of positions along the length of the canal. Zygomaxillare left and right are difficult to locate in patients who do not present with a distinct zygomaxillary notch.

Baumrind and Frantz indicated that the precision (reliability) of landmark placement strongly depends on the morphology of the represented anatomical structure.[29] Anatomical factors including landmark shape, size, contrast with adjacent structures, and anatomical variability all have influence on the accuracy and reliability of 3D landmark placement. Preferred anatomical landmarks include anatomical structures located on sharply pointed bony structures or on sharply curved structures. Tips of teeth apices have been demonstrated to show good reliability and accuracy, but due to the low-density con-

Table 7-1 Examples of traditional and new landmarks that can be used in 3D imaging

Landmark	Special notes	Axial view (xy)	Coronal view (xz)	Sagittal view (yz)
Maxillomandibular skeletal landmarks				
Greater palatine foramen (GPF)	First use the coronal view. Find the orifice at the level of the nasal floor.	Centermost 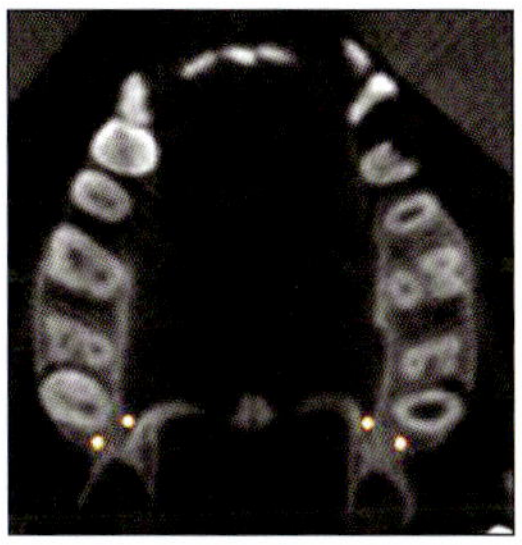	Inferior-centermost 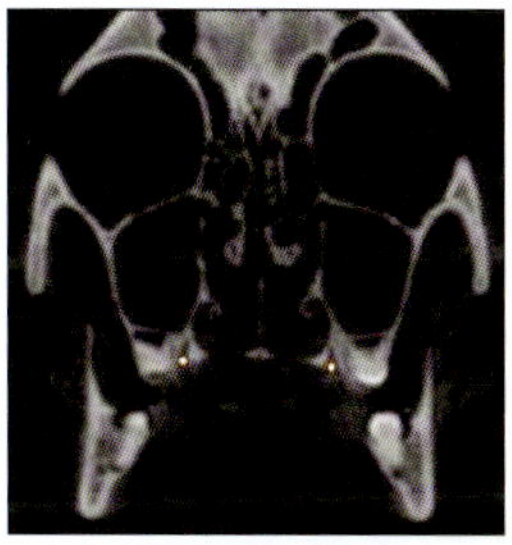	Centermost 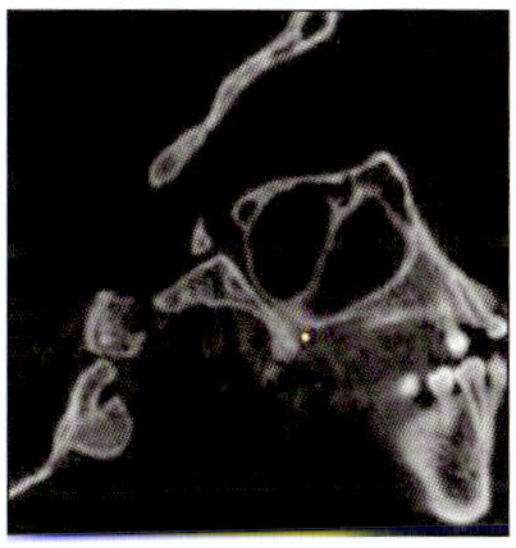
Infraorbital foramen (IORB; anteriormost orifice)	First use the axial and coronal views. Find the orifice along the canal.	Centermost 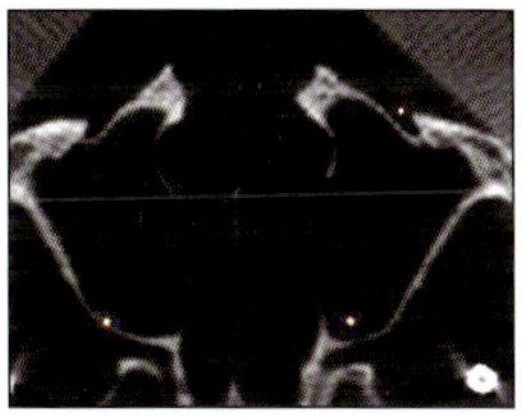	Centermost 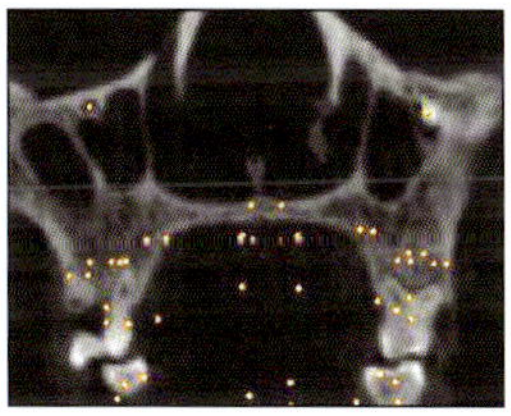	Anterior-centermost 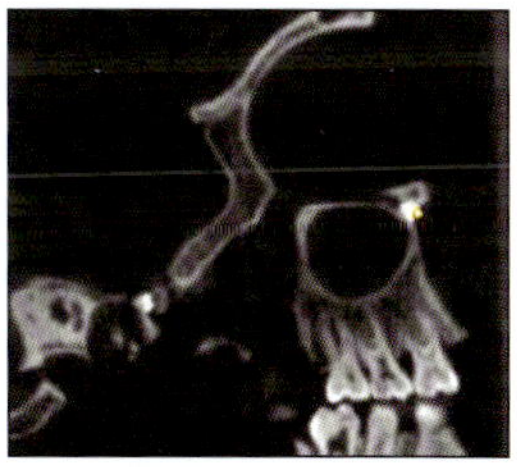
Nasopalatine foramen (NPF)	First use the axial view. Mark the most concave bony cortical rims for both left and right halves.	Most concave and centered 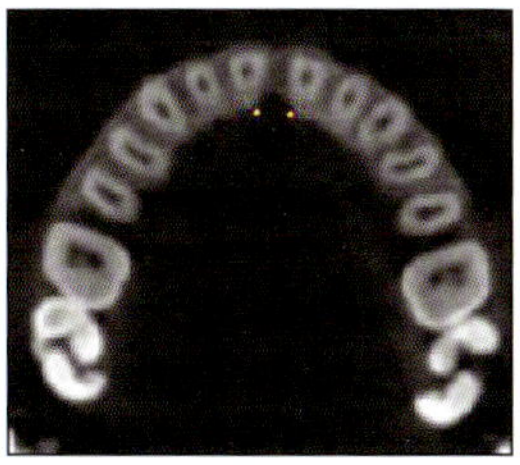	Most concave and centered 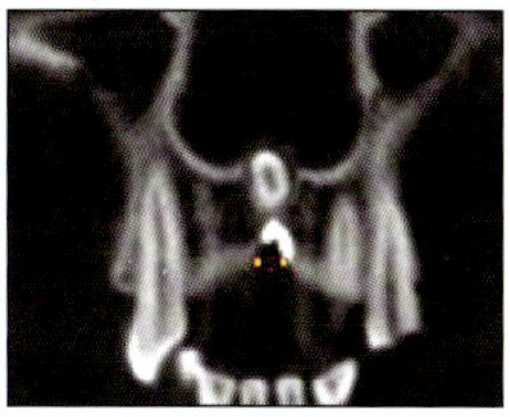	Lateralmost cortical border 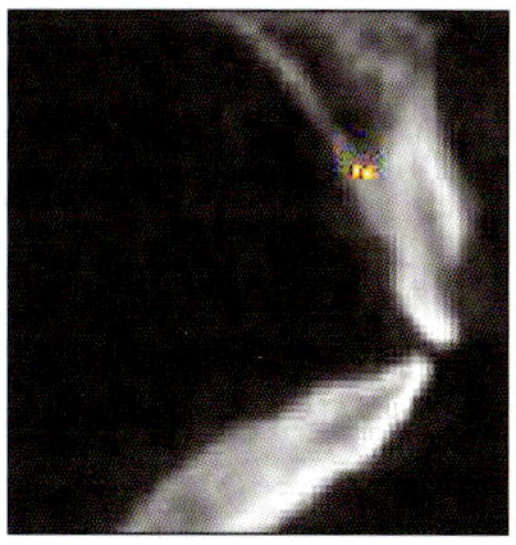
Mental foramen (MF)	First use the coronal view to find the middle slice. Then go to the axial view.	Centermost 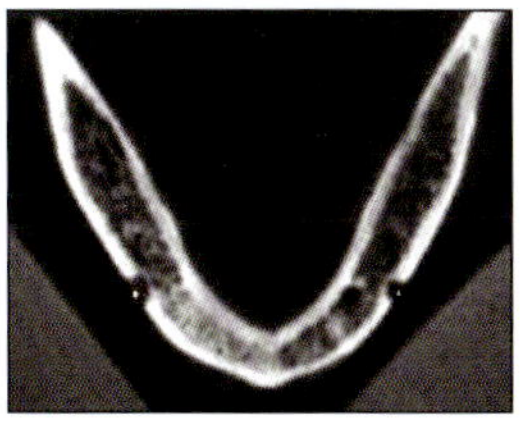	Center-lateralmost 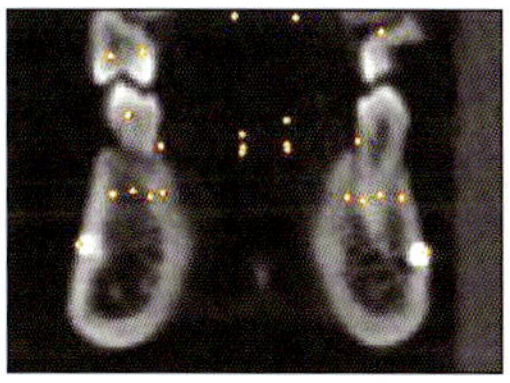	Center-lateralmost 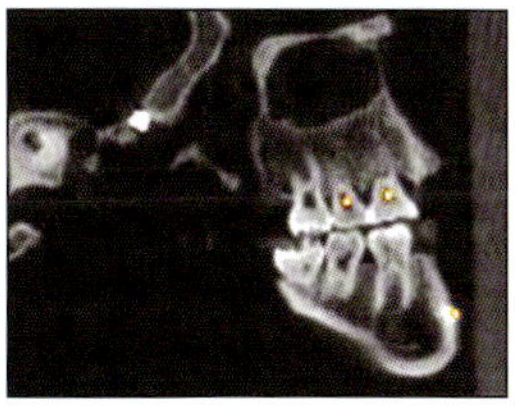
Cranial base skeletal landmarks				
Crista galli (CG)	First use the axial view, then go to the coronal view.	Superiormost tip 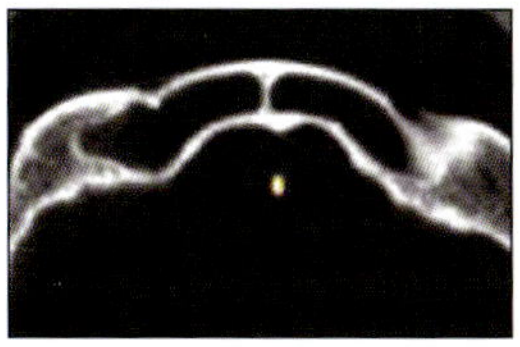	Centermost tip 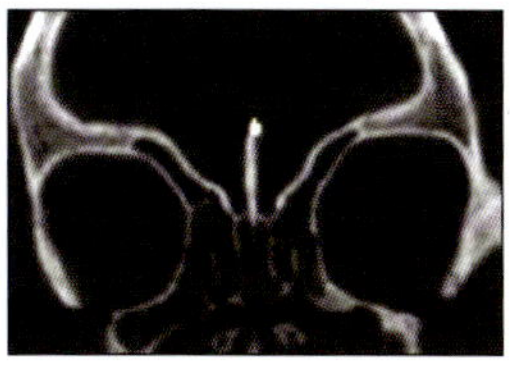	Centermost tip 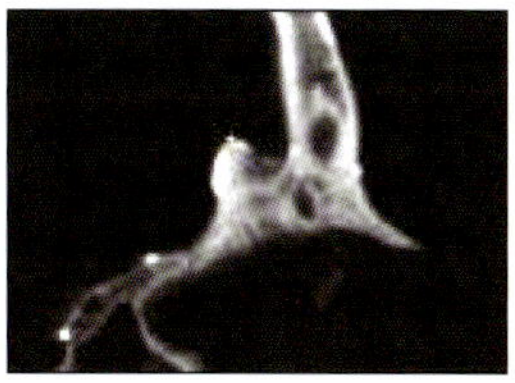

(cont)

Table 7-1 (cont) Examples of traditional and new landmarks that can be used in 3D imaging

Landmark	Special notes	Axial view (xy)	Coronal view (xz)	Sagittal view (yz)
Foramen ovale (OVALE)	First use the axial view, then go to the coronal view.	Centermost 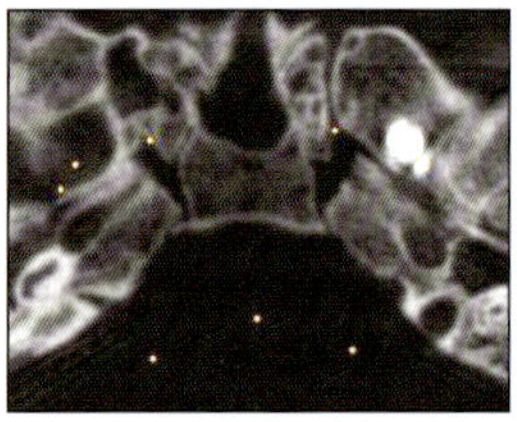	Centermost 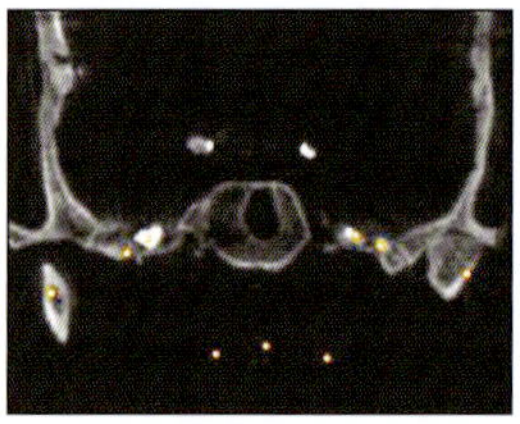	Centermost 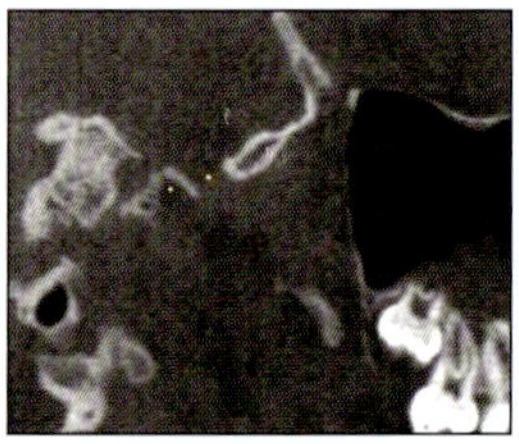
Foramen spinosum (SPIN)	First use the axial view. Use the mandibular condyles and glenoid fossae as guides.	Centermost 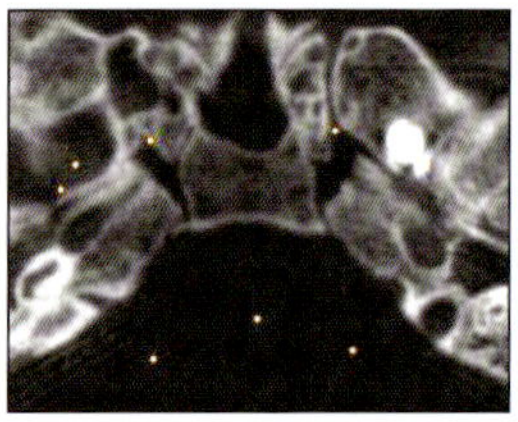	Centermost 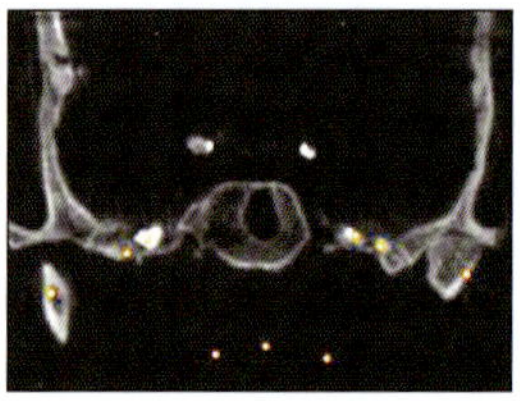	Centermost 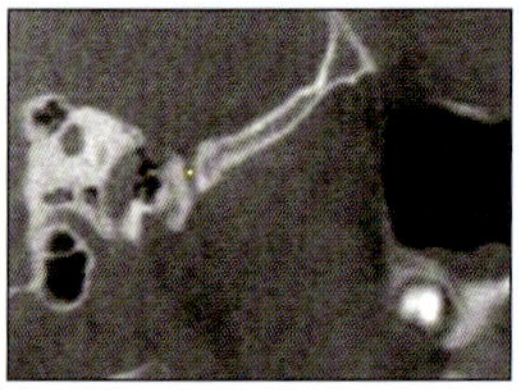
Foramen rotundum (ROTUN)	First use the coronal view, then go to the sagittal and axial views.	Centermost 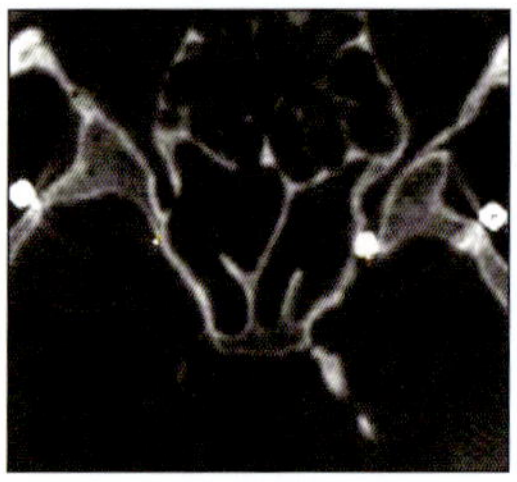	Centermost 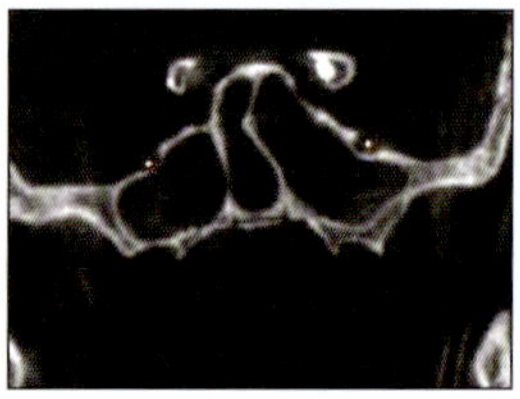	Posteriormost 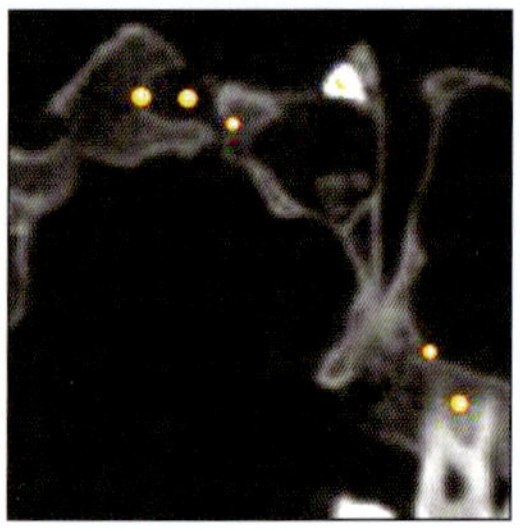
Dorsum foramen magnum (MDFM; mesialmost point when left and right bony cortices first join)	First use the sagittal view, then go to the axial view. Find the mesialmost point (clivus).	Mesial-inferior-posteriormost bony cortex 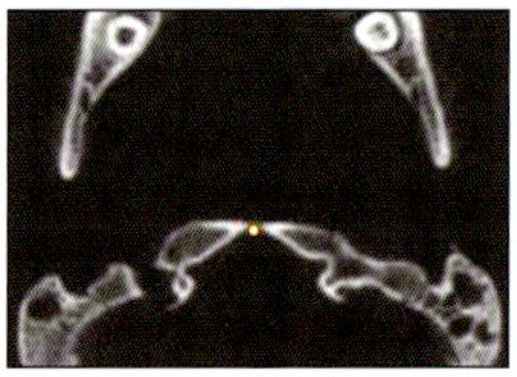	Inferior-centermost 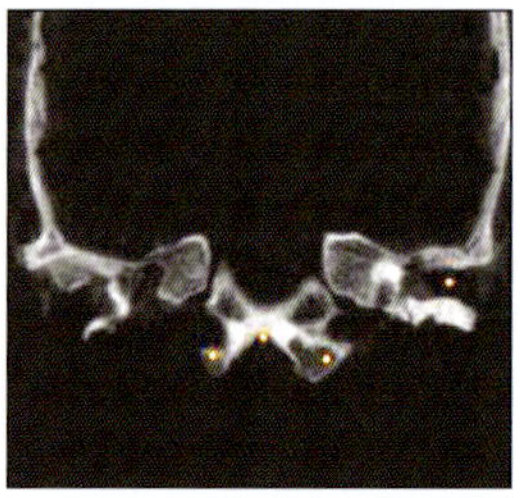	Anterior-inferiormost 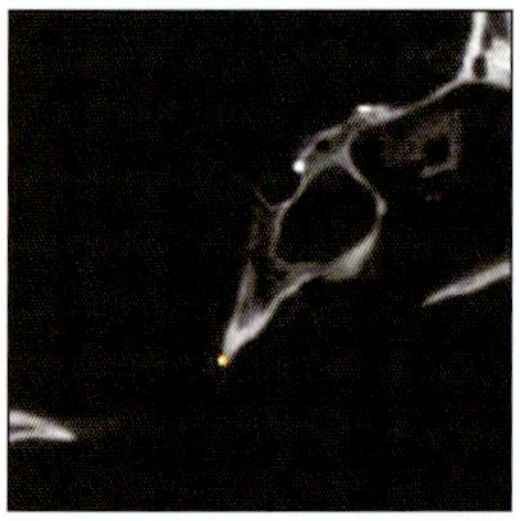
Posterior vidian canals (PVID)	First use the axial view, then go to the coronal view. Use OVALE and SPIN as guides.	Posteriormost 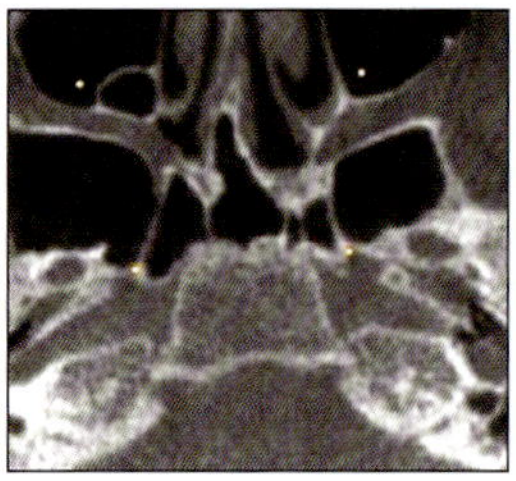	Centermost 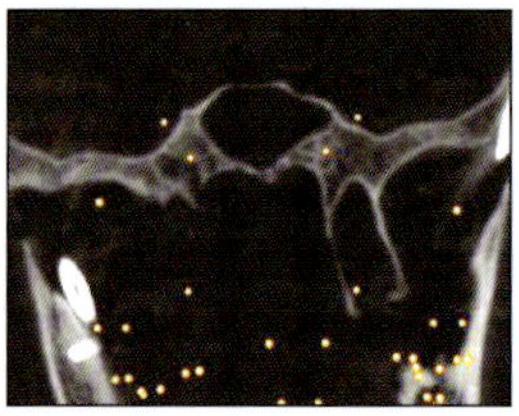	Posteriormost 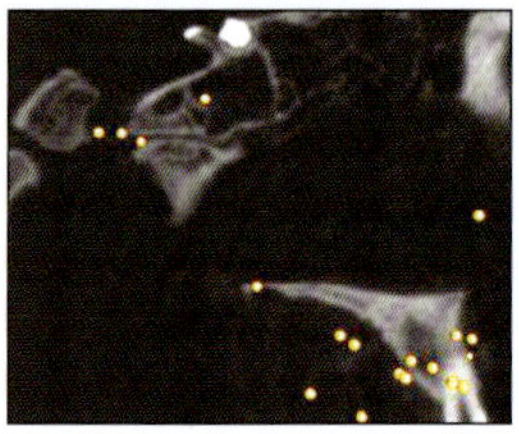

(cont)

Table 7-1 (cont) **Examples of traditional and new landmarks that can be used in 3D imaging**

Landmark	Special notes	Axial view (xy)	Coronal view (xz)	Sagittal view (yz)
Hypoglossal canals (HYPO)	First use the coronal view. Find the medialmost orifice openings.	Medial-centermost 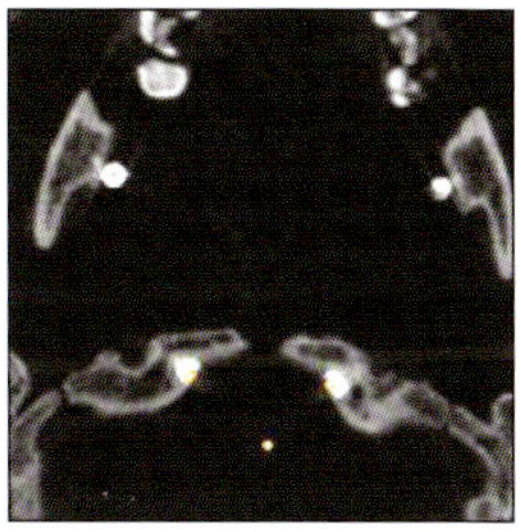	Centermost 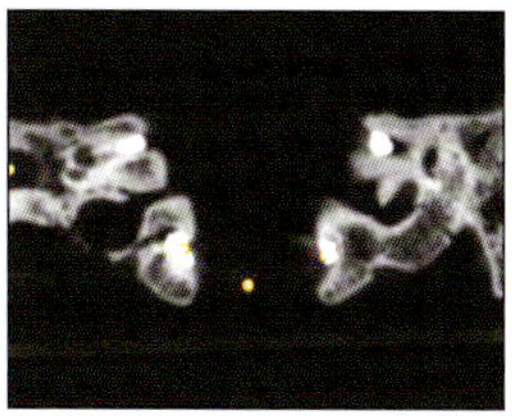	Medial-centermost 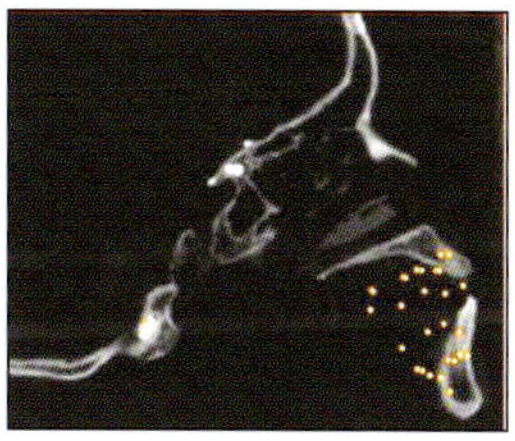
External auditory meatus, left (EAM.L; bony portion)	First use the coronal view.	Centermost 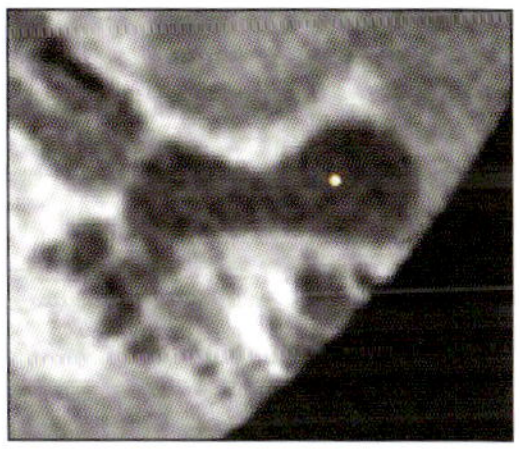	Centermost 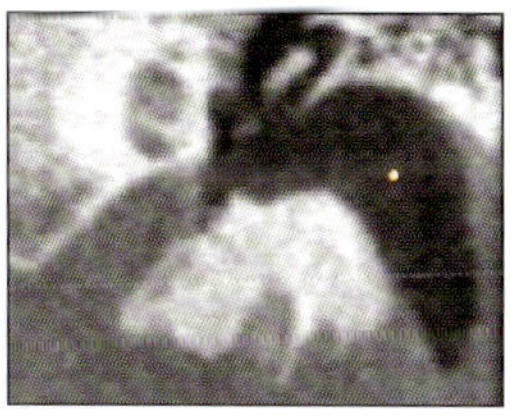	Centermost 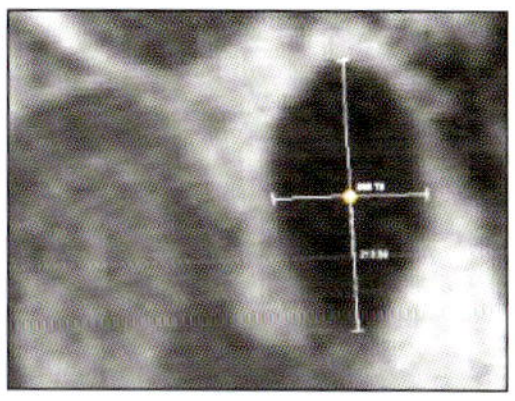
External auditory meatus, right (EAM.R)	First use the coronal view.	Centermost 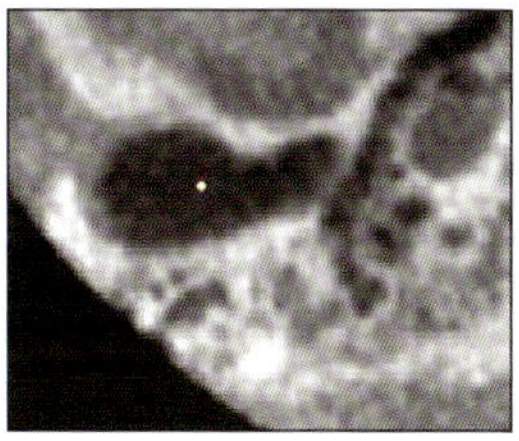	Centermost 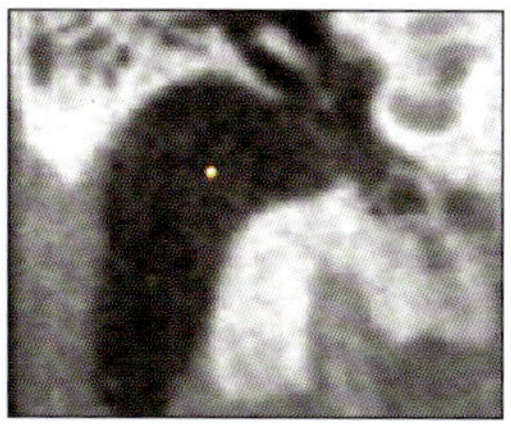	Centermost 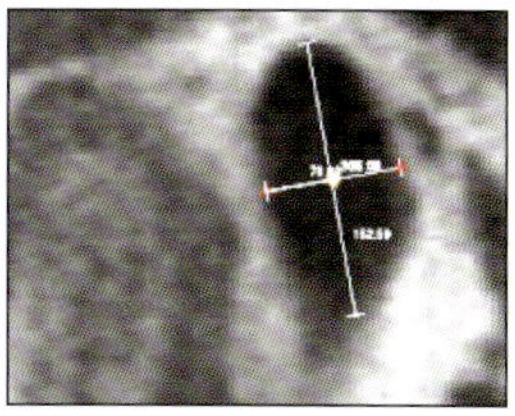
Dental landmarks				
Molar PULP (buccal-mesial tip of pulp horn, maxilla and mandible)		Centermost tip 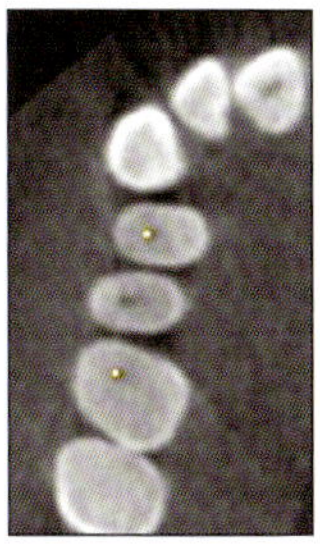		
Premolar PULP (buccal tip of pulp horn, maxilla only)		Centermost tip 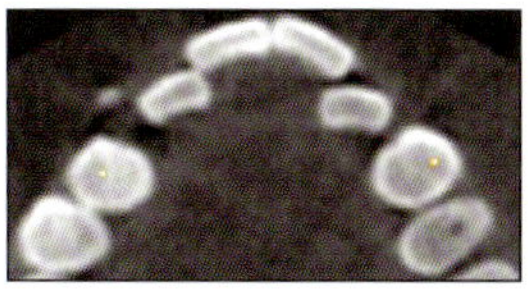		
Canine PULP (buccal tip of pulp horn, maxilla and mandible)		Centermost tip 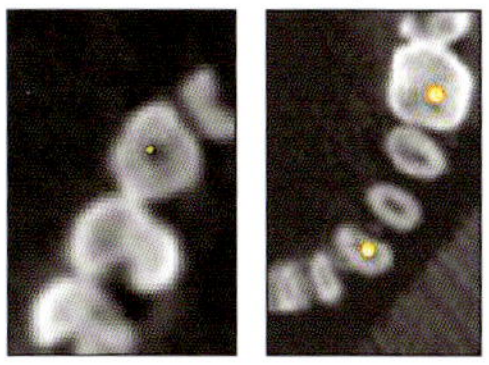		

(cont)

Table 7-1 (cont) Examples of traditional and new landmarks that can be used in 3D imaging

Landmark	Special notes	Axial view (xy)	Coronal view (xz)	Sagittal view (yz)
Tip of mesiobuccal molar APEX, maxilla and mandible		Centermost tip 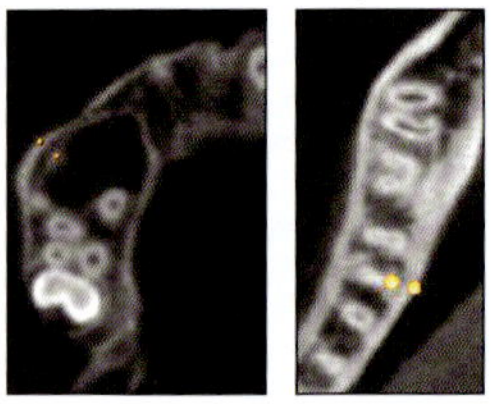		
Buccal alveolar cortical bone of molar (AVBN, maxilla and mandible)		Same level with APEX, along an imaginary parallel line relative to the root canal and center of the root apex 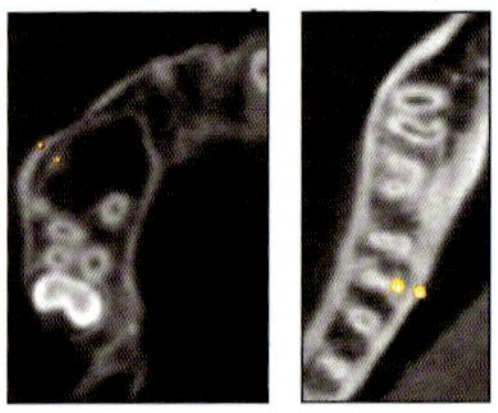		
Tip of buccal root premolar APEX (maxilla only)		Centermost tip 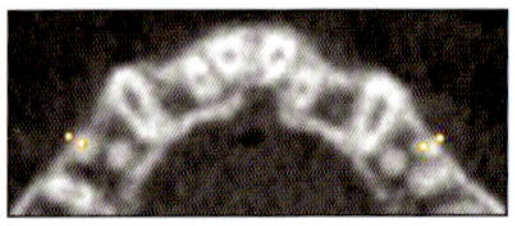		
Buccal alveolar cortical bone of premolar (AVBN, maxilla only)		Same level with APEX, along an imaginary parallel line relative to the root canal and center of the root apex 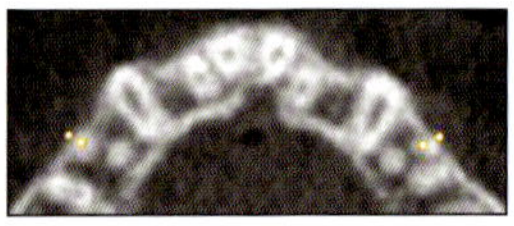		
Tip of canine APEX (maxilla and mandible)		Centermost tip 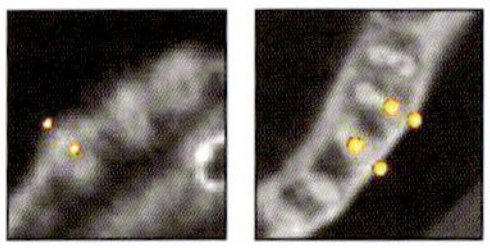		
Buccal alveolar cortical bone of canine (AVBN, maxilla and mandible)		Same level with APEX, along an imaginary parallel line relative to the root canal and center of the root apex 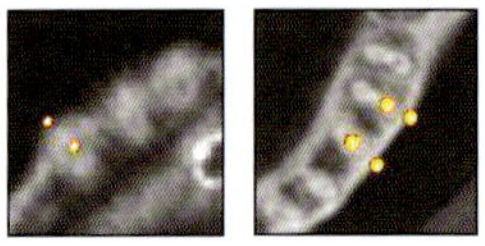		

trast with the adjacent bone, some teeth apices can be difficult to identify and end up being not as accurate as the skeletal landmarks.[49] Bony canals with a tortuous path, an oblique path, or a large diameter can also make it difficult to pinpoint the exact center of the canal or foramen in cross section. This explains why the foramen spinosum had superior accuracy and reliability compared with the landmarks hypoglossal, external auditory meatus, and infra-orbital foramen. In addition, landmarks located within thin bony plates also make visualization difficult. For example, the greater palatine foramen is located in the thin horizontal part of the palatine bone from the axial view. Localization is much easier from the coronal and sagittal view, where the high-density contrast with the floor of the nasal cavity and palatine bone can be used as a guide to aid in visualizing the inferiormost opening of the greater palatine foramen.

3D Landmarks Previously Not Visible on Cephalograms

As mentioned previously, several anatomical landmarks previously not visible on 2D posteroanterior or lateral cephalograms can now be identified with accuracy and reliability using 3D imaging. The greater palatine foramen (GPF) is an elongated foramen in the anteroposterior direction with a small mean diameter of 2 × 4 mm.[20] It is typically located parallel to the mesial or distal surface of the maxillary third molar. Any skeletal changes in the posterior maxilla after rapid maxillary expansion will be reflected as change in the position of the GPF. The GPF is also far enough from the maxillary first molar roots to be affected by potential dentoalveolar changes. The GPF carries the GPF nerves and vessels and has been proved to exist on both sides of the skull. Only one study out of 200 (0.5%) was reported to have a double GPF unilaterally.[20]

The nasopalatine foramen (NPF) is a funnel-shaped opening in the anterior maxilla, immediately behind the maxillary central incisors. In the mesiodistal dimension, it averages 3.5 mm; in the labiopalatal aspect, it averages 2.8 mm.[20] The NPF is an important landmark because it is positioned far away from the maxillary canines, premolars, and molars, which are often moved as a result of rapid maxillary expansion. Excellent reliability and accuracy have been found in measurements between NPF and other dental and skeletal structures.

The infraorbital foramen (IORB) is located in the maxillary bone at a level high above the root apices of the first and second premolars bilaterally. The authors' findings correspond with a similar previous study that reported excellent reliability and an accuracy within 0.7 mm in all three dimensions.[47] However, the obliquity of the IORB and canal as well as the large and variable diameter (3.4 × 2.4 mm ± 1.5 mm) of the IORB contribute to the difficulty in localizing it.[20]

The mental foramen (MF) is located in the mandibular bone inferior to the root apices of the first and second premolars bilaterally. The mean diameter of the foramen is 2.4 × 1.8 mm.[20] The authors' findings correspond with a similar previous study that reported excellent reliability and an accuracy within 0.5 mm in all three dimensions.[47]

Root apices of multirooted teeth can be identified with 3D imaging more easily and with more accuracy than single-rooted apices, most likely because of a narrower diameter at the tip of the apex. However, incompletely formed, curved roots may give rise to misleading results when interpreting transverse measurements; it is questionable whether this is clinically significant.

The center of foramen spinosum (SPIN) has a mean diameter of 2.4 × 2.0 mm[20] and has been shown to be a good landmark to determine skull midlines.[50]

The center of foramen ovale (OVALE) has a large diameter of 7.0 × 3.6 mm[20] and was more difficult to locate than SPIN because of its elongated shape in the anteroposterior dimension (y-axis). Furthermore, the canal runs medial from inferior to superior in the vertical (z) axis, causing difficulty in landmark identification.

The center point of the posteriormost aspect of the vidian canal foramen orifice (PVID) was easy to identify due to its small diameter and consistently round shape in the coronal view. It has a relatively straight canal running parallel to the Frankfort plane and palatal plane, allowing its posteriormost opening to be reliably and easily traced. The authors found this to be a good landmark to use as long as care is taken to avoid confusing it with the adjacent foramina and canals in this area of the cranial base.

Table 7-2 provides additional details regarding the ease of identifying suggested 3D landmarks for cephalometric analysis.

Table 7-2 Additional details regarding the ease of identifying all suggested 3D landmarks

Landmark	Definition	Ease of landmark placement			Reason
		x-axis	y-axis	z-axis	
Cranial base					
SPIN	Center of foramen spinosum	Simple	Simple	Simple	Small diameter and runs fairly perpendicular to the plane of the cranial base
OVALE	Center of foramen ovale	Simple	Difficult	Difficult	Large-diameter, oval, elongated foramen with thin lateral walls
PVID	Center point of the posteriormost aspect of the vidian canal foramen orifice	Simple	Difficult	Simple	Small-diameter, straight canal that runs fairly parallel to the Frankfort horizontal plane and palatal plane (ANS-PNS), but the posteriormost 10 mm of the canal tapers slightly
ROTUN	Centermost point of the posteriormost level of the foramen rotundum orifice	Difficult	Difficult	Simple	Large diameter with thin superior walls that runs obliquely anteroposteriorly
MDFM	Mesialmost point on the anterior-inferior portion of the dorsum foramen magnum (corresponds to clivus/basion)	Simple	Simple	Simple	Clivus can be identified accurately and reliably
CG	Most superior point of the crista galli	Simple	Simple	Simple	Sharp point that allows easy identification
EAM	Center of the bony portion of the external auditory meatus canal	Difficult	Difficult	Difficult	Extremely large-diameter, tortuous canal that blends with cartilage
HYPO	Center point of the medialmost endocranial orifice of the hypoglossal canal	Difficult	Difficult	Difficult	Curved canal with tapered orifice
Maxilla					
GPF	Center point of the inferiormost level of the greater palatine canal foramen orifice	Difficult	Simple	Simple	Thin palatal bone
NPF	Center point of the mesial and distal halves of the inferiormost level of the nasopalatine/incisive canal orifice (oral aspect)	Difficult	Simple	Simple	The most sharply curved portion of the mesial and distal halves posed some difficulty in localization
IORB	Center point of the anteriormost level of the infraorbital canal foramen orifice	Difficult	Difficult	Difficult	Most anterior 15 to 20 mm of the canal orifice tapers obliquely in a medial-inferior direction
PULP (tooth)	Tip of the buccal-mesialmost pulp horn of the specified tooth	Simple	Simple	Simple	Tip was simple to identify
APEX (tooth)	Tip of the buccal-mesialmost root apex of the specified tooth	Simple	Simple	Simple	Tip was simple to identify
AVBN (tooth)	Point on the buccal cortical plate that aligns parallel to and at the same level as the specified root apex of the involved tooth	Simple	Simple	Difficult	In the absence of a reference based on the root apex tip, there is no vertical stop to localize this point
Mandible					
MF	Center point of the lateralmost foramen orifice of the mental canal	Simple	Simple	Difficult	Large, tapered orifice
PULP (tooth)	Tip of the mesial-buccalmost pulp horn of the specified tooth	Simple	Simple	Simple	Tip was simple to identify
APEX (tooth)	Tip of the mesial-buccalmost root apex of the specified tooth	Simple	Simple	Simple	Tip was simple to identify
AVBN (tooth)	Point on the buccal cortical plate that aligns parallel and at the same level as the specified root apex of the involved tooth	Simple	Simple	Difficult	In the absence of a reference based on the root apex tip, there is no vertical stop to localize this point

ANS, anterior nasal spine; PNS, posterior nasal spine.

References

1. Rubin RM. Making sense of cephalometrics. Angle Orthod 1997;67:83–85.
2. Athanasiou AE. Orthodontic Cephalometry. London: Mosby-Wolfe, 1995.
3. Major PW, Johnson DE, Hesse KL, Glover KE. Landmark identification error in posterior anterior cephalometrics. Angle Orthod 1994;64:447–454.
4. DeFranco JC, Koenig HA, Burstone CJ. Three-dimensional large displacement analysis of orthodontic appliances. J Biomech 1976;9:793–801.
5. Chaconas SJ, Caputo AA, Davis JC. The effects of orthopedic forces on the craniofacial complex utilizing cervical and headgear appliances. Am J Orthod 1976;69:527–539.
6. Ayala Perez C, de Alba JA, Caputo AA, Chaconas SJ. Canine retraction with J hook headgear. Am J Orthod 1980;78:538–547.
7. Vannier MW. Craniofacial imaging informatics and technology development. Orthod Craniofac Res 2003;6(suppl):73–81.
8. Maki K, Inou N, Takanishi A, Miller AJ. Computer-assisted simulations in orthodontic diagnosis and the application of a new cone beam X-ray computed tomography. Orthod Craniofac Res 2003;6(suppl):95–101.
9. Beers AC, Choi W, Pavlovskaia E. Computer-assisted treatment planning and analysis. Orthod Craniofac Res 2003;6(suppl):117–125.
10. Meehan M, Teschner M, Girod S. Three-dimensional simulation and prediction of craniofacial surgery. Orthod Craniofac Res 2003;6(suppl):102–107.
11. Moss JP, Ismail SF, Hennessy RJ. Three-dimensional assessment of treatment outcomes on the face. Orthod Craniofac Res 2003;6(suppl):126–131.
12. Baumrind S, Carlson S, Beers A, Curry S, Norris K, Boyd RL. Using three-dimensional imaging to assess treatment outcomes in orthodontics: A progress report from the University of the Pacific. Orthod Craniofac Res 2003;6(suppl):132–142.
13. Miller RJ, Kuo E, Choi W. Validation of Align Technology's Treat III digital model superimposition tool and its case application. Orthod Craniofac Res 2003;6(suppl):143–149.
14. Hannam AG. Dynamic modeling and jaw biomechanics. Orthod Craniofac Res 2003;6(suppl):59–65.
15. Mah J, Hatcher D. Current status and future needs in craniofacial imaging. Orthod Craniofac Res 2003;6(suppl):10–16.
16. Hu L, Zhao Z, Song J, Fan Y, Jiang W, Chen J. The influences of the stress distribution on the condylar cartilage surface by Herbst appliance under various bite reconstruction—A three dimensional finite element analysis [in Chinese]. Hua Xi Kou Qiang Yi Xue Za Zhi 2001;19:46–48.
17. Song J, Zhao Z, Hu L, Jiang W, Fan Y, Chen J. The influences upon the passive tensile of the masticatory muscles and ligaments by Herbst appliance under various bite reconstruction—A three dimensional finite element analysis [in Chinese]. Hua Xi Kou Qiang Yi Xue Za Zhi 2001;19:43–45.
18. Scarfe WC, Farman AG, Sukovic P. Clinical applications of cone-beam computed tomography in dental practice. J Can Dent Assoc 2006;72:75–80.
19. Ziegler CM, Woertche R, Brief J, Hassfeld S. Clinical indications for digital volume tomography in oral and maxillofacial surgery. Dentomaxillofac Radiol 2002;31:126–130.
20. Mah J. 3-dimensional visualization of impacted maxillary cuspids. AADMRT Newsletter, Winter 2003.
21. Kragskov J, Bosch C, Gyldensted C, Sindet-Pedersen S. Comparison of the reliability of craniofacial anatomic landmarks based on cephalometric radiographs and three-dimensional CT scans. Cleft Palate Craniofac J 1997;34:111–116.
22. Lou L, Lagravère MO, Compton S, Major PW, Flores-Mir C. Accuracy of measurements and reliability of landmark identification with computed tomography (CT) techniques in the maxillofacial area: A systematic review. Oral Surg Oral Med Oral Pathol Oral Radiol Endod 2007;104:402–411.
23. Kamoen A, Dermaut L, Verbeeck R. The clinical significance of error measurement in the interpretation of treatment results. Eur J Orthod 2001;23:569–578.
24. Chen YJ, Chen SK, Yao JC, Chang HF. The effects of differences in landmark identification on the cephalometric measurements in traditional versus digitized cephalometry. Angle Orthod 2004;74:155–161.
25. Gravely JF, Benzies PM. The clinical significance of tracing error in cephalometry. Br J Orthod 1974;1:95–101.
26. Cohen AM. Uncertainty in cephalometrics. Br J Orthod 1984;11:44–48.
27. McWilliam JS, Welander U. The effect of image quality on the identification of cephalometric landmarks. Angle Orthod 1978;48:49–56.
28. Houston WJ, Maher RE, McElroy D, Sherriff M. Sources of error in measurements from cephalometric radiographs. Eur J Orthod 1986;8:149–151.
29. Baumrind S, Frantz RC. The reliability of head film measurements. 1. Landmark identification. Am J Orthod 1971;60:111–127.
30. Savage AW, Showfety KJ, Yancey J. Repeated measures analysis of geometrically constructed and directly determined cephalometric points. Am J Orthod Dentofacial Orthop 1987;91:295–299.
31. Waitzman AA, Posnick JC, Armstrong DC, Pron GE. Craniofacial skeletal measurements based on computed tomography: Part II. Normal values and growth trends. Cleft Palate Craniofac J 1992;29:118–128.
32. Matteson SR, Bechtold W, Phillips C, Staab EV. A method for three-dimensional image reformation for quantitative cephalometric analysis. J Oral Maxillofac Surg 1989;47:1053–1061.
33. Tyndall DA, Renner JB, Phillips C, Matteson SR. Positional changes of the mandibular condyle assessed by three-dimensional computed tomography. J Oral Maxillofac Surg 1992;50:1164–1172.
34. Hildebolt CF, Vannier MW, Knapp RH. Validation study of skull three-dimensional computerized tomography measurements. Am J Phys Anthropol 1990;82:283–294.
35. Klinge B, Petersson A, Maly P. Location of the mandibular canal: Comparison of macroscopic findings, conventional radiography, and computed tomography. Int J Oral Maxillofac Implants 1989;4:327–332.
36. Aaron A, Weinstein D, Thickman D, Eilert R. Comparison of orthoroentgenography and computed tomography in the measurement of limb-length discrepancy. J Bone Joint Surg Am 1992;74:897–902.
37. Goldenberg DC, Alonso N, Goldenberg FC, et al. Using computed tomography to evaluate maxillary changes after surgically assisted rapid palatal expansion. J Craniofac Surg 2007;18:302–311.
38. Loddi PP, Pereira MD, Wolosker AB, Hino CT, Kreniski TM, Ferreira LM. Transverse effects after surgically assisted rapid maxillary expansion in the midpalatal suture using computed tomography. J Craniofac Surg 2008;19:433–438.
39. Habersack K, Karoglan A, Sommer B, Benner KU. High-resolution multislice computerized tomography with multiplanar and 3-dimensional reformation imaging in rapid palatal expansion. Am J Orthod Dentofacial Orthop 2007;131:776–781.
40. Garrett BJ, Caruso JM, Rungcharassaeng K, Farrage JR, Kim JS, Taylor GD. Skeletal effects to the maxilla after rapid maxillary expansion assessed with cone-beam computed tomography. Am J Orthod Dentofacial Orthop 2008;134:8–9.
41. Garib DG, Henriques JF, Janson G, Freitas MR, Coelho RA. Rapid maxillary expansion—Tooth tissue-borne versus tooth-borne expanders: A computed tomography evaluation of dentoskeletal effects. Angle Orthod 2005;75:548–557.
42. Swennen GR, Schutyser F, Barth EL, De Groeve P, De Mey A. A new method of 3-D cephalometry Part I: The anatomic Cartesian 3-D reference system. J Craniofac Surg 2006;17:314–325.
43. Tausche E, Hansen L, Hietschold V, Lagravère MO, Harzer W. Three-dimensional evaluation of surgically assisted implant bone-borne rapid maxillary expansion: A pilot study. Am J Orthod Dentofacial Orthop 2007;131(suppl):S92–S99.
44. Major PW, Johnson DE, Hesse KL, Glover KE. Effect of head orientation on posterior anterior cephalometric landmark identification. Angle Orthod 1996;66:51–60.
45. Liu JK, Chen YT, Cheng KS. Accuracy of computerized automatic identification of cephalometric landmarks. Am J Orthod Dentofacial Orthop 2000;118:535–540.
46. Trpkova B, Major P, Prasad N, Nebbe B. Cephalometric landmarks identification and reproducibility: A meta analysis. Am J Orthod Dentofacial Orthop 1997;112:165–170.
47. Naji P, Alsufyani NA, Lagravère MO. Reliability of anatomic structures as landmarks in three-dimensional cephalometric analysis using CBCT. Angle Orthod 2014;84:762–772.
48. Lemieux G, Carey JP, Flores-Mir C, Secanell M, Hart A, Lagravère MO. Precision and accuracy of suggested maxillary and mandibular landmarks with cone-beam computed tomography for regional superimpositions: An in vitro study. Am J Orthod Dentofacial Orthop 2016;149:67–75.
49. Lagravère MO, Gordon JM, Guedes IH, et al. Reliability of traditional cephalometric landmarks as seen in three-dimensional analysis in maxillary expansion treatments. Angle Orthod 2009;79:1047–1056.
50. Marmary Y, Zilberman Y, Mirsky Y. Use of foramina spinosa to determine skull midlines. The Angle Orthod 1979;49:263–268.

8

Cephalometric Airway Analysis

Ahmed Ghoneima, BDS, PhD, MSD
Katherine Kula, MS, DMD, MS

The human *upper airway* could be defined as the airway space extending from the nares of the nose and the stoma of the mouth down to the cricoid cartilage in the larynx. The nasal and oral cavities merge in the area known as the *pharynx*, which is anatomically divided into three sections: the nasopharynx, oropharynx, and hypopharynx (Fig 8-1). The nasopharynx is the superior portion of the pharynx that is located posterior to the nasal cavity and above the soft palate. The oropharynx, below the nasopharynx, can be divided into the retropalatal and retroglossal oropharynx; it acts as a digestive and respiratory conduit and extends to the epiglottis. The hypopharynx or laryngopharynx is that area of the pharynx caudal to the epiglottis and extending to the larynx. The maxillary sinuses are also included in the upper airway, but little is known about the exchange of air between the nasal passages and the sinuses.

The shape and dimensions of upper airway passages influence the volume of air passing through them. The close anatomical relationship of the upper airway with the craniofacial and dental structures dictates their influence on each other. Normal growth and development of craniofacial structures depends on a patent airway and nasal breathing.[1–3] The purpose of this chapter is to provide measures using two-dimensional (2D) and three-dimensional (3D) imaging that allow evaluation of the upper airway.

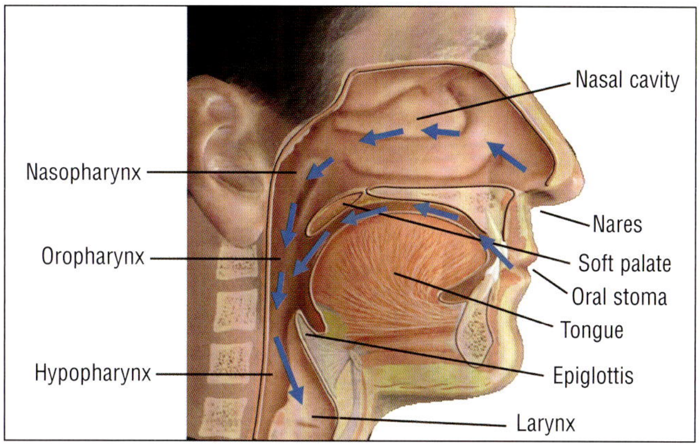

Fig 8-1a Sagittal drawing showing the anatomical sections of the upper airway.

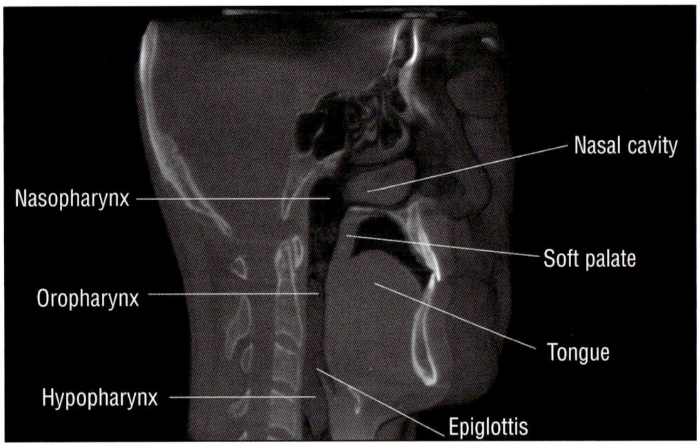

Fig 8-1b Three-quarter CBCT image sliced at the midsagittal section showing the anatomical sections of the upper airway.

2D Versus 3D Evaluation of the Upper Airway

Some common obstructive airway disorders such as asthma and apneas are associated with collapse of the soft tissue structures and subsequent decrease in the volume or flow of air. Alterations in the size of pharyngeal and palatine tonsils or the adenoids also significantly affect airway flow and dynamics (Fig 8-2). Respiratory diseases associated with edema and/or inflammation of the soft tissues cause airway constriction and impact airway patency. The continuous flow of air through the upper airway system is thought to be a stimulus for maxillary lateral growth. Narrowing or alterations in airway dimensions can lead to challenges in breathing. Clinical detection of structural narrowing of the upper airway could allow early recognition of developing dental and skeletal discrepancies, atypical facial morphology, and/or obstructive sleep apnea (OSA).[4–6]

Functional abnormalities and altered patterns of nasal respiration during active growth periods adversely affect the development of the craniofacial skeletal structures. Human and experimental animal studies suggest that morphologic discrepancies in the jaws and craniofacial structures may exist as a result of airway disorders. Severely reduced nasal airflow over time causes developmental changes such as continuous jaw opening during rest, increased interocclusal distance, lowering of tongue and hyoid bone position, incompetent lips, hyperdivergency and backward rotation of the mandible, increased anterior facial height, and even the development of posterior crossbite and a collapsed maxilla. These changes are known as *long face syndrome* or *adenoid facies*. The presentation and effects of these changes vary from mild to severe according to the intensity, onset, and duration of the airway disorder.[7,8]

Because the development of normal occlusion and craniofacial growth are dependent on maintaining normal airway morphology and function, assessment of the airway should be considered an important aspect in orthodontic diagnosis and treatment planning. The preliminary orthodontic screening process provides an appropriate prospect to identify signs of airway disorders. A questionnaire including symptoms or signs of snoring and interrupted sleep together with diagnostic imaging findings discovered during the examination can give indications of possible airway disorders and support the need for referral to a sleep medicine specialist for a comprehensive examination to detect potential sleep-disordered breathing problems.[9,10]

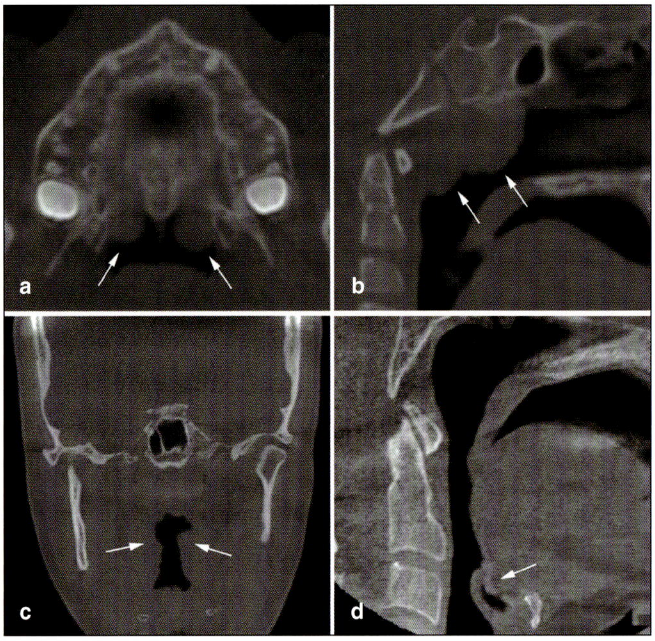

Fig 8-2 *(a)* Axial section showing a thickened mucosa lining the inferior nasal turbinates. *(b)* Sagittal section showing an enlarged pharyngeal tonsil (adenoid). *(c)* Coronal section showing enlarged palatine tonsils. *(d)* Sagittal section showing a mildly enlarged lingual tonsil.

Techniques such as fluoroscopy, acoustic reflection, fiberoptic pharyngoscopy, cephalograms, optical coherence tomography, cone beam computed tomography (CBCT), and magnetic resonance imaging (MRI) have been employed over the years to assess the upper airway.[11–15] Although OSA tests are generally performed overnight in a hospital under the supervision of a sleep medicine physician, physicians now can employ reliable diagnostic equipment designed for home use to diagnose and determine the severity of OSA.[10] The advanced techniques of airway evaluation are considered expensive and may not be available at all health facilities.

Lateral cephalograms are routinely used in orthodontic settings to analyze dental and skeletal structures and relationships as well as soft tissue structures and form. They have also been used to assess the airway in subjects with OSA and are proven to be a simple and helpful method of measuring airway patency. They are considered a reliable and valid method for measuring dimensions of the airway, especially the nasopharyngeal and retropalatal regions.[15–17] Lateral cephalograms provide information about the adenoids, soft palate, tongue, hyoid bone, and pharynx. They also allow visual assessment of airway clearance and/or cloudiness. However, there are several limitations for using them for comprehensive assessment of upper airway structures. Lateral cephalograms only display a

Table 8-1 **Cephalometric landmarks used to assess pharyngeal airway, soft palate dimensions, hyoid bone position, and craniofacial angulation**

Landmark	Definition
Hormion (Ho)	Most anteroinferior contact point of the spheno-occipital synchondrosis, located in the midsagittal plane
Adenoid 1 (ad1)	Point of intersection of the posterior nasopharyngeal wall and a line from PNS to Ba
Adenoid 2 (ad2)	Point of intersection of the line PNS perpendicular to SBa and the posterior nasopharyngeal wall
Posterior pharyngeal wall (ppw)	Point of intersection between the posterior pharyngeal wall and the occlusal plane
Posterior pharyngeal wall 1 (ppw1)	Point of intersection between the posterior pharyngeal wall and the palatal plane
Posterior pharyngeal wall 2 (ppw2)	Point of intersection between the posterior pharyngeal wall and the line connecting hyoid (hy) and the most inferoanterior point on CV2
Posterior pharyngeal wall 4 (ppw4)	Point of intersection between the posterior pharyngeal wall and the line connecting hy and the most inferoanterior point on CV4
Anterior pharyngeal wall 2 (apw2)	Point of intersection between the anterior pharyngeal wall and the line connecting hy and the most inferoanterior point on CV2
Anterior pharyngeal wall 4 (apw4)	Point of intersection between the anterior pharyngeal wall and the line connecting hy and the most inferoanterior point on CV4
Superior pharyngeal wall (spw)	Point of intersection between the superior pharyngeal wall and a perpendicular line to the palatal plane passing through PNS
Atlas vertebra (AA)	Most anterior point on the anterior arch of the atlas vertebra (C1), located on the median sagittal plane
Second cervical vertebra (CV2ia)	Most inferoanterior point on the body of the second cervical vertebra
Third cervical vertebra (CV3ia)	Most inferoanterior point on the body of the third cervical vertebra
Fourth cervical vertebra (CV4ia)	Most inferoanterior point on the body of the fourth cervical vertebra
CV2ap	Point at the apex of the odontoid process of the second cervical vertebra
CV2tg	Posterior tangent point of the odontoid process of the second cervical vertebra
CV2ip	Most inferoposterior point on the body of the second cervical vertebra
CV4ip	Most inferoposterior point on the body of the fourth cervical vertebra
Opisthion (Op)	Most anteroinferior point of the posterior margin of the foramen magnum
Epiglottis base (Eb)	Most inferior and anterior point of the epiglottis (the deepest point of the epiglottis representing the base of the epiglottis)
Epiglottis tip (Et)	Tip of the epiglottis (its most superior point)
Uvula tip (U)	Most inferior tip of the soft palate (tip of the uvula)
Tongue (t)	Point at the intersection between the dorsal tongue surface and the occlusal plane
Tongue base (tb)	Point at the intersection between B-point–gonion line and the base of the tongue
Hyoid (hy)	Most superior and anterior point on the body of the hyoid bone

PNS, posterior nasal spine; Ba, basion; SBa, sella-basion.

2D view of a 3D object. Volume and cross-sectional area cannot be assessed. Measurement error can vary greatly with any given landmark due to problems in landmark identification. In addition to the inherent structure overlap and projection, magnification, and distortion errors, patient positioning significantly affects the shape and size of the airway passage being assessed.[17–20] OSA generally occurs while sleeping in a prone position, whereas lateral cephalograms are taken with a patient awake and in an upright position. Central problems can also cause other sleep-disordered breathing that might not be apparent on a lateral cephalogram.

On the other hand, 3D CT and CBCT imaging are currently available worldwide. They are relatively inexpensive and have improved diagnostic capacities compared with traditional 2D radiography. 3D images allow accurate identification of anatomical landmarks, making visualization and volumetric analysis of the airway details more reliable. CBCT imaging tends to be less expensive than CT imaging and has a lower radiation dose. MRI is another technique for evaluating the airway three-dimensionally and for assessment of ventilation differences in respiratory diseases. However, most clinicians and researchers consider CBCT imaging to be a faster, easier, and more accurate method for visualizing and measuring airway structures than MRI.[21]

Cephalometric Measures of Airways

Early studies that focused on evaluating the airway to determine when its morphologic characteristics and dimensions might relate to functional disorders, such as with restricted airways that induce mouth breathing or OSA, were not diagnosed with imaging. Currently, imaging plays an essential role in anatomical assessment of the airway and the adjacent structures, allowing clinicians to identify patients who are at risk. Table 8-1

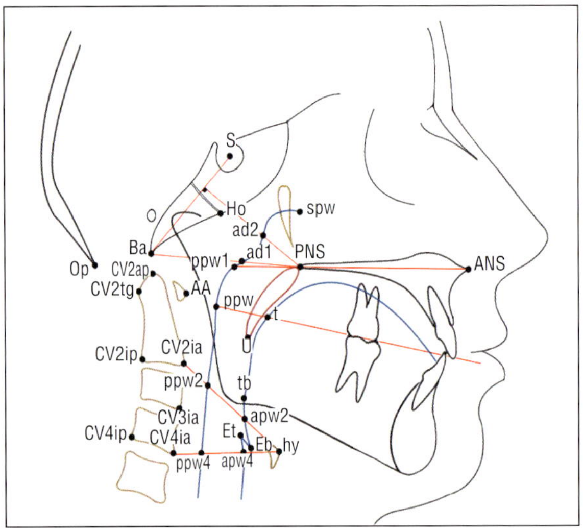

Fig 8-3 CBCT sagittal view image showing the anatomical landmarks of airway structures.

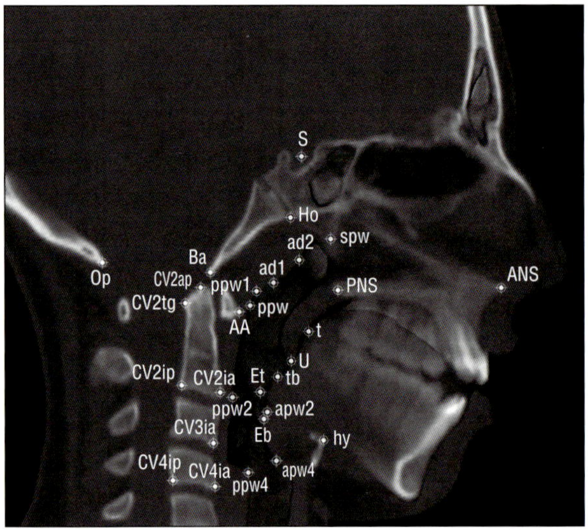

Fig 8-4 Cephalometric landmarks for pharyngeal airway, soft palate, hyoid bone, and craniofacial angulation assessment.

and Figs 8-3 and 8-4 describe the cephalometric landmarks commonly used for airway assessment along with multiple related structures such as soft palate position and size, hyoid bone position, and craniofacial angulations. Many of the landmarks are based on planes connecting facial hard tissue structures (eg, palatal plane, occlusal plane, and many other planes). These planes need to be constructed first to identify the airway landmarks.

Cephalometric assessment of airway structure can be performed either manually or using one of the cephalometric tracing software programs in either the anteroposterior (AP) or vertical dimension (Table 8-2 and Figs 8-5 to 8-8). Linear measurements in the AP dimension allow evaluation of the width and depth of the airway passage, while linear measurements in the vertical dimension allow evaluation of the length of the airway structure. Angular measurements could also be used to determine the AP and vertical positions of both soft tissue and hard tissue structures related to the airway.[22] Soft tissue measures provide information about soft tissue effects on airway constrictions.

Factors such as soft palate size, hyoid bone position, and cervical vertebra angulations are closely related to the airway structures and can significantly affect the airway size (Tables 8-3 and 8-4 and Figs 8-9 to 8-12). The sagittal depth of the nasopharynx is measured as the shortest distance between the outer margin of the soft palate and the posterior pharyngeal wall. This distance is considered a measure of patency of the upper respiratory region. Whether using 2D or 3D imaging to assess the airway size, it is crucial to take the radiograph while the soft palate is in the normal position. If the patient is swallowing or breathing from the mouth during the scanning, the soft palate will change its size and shape and will assume a different location, affecting pharyngeal airway measurements.[23]

Factors affecting cephalometric measures

Head posture, which can influence airway constriction, can be evaluated by assessing the craniocervical angulations using lateral cephalometric radiographs.[2,5,24] Cephalometric head holder (ear rod) position and natural head (mirror) position are the two most common methods of head positions. Natural head position (NHP) is a standardized and reproducible position of the head in an upright posture. Subjects stand in the cephalostat machine with forehead support, with no interference from ear rods, and focus on a point that is in the distance at eye level. Their visual axis should be horizontal to the floor.

Cephalometric results can sometimes be misleading in the diagnosis of craniofacial discrepancies because traditional cephalometric methods usually rely on intracranial reference lines. A rather reliable and stable reference plane is required to accurately compare deviations from the norm or to follow up with the treatment outcomes over time. This is also important for long-term evaluation of craniofacial growth and development. The landmarks defining these lines are subject to change undoubtedly during growth and may vary greatly among different individuals. An extracranial reference plane such as NHP may be able to overcome these problems. The literature also indicates that cranial base structures can be considered stable reference landmarks. Consequently, the sella-nasion plane (SN plane) and the Frankfort horizontal plane (FH plane) have been most commonly used as horizontal reference planes. However, some authors have reported individual variations of intracranial landmarks.[25,26]

Currently available 3D imaging software programs make it possible to evaluate, simulate, and quantify the upper airway

Table 8-2 Parameters used for cephalometric assessment of pharyngeal airway space

Parameter	Definition
Ba-ad1	Thickness of soft tissue of the posterior pharyngeal wall behind ad1
Ba-ad2	Thickness of soft tissue of the posterior pharyngeal wall behind ad2
Ba-PNS	Depth of the bony nasopharynx along line PNS-Ba
PNS-ppw1	Sagittal depth of the nasopharyngeal airway
PNS-ad1	Sagittal depth of the nasopharyngeal airway at the level of ad1 along line PNS-Ba
PNS-ad2	Sagittal depth of the nasopharyngeal airway at the level of ad2
AA-PNS	Anteroposterior dimension of the upper pharyngeal space
PNS-spw	Height of the nasopharynx represented by the linear distance between a perpendicular line to the palatal plane at PNS to the superior wall of the nasopharynx (spw)
apw2-ppw2	Sagittal depth of the oropharynx represented by the linear distance between the anterior and posterior walls of the airway along a line from hy to CV2ia
apw4-ppw4	Sagittal depth of the hypopharynx represented by the linear distance between the anterior and posterior walls of the airway along a line connecting hy and CV4ia
t-ppw	Linear distance between the dorsal tongue surface and the posterior pharyngeal wall intersecting with the occlusal plane
PNS-Eb	Vertical airway length measured as the linear distance between PNS and the most inferoanterior point of the epiglottis
PAS	Posterior airway space diameter behind the most dorsal part of the root of the tongue along a line passing through the reference points B-point and gonion
Ho ⊥ ANS-PNS	Linear distance between the most inferior point of the spheno-occipital synchondrosis (Ho) perpendicular on the palatal plane representing the height of the bony nasopharynx
Ho ⊥ Ba-PNS	Linear distance between a line from Ho perpendicular on the Ba-PNS representing the height of the bony nasopharynx
NS-PTM	Angle representing the shape of the anterior bony nasopharyngeal space
PTM-SBa	Angle representing the shape of the posterior bony nasopharyngeal space
BaS-PNS	Used to determine the horizontal position of the hard palate and soft palate as well as the cause of airway obstruction; measured by the angle formed by the planes BaS and S-PNS (norm, 63 ± 2.5 degrees)
Upper pharyngeal airway space (UP)	Distance from a point on the posterior outline of the soft palate to the closest point on the pharyngeal wall; the average upper pharyngeal space is approximately 15 to 20 mm in width (a width of 2 mm or less in this region may indicate airway impairment); airway obstruction should be confirmed by an otorhinolaryngologist
Lower pharyngeal airway space (LP)	Distance from a point of intersection of the posterior border of the tongue and the inferior border of the mandible to the closest point on the posterior pharyngeal wall; the average lower pharyngeal space is approximately 11 to 14 mm in width (smaller values indicate obstruction at this area and need to be medically confirmed to determine if true airway obstruction is present)

Ba, basion; PNS, posterior nasal spine; PTM, pterygomaxillary fissure; S, sella. For other landmark abbreviations and definitions, see Table 8-1.

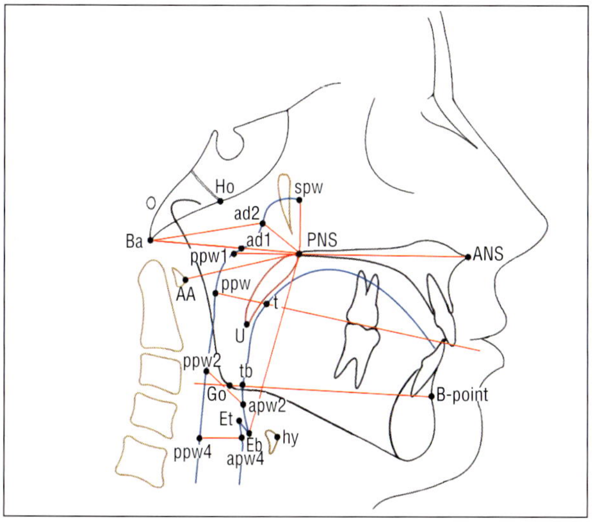

Fig 8-5 Cephalometric assessment of the pharyngeal airway space in width and height.

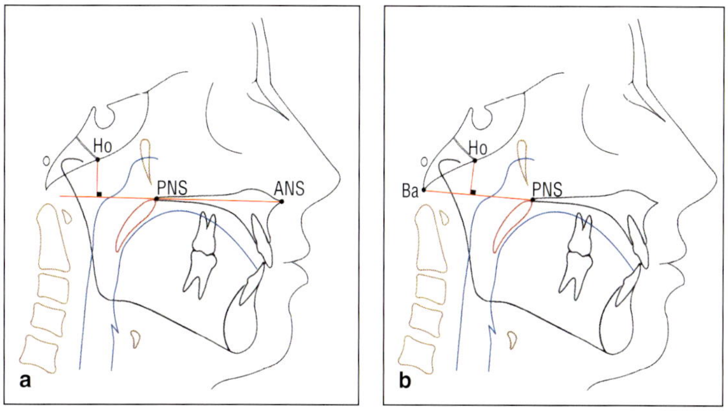

Fig 8-6 Cephalometric assessment of the height of the bony nasopharynx using *(a)* Ho perpendicular to the palatal plane or *(b)* Ho perpendicular to Ba-PNS line.

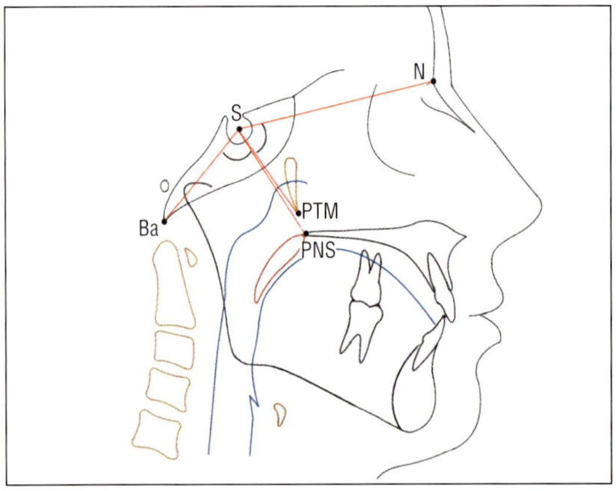

Fig 8-7 Cephalometric assessment of the shape of the bony nasopharynx and the position of the hard palate.

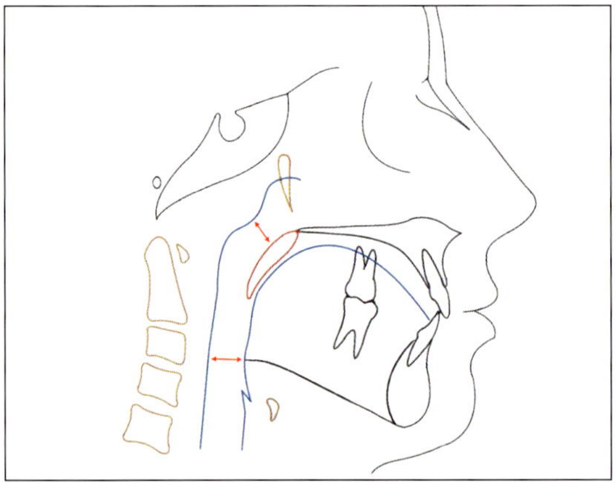

Fig 8-8 Cephalometric assessment of the upper and lower pharyngeal airway space (McNamara analysis).

Table 8-3 Parameters for cephalometric assessment of soft palate size and hyoid bone position

Parameter	Definition
Soft palate length	Distance from posterior nasal spine to the tip of the soft palate (U)
Soft palate thickness	Measured through the widest area between the anterior and posterior border of the soft palate
hy-apw2	Linear distance between point hy and the anterior pharyngeal wall on point apw2
hy-apw4	Linear distance between point hy and the anterior pharyngeal wall on point apw4
C3-hy	Anteroposterior position of the hyoid linear distance between C3 and hy
hy-MPhy-H′	Vertical position of the hyoid bone
hy-m	Linear distance between point hy and the most posterior point on the mandibular symphysis (m); it represents the anteroposterior position of the hyoid bone
hy-Gnpost	Linear distance between point hy and the most posteroinferior point on the mandibular symphysis (retrognathion: Gnpost); it represents the horizontal position of the hyoid bone
hy-MP	Vertical position of hy (distance along a perpendicular from hy to the mandibular plane)
hy-OP	Vertical position of hy (distance along a perpendicular from hy to the occlusal plane)
hy-PP	Vertical position of hy (distance along a perpendicular from hy to the palatal plane)
hy-SN	Vertical position of hy (distance along a perpendicular from hy to the anterior cranial base [sella-nasion])

Table 8-4 Parameters used for cephalometric assessment of craniocervical angulation (head posture angles)

Parameter	Definition
CVT-HOR	Inclination of the cervical column to the true horizontal represented by the angle between CVT and the true horizontal (HOR) line; CVT is the plane that connects the posteriormost and superiormost point of the second vertebra (CV2tg) with the inferiormost point of the fourth vertebra (CV4ip)
CVT-MP	Head position in relation to the cervical column represented by the angle between CVT and the mandibular plane (MP)
CVT-PP	Head position in relation to the cervical column represented by the angle between CVT and the palatal plane (PP)
CVT-FH	Inclination of the cervical column in relation to the Frankfort horizontal (FH) line represented by the angle between CVT and the FH plane
CVT-SN	Head position in relation to the cervical column represented by the angle between CVT and the anterior cranial base (SN) plane
CVT-RP	Head position in relation to the cervical column represented by the angle between CVT and the ramus plane (RP)
OPT-HOR	Inclination of the cervical column to the true horizontal line represented by the angle between odontoid process tangent (OPT) and HOR; OPT is the plane that connects the posterior tangent (CV2tg) to the odontoid process through CV2ip
OPT-MP	Head position in relation to the cervical column represented by the angle between OPT and MP
OPT-PP	Head position in relation to the cervical column represented by the angle between OPT and PP
OPT-FH	Inclination of the cervical column in relation to the Frankfort horizontal line represented by the angle between OPT and the FH plane
OPT-SN	Head position in relation to the cervical column represented by the angle between OPT and the anterior cranial base (SN) plane
OPT-RP	Head position in relation to the cervical column represented by the angle between OPT and RP
OPT-CVT	Inclination of the two cervical reference lines to each other (ie, the cervical curvature represented by the angle between OPT and CVT)
CV2ap-CV4ip	Length of the cervical column represented by the linear distance between the points CV2ap and CV4ip

SN, sella-nasion.

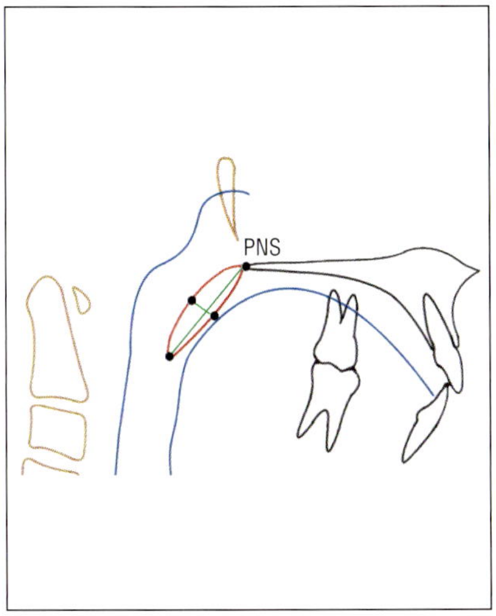

Fig 8-9 Cephalometric assessment of the soft palate length and width.

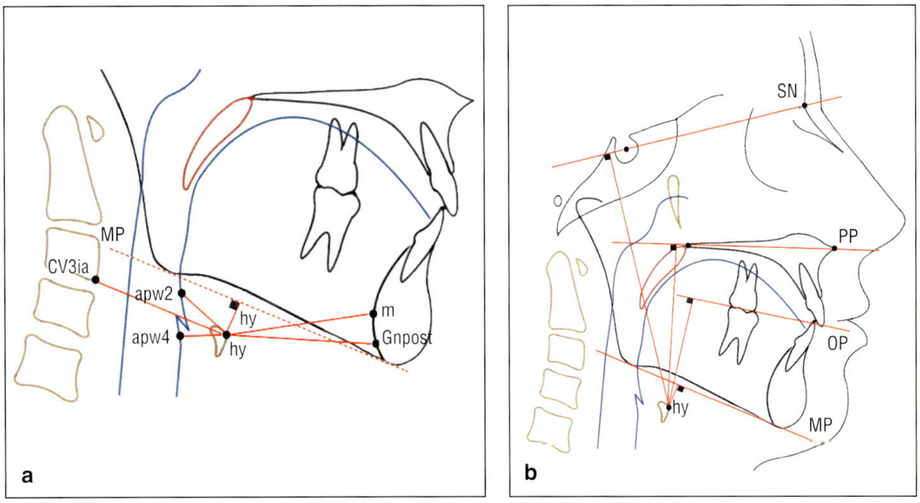

Fig 8-10 *(a and b)* Cephalometric assessment of hyoid bone position.

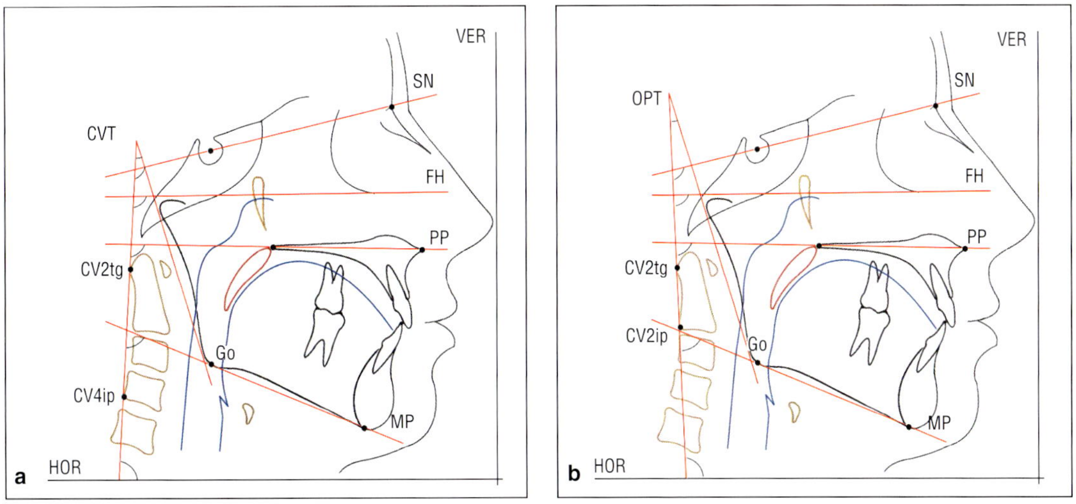

Fig 8-11 Cephalometric assessment of craniocervical angulations taken with *(a)* the cervical vertebra tangent (CVT) and *(b)* the odontoid process tangent (OPT).

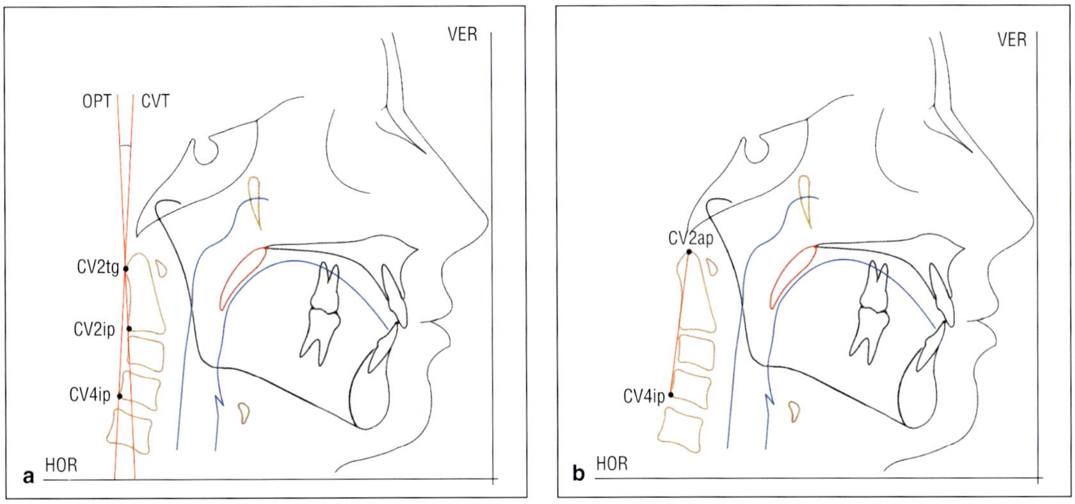

Fig 8-12 *(a)* The cervical curvature represented by the inclination of the OPT and the CVT to each other. *(b)* The length of the cervical column represented by the linear distance between CV2ap and CV4ip.

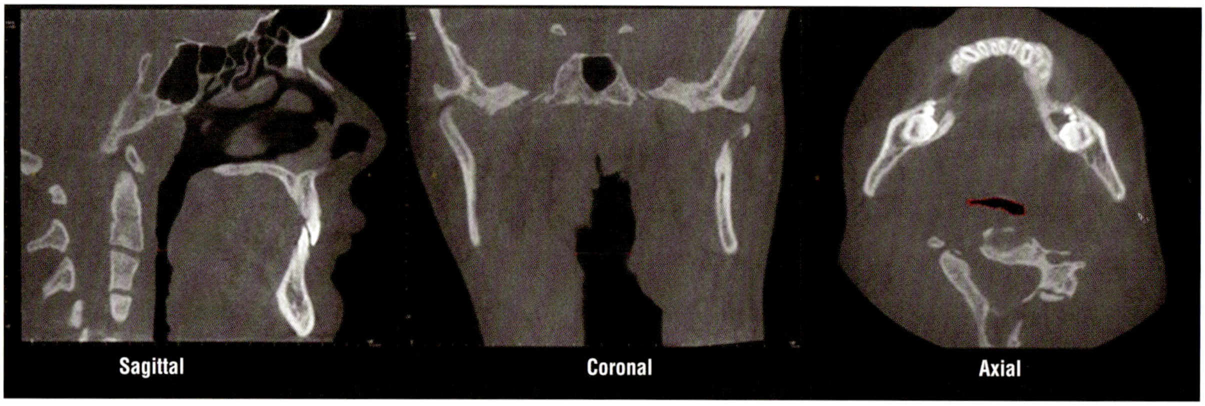

Fig 8-13 Airway structures from the sagittal, coronal, and axial sections. The sagittal view of the airway provides an indication of airway constriction while the coronal gives an indication of airway width. The cross-section view of the axial slice is the only section that can be used to measure the airway circumference.

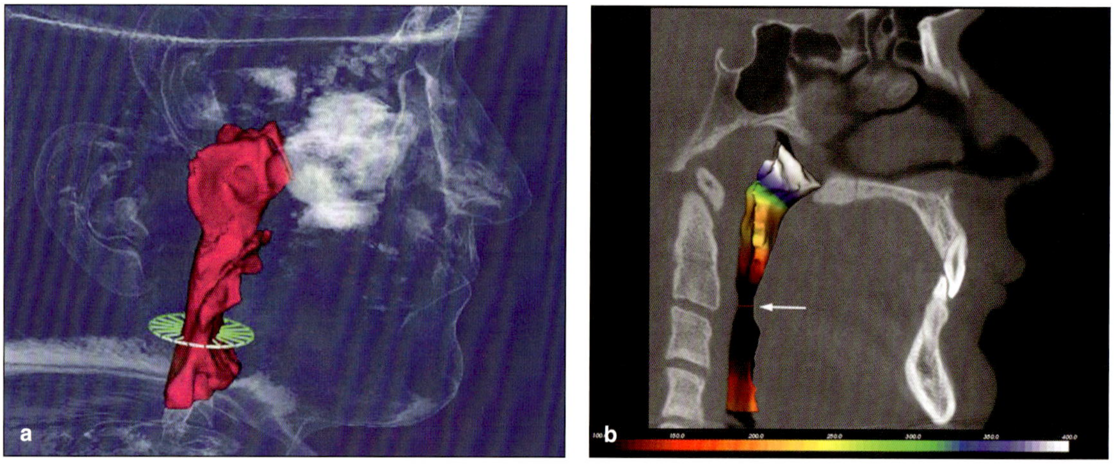

Fig 8-14 The most constricted area (MCA) of the airway can be detected and measured automatically using certain software programs. MCA is demarcated by the *green ring (a)* or the *red line (b)*.

morphology both in cross-sectional and longitudinal studies. The effects of growth and treatment on the airway shape and size can now be evaluated. These programs allow linear and angular measurements to assess airway length and width and also allow clinicians to obtain accurate surface area and volumetric measurements. The cross-sectional area of any portion of the upper airway can be evaluated merely using the axial slices of CBCT images (Fig 8-13), and the software can identify the most constricted area specifically (Fig 8-14). The cross-sectional area shows the circumference of the airway border (Fig 8-15) and provides the additional z-dimension to best assess airway volume. The axial view also has the advantage of visualizing the whole border of the airway, which cannot be done using the coronal and sagittal images. Currently, extensive literature confirms that CBCT and 3D imaging software programs can accurately assess the airway volume and can identify and measure the size of the most constricted area of the airway[27–31] (see Fig 8-14).

Several variables can affect the reliability of using CBCT in airway evaluation. These variables should be considered when using CBCT for airway assessment. There could be human-related factors such as scanning patients with inaccurate positions of the head, jaws, hyoid bone, soft palate, or epiglottis. Breathing, swallowing, and improper tongue positions during the scanning time can impinge on the posterior airway area. Opening the jaws can significantly affect numerous upper airway measures (eg, most constricted area, palatal area, nasopharynx volume, and oropharynx volume).[32] These changes suggest that having the mouth open for extended periods of time (eg, sleeping, dental treatment) can decrease airway volume and affect breathing. Definitively, they indicate that positions of the head and the jaw must be standardized when lateral cephalograms or CBCT studies are performed for accurate and reliable measures. These variables are basically attributed to the fact that the evaluation process entails an attempt to evaluate dynamic structure using static images. A second group of variables include scanner machine–related factors such as distortion, resolution, and inconsistent scanning settings (eg, voxel size, Kv, mA, and variable scanning time or use of different machines). Another variable that can affect values is differing or inconsistent software settings (eg, threshold or sensitivity of airway segmentation).[25]

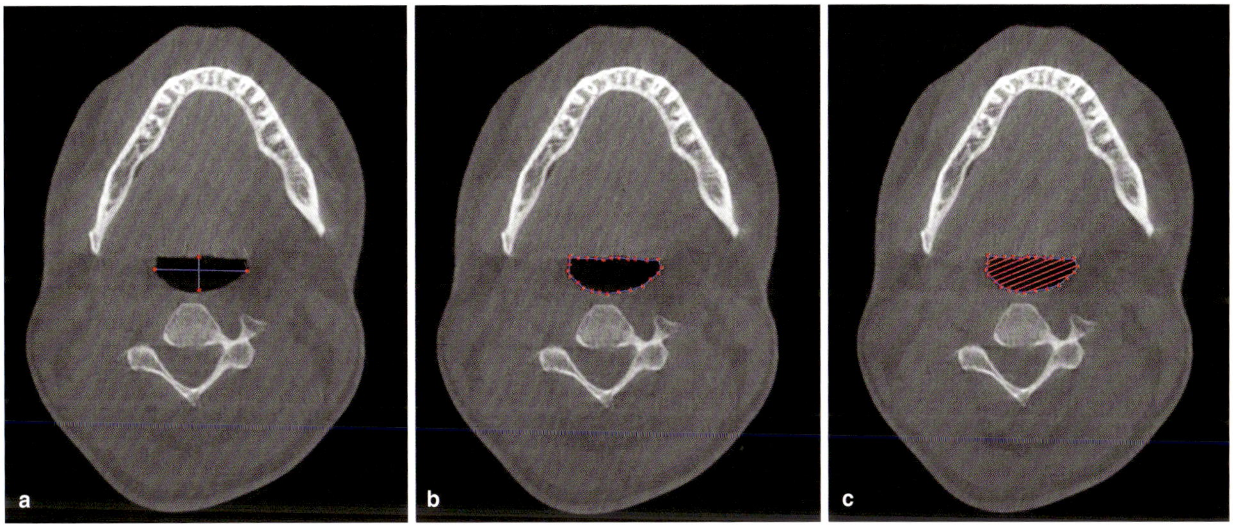

Fig 8-15 Airway structures can be measured in *(a)* width and depth, *(b)* circumference, and *(c)* surface area using the axial sections of the CBCT scan.

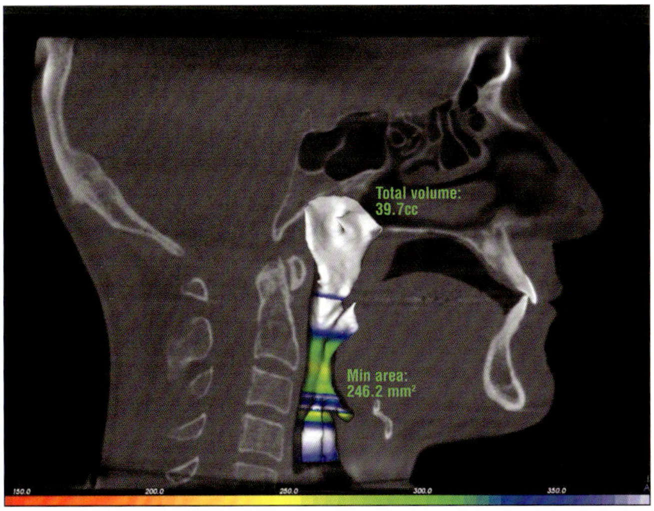

Fig 8-16 3D CBCT image showing airway segmentation of the pharynx.

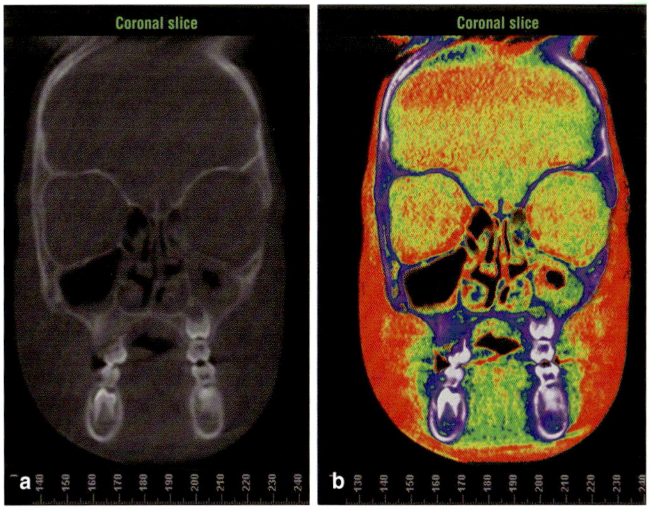

Fig 8-17 3D CBCT coronal section showing the difference between intensities of voxels representing bone, soft tissue, and air in the sinuses of a patient with cleft palate: *(a)* in shades of gray; *(b)* with the intensities of gray translated to color. *Black* represents air; *red, yellow,* and *green* represent soft tissue; and *blue* and *purple* represent bone.

Process of Airway Segmentation

One of the unique tools of 3D technology is the ability to perform airway segmentations (Fig 8-16). The segmentation process depends on the fact that tissues with different density values and different shades of gray levels (dynamic range) should also have different threshold values (Fig 8-17). By adjusting the threshold values, hard tissue (bone and teeth), soft tissue, and airway structures can be identified and segmented. Software programs also have different segmentation techniques based on the algorithm they use. The segmented airway structure can then be quantified by using the volumetric measuring tools available in several software programs. This tool calculates the volume (cubic millimeter or mm^3) of the segmented part of the airway, identifies the location of the most constricted area (the minimal airway area), and calculates the surface area (square millimeter or mm^2).

To assess airway volume, the airway can be segmented into nasal cavity, nasopharynx, oropharynx, and hypopharynx (Fig 8-18). Even the airway volume of maxillary sinuses can be determined using segmentation, although the threshold values might need to be adjusted to differentiate between air space and mucous or inflamed tissue.[33] Each segment has to be defined and outlined in the sagittal and coronal dimensions for the software to calculate the volume. Multiple landmarks are utilized to outline the airway segments.

Using the sagittal section showing the midsagittal plane, the nasal cavity can be outlined inferiorly by drawing a line repre-

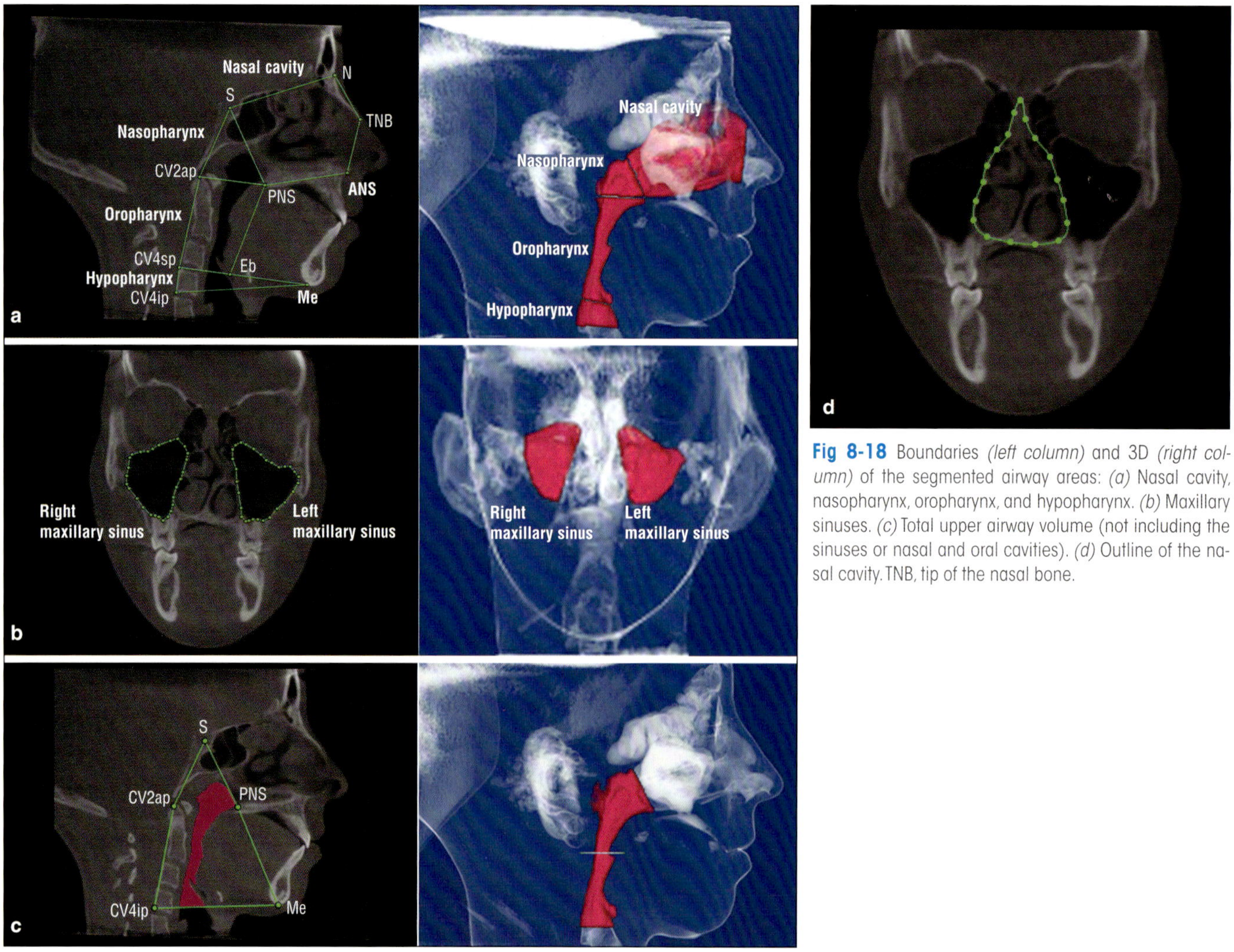

Fig 8-18 Boundaries *(left column)* and 3D *(right column)* of the segmented airway areas: *(a)* Nasal cavity, nasopharynx, oropharynx, and hypopharynx. *(b)* Maxillary sinuses. *(c)* Total upper airway volume (not including the sinuses or nasal and oral cavities). *(d)* Outline of the nasal cavity. TNB, tip of the nasal bone.

senting the palatal plane from the posterior nasal spine (PNS) to the anterior nasal spine (ANS), anteriorly by drawing a line connecting ANS to the tip of the nasal bone (TNB) to nasion (N) point, superiorly by extending a line from N to sella (S), and posteriorly by drawing a line from S to PNS. The nasal cavity should be outlined on the coronal section by drawing a line all the way along the outline of the nasal cavity (see Fig 8-18d).

The nasopharynx can be outlined anteriorly by extending a line from PNS to S, posteriorly by extending a line from S to the tip of the odontoid process (CV2tp), and inferiorly by drawing a line from CV2tp to PNS. This segment is usually triangular in shape.

The oropharynx can be outlined anteriorly by extending a line from PNS to the base of the epiglottis (Eb), inferiorly by extending a line from Eb to CV4sp, posteriorly by extending a line from the posterosuperior border of CV4 (CVsp) to CV2tp, and superiorly by extending a line from CV2tp to PNS. The oropharynx shares borders with the nasopharynx and the hypopharynx.

The hypopharynx can be outlined anteriorly by drawing a line from Eb to menton (Me) point, inferiorly by extending a line from Me to CV4ip, posteriorly by extending a line from CV4sp to the posterior inferior corner of CV4ip, and superiorly by extending a line from CV4sp to Eb.

The maxillary sinuses can be outlined individually by drawing a line on the sagittal midline section all the way around the superior, inferior, medial, and lateral walls of each maxillary sinus. This process is repeated on a coronal section showing the widest area of the maxillary sinus.

The software algorithm can measure volume or area by segmenting the airway using the growing seed point that is placed into a specific segment or total airway by the researcher/clinician. The sensitivity of the airway segmentation is based on the intensity of the selected voxel range and is adjustable. The volume is determined by multiplying the number of voxels with similar intensity by the size of the voxel. If the segmentation threshold is changed, the number of voxels with similar intensity can change, which can in turn change the measurement. The voxels of air, soft tissue or fluid, and hard tissue generally have different, although variable, intensities, which means that unless sensitivity is kept consistent, air space measures can vary for that patient or among patients.[33]

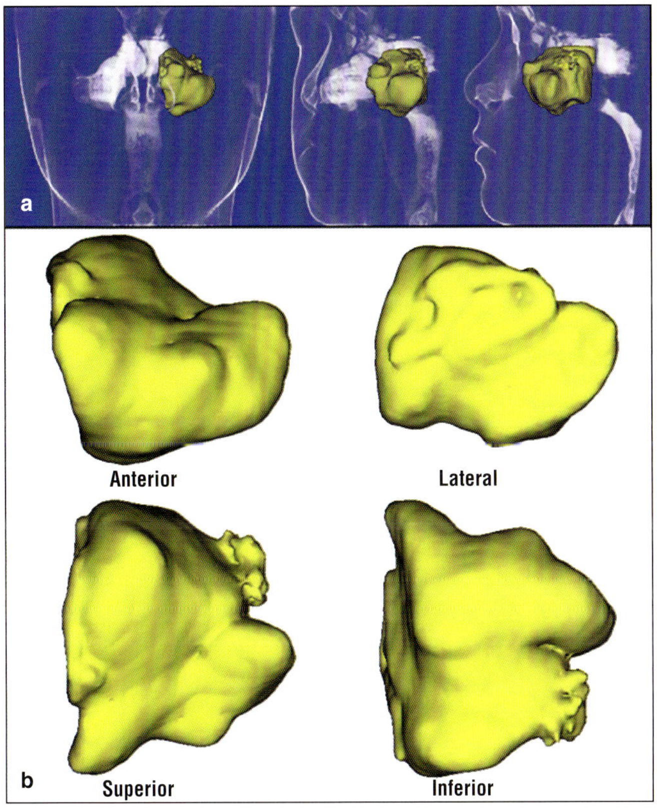

Fig 8-19 *(a)* 3D segmentation of the left sinus seen from three different views. *(b)* 3D model of the left sinus seen from anterior, lateral, superior, and inferior views. (Reprinted and recolored with permission from Kula et al.[33])

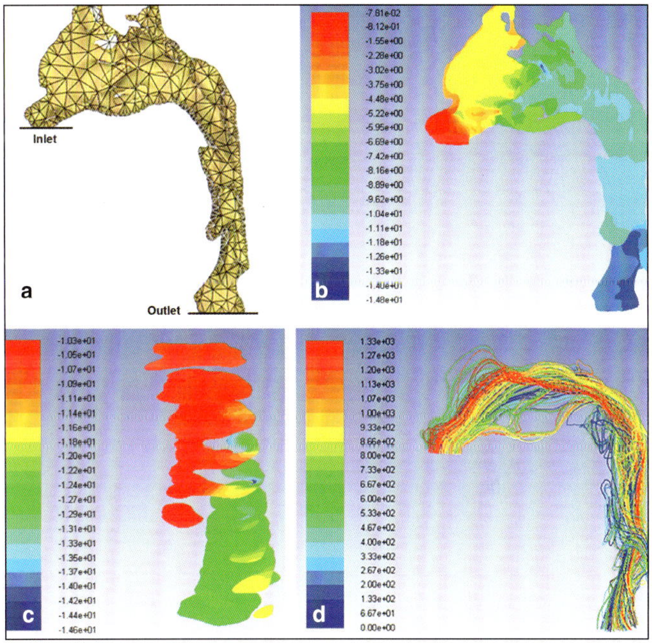

Fig 8-20 *(a)* Finite element model of upper airway structures. *(b)* Fluid dynamic analysis shows the pressure distribution of airflow along the upper airway structures. *(c)* Pressure of airflow at the cross sections of airway structures. *(d)* Stream lines of the laminar flow.

3D models of the airway can be constructed and viewed from all angles using the software (Fig 8-19), but they are influenced by the sensitivity of the settings. In other words, the shape of the model is influenced by soft tissue and fluids in the surrounding area.[33]

Computational fluid dynamics

Computational fluid dynamics (CFD) is a technique using finite element analysis to simulate the internal flow dynamics of the upper airway. This technique evaluates the airflow in the nasal, nasopharyngeal, and oropharyngeal areas using airway models developed from the patient's 3D CBCT or CT scan (Fig 8-20). CFD also provides accurate simulation of the magnitudes of air pressure and velocity and is thus considered an appropriate assessment tool for the evaluation of airway function. Studies using CFD confirmed that in children with OSA, the pharyngeal airway pressure during inspiration decreases with the reduction of nasal resistance by rapid maxillary expansion.[34–36]

Conclusion

Dental clinicians and especially orthodontists have long been interested in airway analysis because of the potential importance to normal development of the craniofacial region as well as their involvement in diagnosing and treating mouth breathing and sleep disorders. It is important for clinicians to evaluate the upper airway objectively and identify the normal and abnormal anatomical boundaries and dimensions. Although 2D lateral cephalograms have been used for decades to evaluate airway shape, size, position, and relations with other anatomical structures, they lack the information to illustrate the anatomically complex airway structure in three dimensions. Lateral cephalograms could be used as an initial screening method to evaluate the airway, but 3D CBCT images provide a more reliable and comprehensive tool for airway assessment and volumetric measurements. Findings of snoring and interrupted sleep together with diagnostic images taken during the dental examination can give indications of possible airway disorders and support the need for referrals to a medical specialist. Sleep medicine physicians can provide comprehensive examinations to definitively diagnose sleep-disordered breathing problems.

References

1. Pierce RJ, Worsnop CJ. Upper airway function and dysfunction in respiration. Clin Exp Pharmacol Physiol 1999;26:1–10.
2. Solow B, Siersbaek-Nielsen S, Greve E. Airway adequacy, head posture, and craniofacial morphology. Am J Orthod 1984;86:214–223.
3. McNamara J. Influence of respiratory pattern on craniofacial growth. Angle Orthod 1981;51:269–300.
4. Ricketts RM. Respiratory obstruction syndrome. Am J Orthod 1968;54:495–507.
5. Wenzel A, Höjensgaard E, Henriksen J. Craniofacial morphology and head posture in children with asthma and perennial rhinitis. Eur J Orthod 1985;7:83–92.
6. Grauer D, Cevidanes LS, Styner MA, Ackerman JL, Proffit WR. Pharyngeal airway volume and shape from cone-beam computed tomography: Relationship to facial morphology. Am J Orthod Dentofacial Orthop 2009;136:805–814.
7. Kerr WJ. The nasopharynx, face height, and overbite. Angle Orthod 1985;55:31–36.
8. Quick CA, Gundlach KK. Adenoid facies. Laryngoscope 1978;88:327–333.
9. Schulhof RJ. Consideration of airway in orthodontics. J Clin Orthod 1978;12:440–444.
10. Ghoneima A, Bodkin C, Stewart K, Perlow MJ, Starbuck J, Kula K. Mandibular advancement appliance effects on obstructive sleep apnoea: A prospective three-dimensional computed tomography study. Australas Orthod J 2017;33:114–123.
11. Aboudara C, Nielsen I, Huang JC, Maki K, Miller AJ, Hatcher D. Comparison of airway space with conventional lateral headfilms and 3-dimensional reconstruction from cone-beam computed tomography. Am J Orthod Dentofacial Orthop 2009;135:468–479.
12. Arens R, McDonough JM, Costarino AT, et al. Magnetic resonance imaging of the upper airway structure of children with obstructive sleep apnea syndrome. Am J Respir Crit Care Med 2001;164:698–703.
13. Guttal KS, Burde KN. Cephalometric evaluation of upper airway in healthy adult population: A preliminary study. J Oral Maxillofac Radiol 2013;1:55–60.
14. Armstrong JJ, Leigh MS, Sampson DD, Walsh JH, Hillman DR, Eastwood PR. Quantitative upper airway imaging with anatomic optical coherence tomography. Am J Respir Crit Care Med 2006;173:226–233.
15. Guijarro-Martinez R, Swennen GR. Cone-beam computerized tomography imaging and analysis of the upper airway: A systematic review of the literature. Int J Oral Maxillofac Surg 2011;40:1227–1237.
16. Major MP, Flores-Mir C, Major PW. Assessment of lateral cephalometric diagnosis of adenoid hypertrophy and posterior upper airway obstruction: A systematic review. Am J Orthod Dentofacial Orthop 2006;130:700–708.
17. Susarla SM, Abramson ZR, Dodson TB, Kaban LB. Cephalometric measurement of upper airway length correlates with the presence and severity of obstructive sleep apnea. J Oral Maxillofac Surg 2010;68:2846–2855.
18. Baumrind S, Frantz RC. The reliability of head film measurements. 1. Landmark identification. Am J Orthod 1971;60:111–127.
19. Baumrind S, Frantz RC. The reliability of head film measurements: 2. Conventional angular and linear measures. Am J Orthod 1971;60:505–517.
20. Brown AA, Scarfe WC, Scheetz JP, Silveira AM, Farman AG. Linear accuracy of cone beam CT derived 3D images. Angle Orthod 2009;79:150–157.
21. Stratemann S, Huang JC, Maki K, Hatcher D, Miller AJ. Three-dimensional analysis of the airway with cone-beam computed tomography. Am J Orthod Dentofacial Orthop 2011;140:607–615.
22. Hatcher DC. Cone beam computed tomography: Craniofacial and airway analysis. Dent Clin North Am 2012;56:343–357.
23. McNamara JA Jr. A method of cephalometric evaluation. Am J Orthod 1984;86:449–469.
24. Wenzel A, Williams S, Ritzau M. Relationships of changes in craniofacial morphology, head posture, and nasopharyngeal airway size following mandibular osteotomy. Am J Orthod Dentofacial Orthop 1989;96:138–143.
25. Moorrees CF. Natural head position. In: Jacobson A, Caufield PW (ed). Introduction to Radiographic Cephalometry. Philadelphia: Lea & Febiger, 1985:84–89.
26. Lundström F, Lundström A. Natural head position as a basis for cephalometric analysis. Am J Orthod Dentofacial Orthop 1992;101:244–247.
27. Tso HH, Lee JS, Huang JC, Maki K, Hatcher D, Miller AJ. Evaluation of the human airway using cone-beam computerized tomography. Oral Surg Oral Med Oral Pathol Oral Radiol Endod 2009;108:768–776.
28. Schendel SA, Hatcher D. Automated 3-dimensional airway analysis from cone-beam computed tomography data. J Oral Maxillofac Surg 2010;68:696–701.
29. El H, Palomo JM. Measuring the airway in 3 dimensions: A reliability and accuracy study. Am J Orthod Dentofacial Orthop 2010;137(4, suppl):S50.e1–S50.e9.
30. Lenza MG, Lenza MD, Dalstra M, Melsen B, Cattaneo PM. An analysis of different approaches to the assessment of upper airway morphology: A CBCT study. Orthod Craniofac Res 2010;13:96–105.
31. Ghoneima A, Kula K. Accuracy and reliability of cone-beam computed tomography for airway volume analysis. Eur J Orthod 2011;35:256–261.
32. Glupker L, Kula K, Parks E, Babler W, Stewart K, Ghoneima A. Three-dimensional computed tomography analysis of airway volume changes between open and closed jaw positions. Am J Orthod Dentofacial Orthop 2015;147:426–434.
33. Kula K, Hale LN, Ghoneima A, Tholpady S, Starbuck JM. Cone-beam computed tomography analysis of mucosal thickening in unilateral cleft lip and palate maxillary sinuses. Cleft Palate Craniofac J 2016;53:640–648.
34. Mylavarapu G, Murugappan S, Mihaescu M, Kalra M, Khosla S, Gutmark E. Validation of computational fluid dynamics methodology used for human upper airway flow simulations. J Biomech 2009;42:1553–1559.
35. Iwasaki T, Saitoh I, Takemoto Y, et al. Improvement of nasal airway ventilation after rapid maxillary expansion evaluated with computational fluid dynamics. Am J Orthod Dentofacial Orthop 2012;141:269–278.
36. Ghoneima A, AlBarakati S, Jiang F, Kula K, Wasfy T. Computational fluid dynamics analysis of the upper airway after rapid maxillary expansion: A case report. Prog Orthod 2015;16:10.

9

Radiographic Superimposition: From 2D to 3D

Mohamed Bazina, BDS, MSD
Juan Martin Palomo, DDS, MSD

One of the most difficult challenges in orthodontics is to discern between normal craniofacial growth and treatment effects and to evaluate treatment outcome. Superimposition of two-dimensional (2D) lateral cephalograms has been the standard in quantification of growth and treatment outcome in orthodontics for decades. Superimposing serial cephalograms has taught us about craniofacial growth and development as well as the treatment effects produced by various orthodontic, orthopedic, and surgical procedures.

For a superimposition to be accurate, it needs to be based on areas that have not changed between time points. This includes changes due to growth or treatment. The superimposition of serial cephalograms on metallic implants is considered the most precise and reliable technique to monitor growth and adaptation in the craniofacial region.[1] Implant studies, the most famous being the ones from Björk,[2,3] have provided the basic information on craniofacial growth in humans.

Traditionally, a superimposition analysis includes an overall assessment to evaluate maxillary growth and overall facial and profile changes, as well as two regional assessments, one to evaluate maxillary dental changes and another to evaluate mandibular dental changes and mandibular growth.

Cranial Base Superimposition

Anatomically speaking, the cranial base consists of three regions: anterior, middle, and posterior cranial base. The anterior cranial base is composed of the frontal (which includes nasion), ethmoid, sphenoid, and sella turcica (which includes sella) regions. The cranial base is initially formed in cartilage (endochondral ossification), with ossification centers appearing early in embryonic life; with time, the cartilage is progressively replaced with bone. However, some cartilaginous growth centers called *synchondroses* remain active between ossified

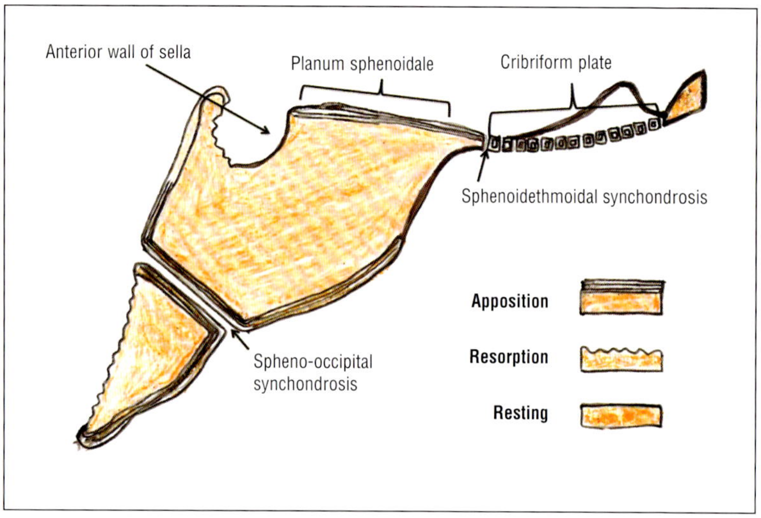

Fig 9-1 Diagram showing the midsagittal anatomy of the cranial base and its stability.

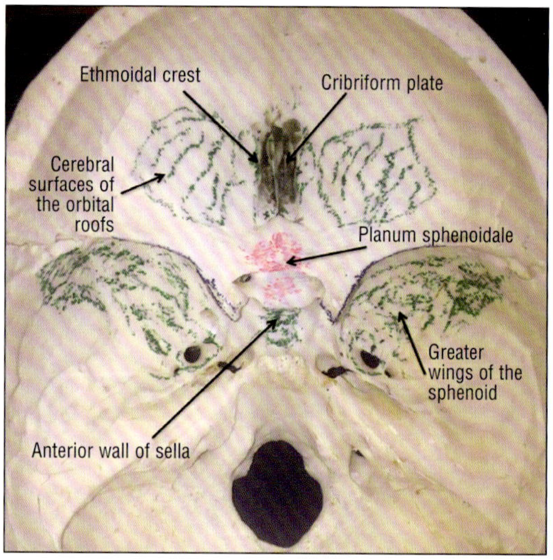

Fig 9-2 Superior view of a dry skull showing areas of the cranial base with different degrees of stability. The areas in green are stable after age 7 years. The area in pink has minimal growth after age 6 years and shows no growth after age 14 years.

areas and mature at different times of life. The anterior cranial base is considered to have completed its most significant growth before other facial skeletal structures.

Melsen found the internal surface of the frontal bone and cribriform plate to be stable after the age of 6 to 7 years in both sagittal and vertical planes, with the anterior part of sella turcica being by far the most stable structure after the age of 5 years.[4] Arat et al found that basion was the most variable landmark (0% stability) followed by nasion (16% stability) in both horizontal and vertical directions due to spheno-occipital synchondrosis and frontal sinus development.[5] Based on the studies evaluated by Afrand et al in their systematic review, the sphenoid and ethmoid regions reach their full development potential before the usual orthodontic age, more specifically by age 7 years for the sphenoid and age 4 years for the ethmoid regions. Nasion moves forward due to an increase in size of the frontal sinus, whereas sella turcica moves backward.[6]

In conclusion, the anterior cranial base has long been considered a stable craniofacial area, suitable to be used for cephalometric superimposition during the usual orthodontic treatment age range (Figs 9-1 and 9-2). Clinicians and researchers have recommended various methods to superimpose the cranial base.

Methods for 2D cranial base superimposition

Broadbent's 1931 introduction of the cephalometer (cephalostat) created a standardized method for taking radiographs, allowing the creation of growth collections, time point and interpatient comparisons, and superimpositions. Broadbent introduced the use of the Bolton-nasion line with registration at point R as a stable reference for superimposition. Point R is the midpoint on a line that is perpendicular from sella to the Bolton-nasion plane (Fig 9-3). The Bolton landmark was primarily used because Broadbent's radiographs did not show porion and the condyle area due to hardware blockage. He based his method on observations of dry skulls and a comparative study of cranial base planes (Bolton-nasion, porion-nasion, sella-nasion) in persons 3 to 18 years of age.[7]

In 1953, Steiner used the sella-nasion line with the registration point at sella to evaluate sagittal changes in mandibular positions and the registration point at nasion to evaluate the position of the maxilla[8] (see Fig 9-3). This was a landmark article for cephalometrics, making it popular and easy to use.

In 1951, Björk started using small, inert metallic implants as radiographic markers in the jaws of a small number of children to study craniofacial growth and development. Shortly after, he published results of a study of 110 Danish schoolchildren of both sexes.[2,3] For the cranial base superimposition of the lateral cephalograms, he concluded that the most stable areas were *(1)* the contours of the anterior wall of sella turcica, *(2)* the anterior contours of the median cranial fossa, *(3)* the intersection of the anterior contour of sella and tuberculum sellae, *(4)* the inner surface of the frontal bone, *(5)* the contours of the cribriform plate, *(6)* the contours of the bilateral frontoethmoidal crests, and *(7)* the contour of the median border of the cerebral surfaces of the orbital roofs (see Figs 9-1 and 9-2). Björk's structural superimposition is considered the gold standard because it has high validity and moderate to high reproducibility.[9] However, it requires high-quality radiographs, time, and effort.

Ricketts advocated the use of the basion-nasion plane for cranial base superimposition (see Fig 9-3). He suggested that the cranial base angle exhibits a change of 5 degrees in either

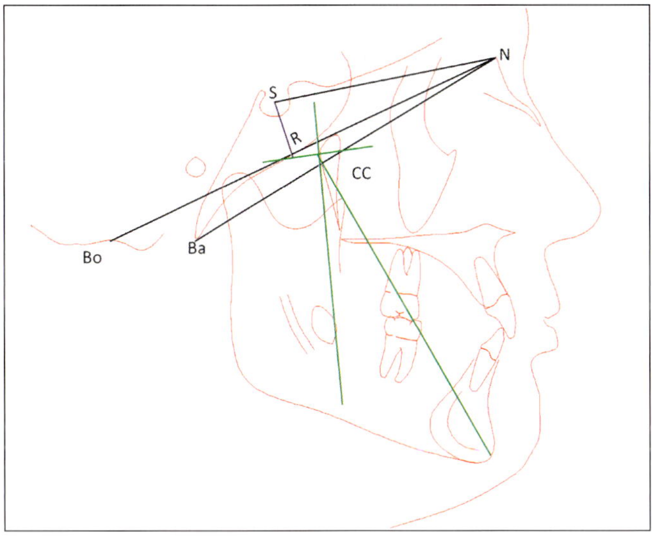

Fig 9-3 Different 2D cranial base superimposition methods. Broadbent recommended the use of the Bolton-nasion (BoN) line with registration point R, Steiner used the sella-nasion (SN) line, and Ricketts used the basion-nasion (BaN) line and point CC as a center for registration.

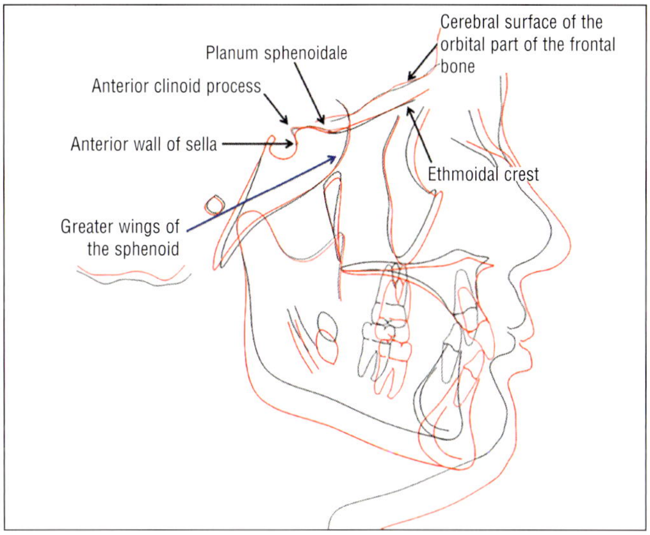

Fig 9-4 2D cranial base superimposition using the reference areas recommended by the ABO: the anterior wall of sella, the anterior clinoid process, planum sphenoidale, the ethmoidal crest, the cerebral surface of the orbital part of the frontal bone, and the greater wings of the sphenoid.

direction over a 3-year period, so he recommended that the use of basion instead of sella helps take into account some of the extremes in divergent growth conditions.[10,11] The reliability of this line is doubtful because of the variability of the growth at nasion, the remodeling at the anterior part of the foramen magnum, and the growth in the spheno-occipital synchondrosis, which affects basion.

Many studies have compared the different superimposition methods. In 1976, Baumrind, Miller, and Molthen compared the superimposition on sella-nasion (SN), registered at sella, with the best-fit superimposition and concluded that rotational errors were somewhat smaller in the best-fit method than with the SN superimposition.[12] Conversely, in 1984, Pancherz and Hansen found the effect of the registration error of the SN method to be less than that of the best-fit method.[13] In 1987, Ghafari et al compared four different superimposition methods and concluded that the best-fit method may be better than the others because it takes into account the detailed individual anatomy of the cranial base, rather than simplifying this anatomy into lines or planes that may change during growth.[14]

In 2003, Arat et al used the superimposition methods of Björk, Steiner, and Ricketts to evaluate the direction and degree of displacement of reference landmarks on the cranial base and face. The landmarks used as references showed significant changes (sella, nasion, basion, pterygomaxillare), indicating that differences in superimposition method should be considered when analyzing changes as a result of treatment.[15]

The American Board of Orthodontics (ABO) has a complete protocol for assessing discrepancy and treatment outcomes, including a superimposition assessment. As reference structures for cranial base superimposition, the ABO recommends the use of the anterior wall of sella, its intersection with the inferior portion of the anterior clinoid process, planum sphenoidale, the greater wings of the sphenoid, the cribriform plate, the ethmoidal crest, and the cerebral surface of the orbital part of the frontal bone[16] (Fig 9-4).

Accuracy of 2D superimposition

2D radiography has been extensively used in orthodontics. However, orthodontics and dentofacial orthopedic problems involve all three dimensions. 2D images are subject to geometric, rotational, and head-positioning errors that can lead to the area of interest being altered.[17]

2D cephalometric analysis also has other limitations with respect to accuracy and reliability. The error involved in landmark identification is indisputably the most important. Landmarks that are placed on anatomically formed edges or corners are easy to identify, whereas those that are placed on curves with wide radii show proportionally greater errors of measurement.[18,19] Houston et al stated that the greatest contribution to the error variance is from the tracings.[20] Researchers who have studied the accuracy of landmark identification have concluded that every attempt to digitize the same landmark, even on the same cephalogram, will result in a different position.[21] The Frankfort horizontal (FH) plane and SN plane are standard for most superimposition methods.[2,8] However, these planes are difficult to construct on 2D cephalometric images, and the error may be magnified depending on facial structure. Several studies have evaluated the accuracies of different superimposition methods and have found that superimposition methods using the SN and FH planes were not accurate and had poor reproducibility.[13,14–23]

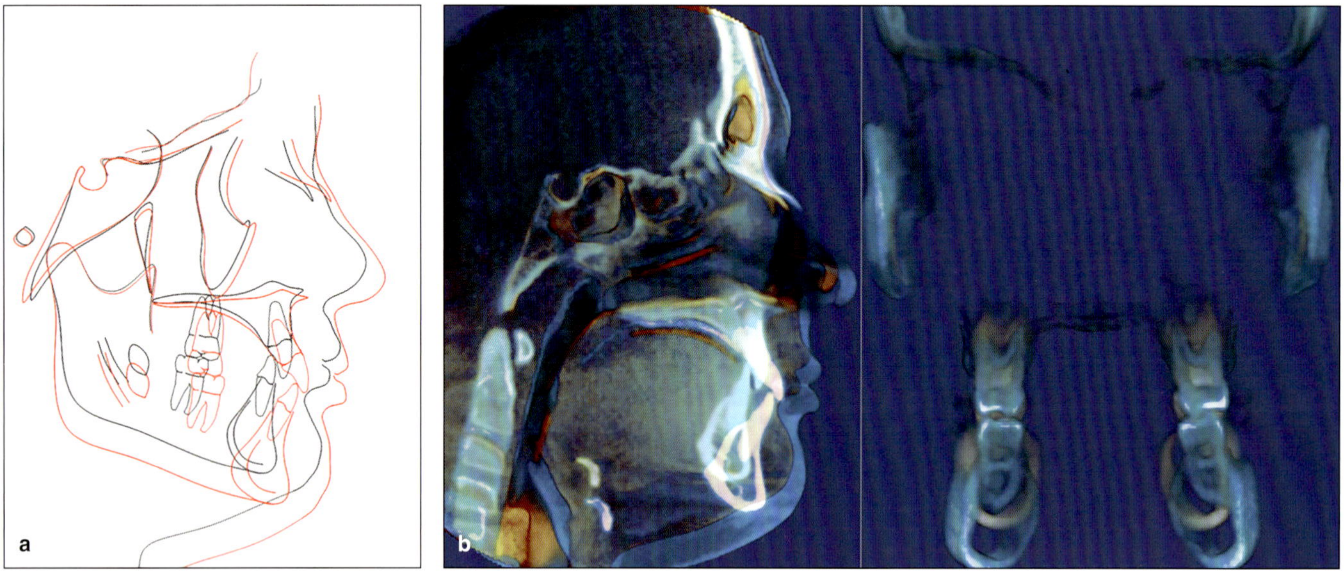

Fig 9-5 2D *(a)* and 3D *(b)* cranial base superimposition of a treated growing patient showing growth and treatment effects.

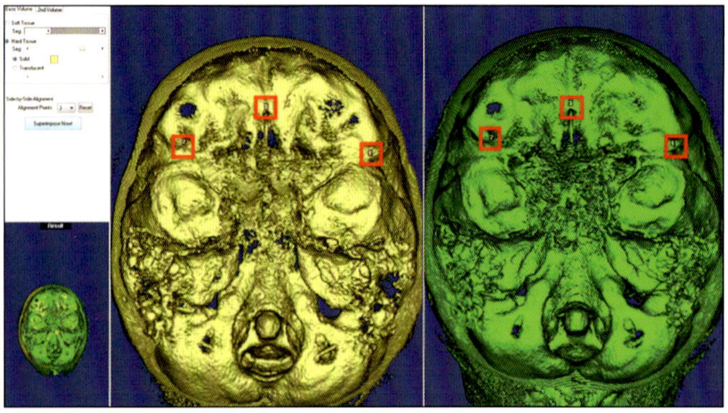

Fig 9-6 Landmark-based superimposition using cranial base reference points (Dolphin Imaging software, Patterson Dental).

Methods for 3D cranial base superimposition

The use of cone beam computed tomography (CBCT) in dentistry, introduced in the late 1990s, has increased dramatically over the last decade. CBCT images increase the clinician's confidence in orthodontic diagnosis and treatment planning and have shown clinical efficacy in several clinical situations.[24–26] When Heymann et al used three-dimensional (3D) superimposition to evaluate the changes after maxillary protraction using miniplates, they concluded that 3D data from CBCT allowed a more comprehensive evaluation of treatment changes.[27]

Based on the information obtained from 2D cephalometry regarding the stable areas for superimposition, different methods have been used for the superimposition (registration) of 3D images (Fig 9-5). These include landmark-based superimposition, surface-based superimposition, and voxel-based superimposition. The accuracy of the first two methods depends on the accuracy of landmark identification and the quality of the surface models. Voxel-based superimposition was developed to avoid operator error.

Landmark superimposition is similar to 2D lateral cephalometric superimposition, and it is the initial method used for 3D superimposition (Fig 9-6). The locations of landmarks in 2D radiographs are somewhat easily identified with a small envelope of error, but that is not the case in the curved surfaces of 3D images. Analysis of 3D images is much more complex than analysis of 2D cephalometric radiographs.[28–30]

Surface-based superimposition is another method to superimpose 3D images. Surface-based superimposition deals with the shell covering the 3D structure, and it requires high-quality surface models in order to get accurate results (Fig 9-7). Ong et al used 3D surface models to quantify and visualize the immediate changes of the midface following rapid maxillary expansion. They concluded that the use of 3D surface models allows quantification and visualization of the 3D changes in the midfacial skeleton at anatomical sites distant to the rapid maxillary expander activation.[30,31] Gkantidis et al evaluated five superimposition techniques using surface models (3P, three-point registration; AC, anterior cranial base; AC+F, anterior cranial base + foramen magnum; BZ, both zygomatic arches; and 1Z, one zygomatic arch). They found that the AC+F technique was the most accurate, followed by AC and BZ superimpositions. BZ superimposition has the additional advantage of being applicable in smaller–field-of-view (FOV) scans, which require less radiation dose and cost. 3P and 1Z were the least accurate superimpositions. Gkantidis et al concluded that superimposition of 3D images using surface models can provide accurate, precise, and reproducible results.[32]

In 2005, a new method for superimposition known as *voxel-based superimposition* was introduced to the medical research field by Cevidanes et al.[28] It has been widely used

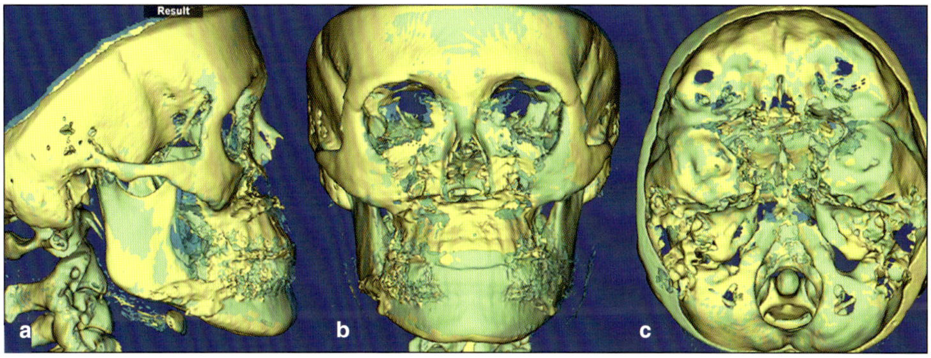

Fig 9-7 Dolphin 3D surface-based superimposition using the cranial base as reference structures. The patient underwent Le Fort I maxillary advancement with asymmetric mandibular setback. The *light blue* represents the presurgical scan, and the *yellow* represents the postsurgical scan. *(a)* Side view. *(b)* Frontal view. *(c)* Superior view.

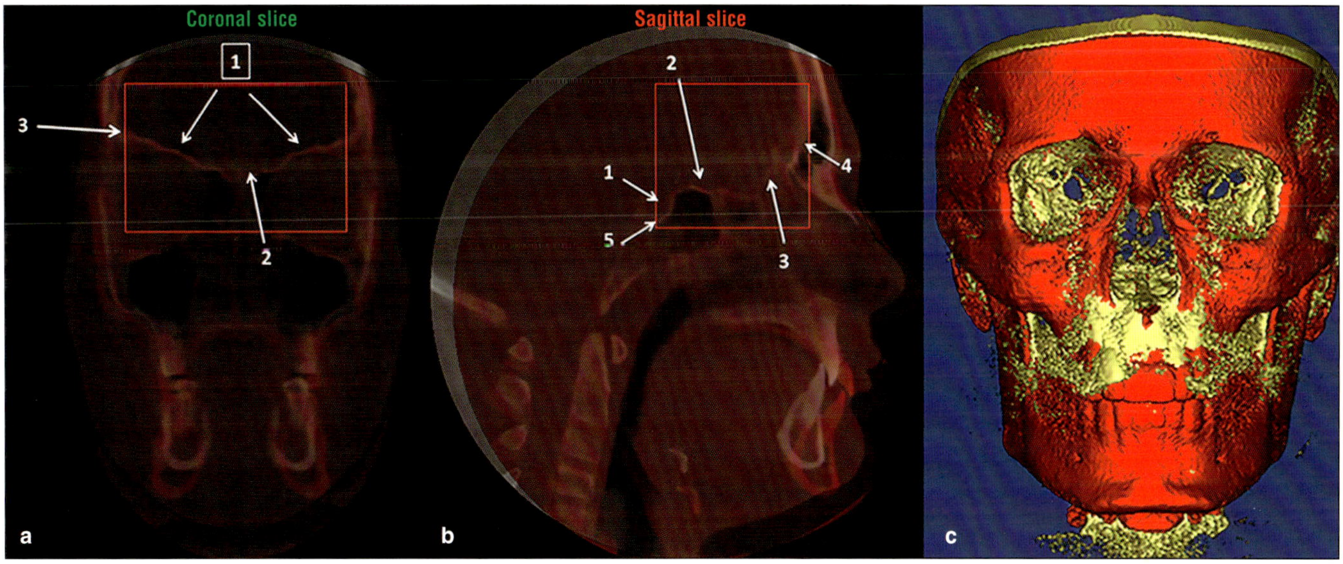

Fig 9-8 Dolphin 3D voxel-based superimposition on the cranial base (growing patient). The *red box* is used to define, in three dimensions, the area of the cranial base to be used as a reference for the superimposition. *(a)* Coronal slice showing the areas of registration included in the red box: *(1)* the cerebral surfaces of the orbital roofs and *(2)* the cribriform plate. *(3)* The lateral limit of the red box stops before it meets the vertical cortices. *(b)* Sagittal slice showing the areas of registration included in the red box: *(1)* the anterior wall of sella turcica, *(2)* planum sphenoidale, *(3)* the cribriform plate, and *(4)* the inner cortex of the frontal sinus. *(5)* The inferior limit of the box is defined by the inferior wall of sella turcica. *(c)* The 3D rendering of the superimposed images. *Yellow* is the initial image, while *red* is the final image.

for various medical applications and research purposes. Voxel-based superimposition utilizes the grayscale of the voxels to align the two DICOM (Digital Imaging and Communications in Medicine) images to the best superimposition, indicated by the least total grayscale density difference between the two images (Fig 9-8). Voxel-based superimposition uses the intensities throughout the entire selected volume, therefore using the image content as the basis of the registration. This method is useful where it is difficult to detect distinct surface topography features, which are the basis for surface-based superimposition. Voxel-based registration can be classified into two main types: rigid and nonrigid. Rigid registration uses translation and rotation tools to register the two images, while nonrigid registration uses translation, rotation, scale, and affine properties, which might lead to some image deformation. Rigid registration is used in dentistry because it maintains the 3D image dimensions, a requirement for quantitative purposes.[28,33–35]

Whereas voxel-based registration uses the raw information of the 3D image to compare the grayscale intensity of the voxels, surface-based registration requires an extra step involving 3D model rendering to generate a 3D surface model. This step may introduce a possible source of error because the algorithm used for segmenting the 3D model depends on the grayscale value of the DICOM images. This extra step also increases processing time. Surface-based registration therefore demonstrates a higher variability in superimposition than does voxel-based registration. For hard tissue superimposition, surface-based registration is as accurate and consistent as voxel-based registration, but voxel-based registration produces a more accurate representation of the soft tissue changes compared with surface-based registration.[36] The voxel-based superimposition method developed by Cevidanes uses two different open-source programs[37] and is time-consuming, so it cannot be used in the clinical setting. However, a few commercially available imaging software programs (Dolphin Imaging [Patterson Dental], Invivo [Anatomage], and OnDemand3D [Cybermed]) recently developed fast, user-friendly algorithms that allow clinicians to use this method in orthodontic practice to evaluate their patients.

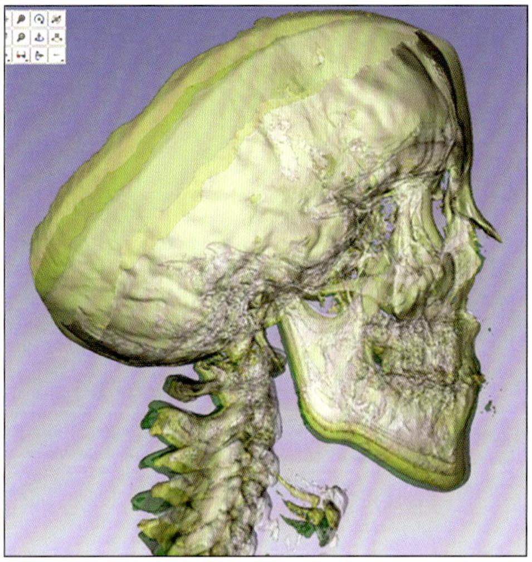

Fig 9-9 Registered 3D surface models of a patient with a repaired unilateral cleft lip and palate showing growth and treatment effects.

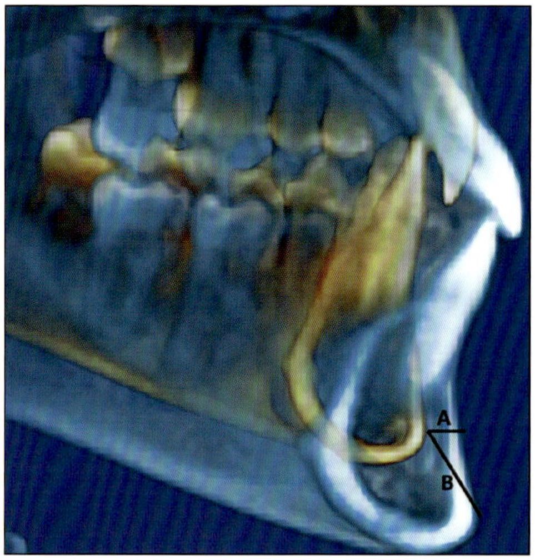

Fig 9-10 Semitransparent 3D models of a growing patient superimposed on the cranial base. A, the line representing the closest-points measurement between the two surfaces that can be achieved by a closest-points algorithm. B, the line representing the correspondent-points measurement that can be achieved by a correspondent-points algorithm.

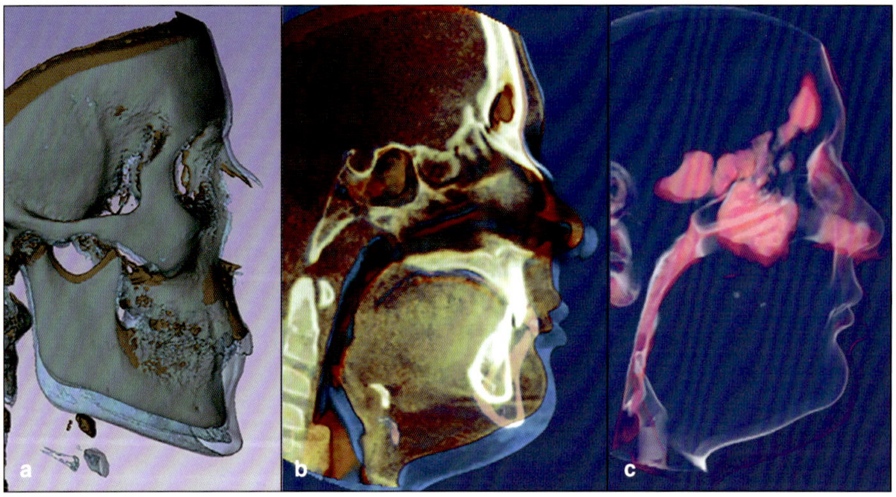

Fig 9-11 Visual evaluation of 3D superimposition of a growing patient. *(a)* 3D rendering of semitransparent superimposed models. *(b)* Midsagittal slice of semitransparent 3D images showing both soft tissue and hard tissue changes. *(c)* Semitransparent 3D models of the soft tissues and airways.

Once the images from different time points are registered, they share the same coordinate system. The idea of using registered images in the dental research field is new. It facilitates the longitudinal evaluation of changes, because all the registered 3D images have the same spatial location as that of the initial image. The registration techniques allow the comparison of different time points directly from the overlay of 3D surface models (Fig 9-9).

Quantification of change in 3D images

There are three ways to quantify changes in 3D models:

1. The use of linear and angular measurements that apply the same concepts used routinely in 2D cephalometry to 3D images.
2. The use of closest-points algorithms that analyze the smallest displacements between two surface files but do not take into account the shape change. These algorithms measure the distance between surface landmarks (eg, from pogonion on the first image to the closest point on the second image) (Fig 9-10).
3. The use of shape correspondence in which researchers can correlate the displacement of the same landmarks from two or more time points and through color-coded maps and vectors depict the magnitude direction of the movement. The main challenges of shape correspondence involve the representation of a population (see Fig 9-10).

Because landmark-based measurements present errors related to landmark identification and the visual evaluation of superimpositions requires professional experience and can present some subjectivity (Fig 9-11), Gerig et al proposed the use

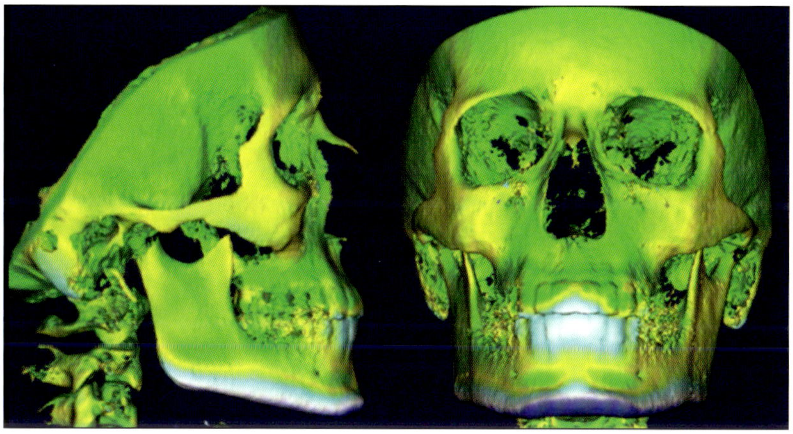

Fig 9-12 Closest-points color maps of the initial and final 3D images of a treated patient showing growth and treatment effects: *yellow*, 2-mm difference; *light blue*, 4 mm; *white*, 6 mm; *dark blue*, 8 mm

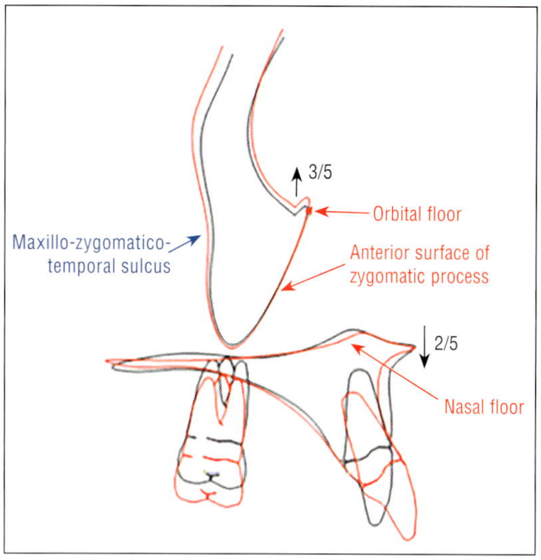

Fig 9-13 2D maxillary regional superimposition using the reference areas recommended by the ABO: the anterior surface of the zygomatic process, the maxillo-zygomaticotemporal sulcus, the orbital floor, and the nasal floor.

of color maps from surface models.[38] The color maps indicate the amount and direction of the displacement between overlaid structures (Fig 9-12).

Accuracy of 3D superimposition

Errors in 3D superimposition techniques are not significant enough to question their application in clinical practice. The mean accuracy of superimposition techniques for 3D data sets varies slightly among different studies. Cevidanes et al evaluated the superimposition of CBCT images of growing patients and reported that the range of interobserver errors for each anatomical region was 0.4 mm for the zygomatic process of the maxilla, chin, condyles, posterior border of the rami, and inferior border of the mandible and 0.5 mm for the anterior maxilla, soft tissue, and upper lip. They concluded that this method is a valid and reproducible assessment of treatment outcomes for growing subjects.[35] In 2012, using an image fusion method to superimpose CT images of human dry skulls with different spatial conditions, Lee et al reported an error of 0.396 mm, which was not affected by positional change.[39] Nada et al in 2011 tested the reliability of another commercial voxel-based method using Maxilim software (Medicim) for CBCT superimposition on the anterior cranial base and zygomatic arch of 16 surgical orthodontic patients. The authors reported a small average of superimposition errors.[40] Weissheimer et al recently evaluated a fast method of 3D voxel-based superimposition using OnDemand3D software. They concluded that the mean superimposition error was less than 0.5 mm in growing and nongrowing patients.[41] Bazina et al evaluated the precision and reliability of the Dolphin 3D voxel-based superimposition method, a user-friendly method that can be used in the clinical setting, and concluded that it is accurate and reliable.[42]

Regional Superimposition

Maxillary superimposition

Several studies have attempted to understand the complex mechanism of maxillary growth and remodeling. Serial cephalometric radiographs have been used to understand facial growth and to determine the stable areas of reference to evaluate maxillary changes during growth. Superimposition on stable maxillary structures can be used to evaluate growth and treatment effects in the maxillary dentoalveolar complex. Multiple maxillary registration methods have been proposed in the literature.[43–46] McNamara proposed the use of the best fit of the internal palatal structures for maxillary superimposition.[43] However, the metallic implants method reported by Björk and Björk and Skieller still remain the gold standard.[44,45] The ABO recommends the use of the anterior surface of the zygomatic process as a primary anteroposterior (AP) structure and the maxillo-zygomaticotemporal sulcus as a secondary AP structure for registration (Fig 9-13). Vertically, the use of the orbital floor and the nasal floor is recommended (the ratio is 3/5 apposition at the floor of the orbit and 2/5 resorption at the floor of the nose).[16]

As discussed earlier, 3D superimposition offers many advantages over 2D superimposition, including larger volumes or areas of registration rather than lines or points, which improves the reliability of the registration and results in less distortion and fewer head-positioning errors. 3D superimposition also allows the clinician to evaluate structures that were previously obstructed on lateral cephalograms as well as unilateral or asymmetric changes due to growth or treatment. However, anatomical structures reported to be stable on a lateral cephalogram may not be reliable for 3D analysis, which involves the

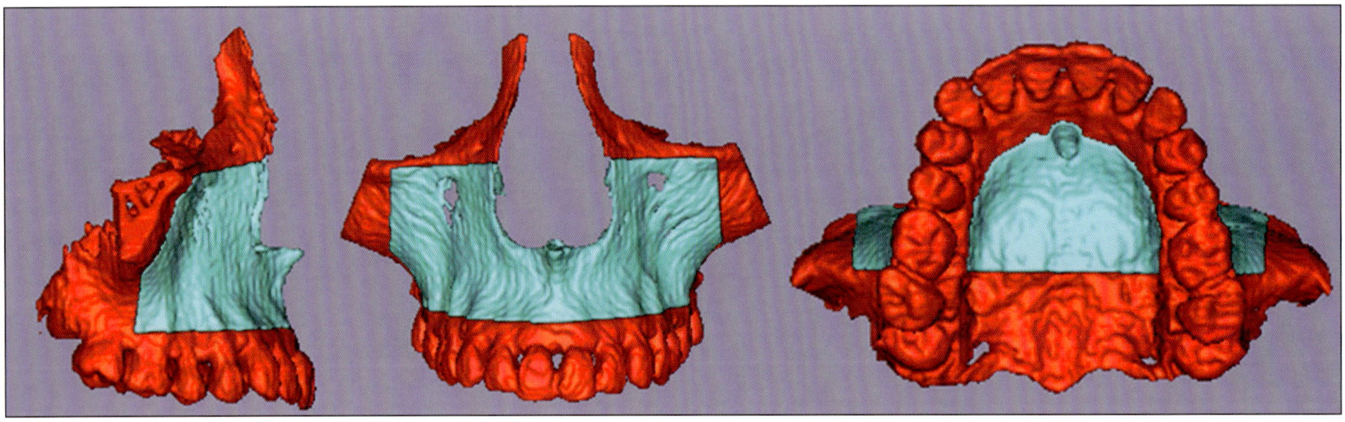

Fig 9-14 3D model of a maxilla showing the region of reference *(blue)* used for maxillary voxel-based registrations as recommended by Ruellas et al.[47] (Courtesy of Dr Antonio Carlos de Oliveira Ruellas, Rio de Janeiro, Brazil.)

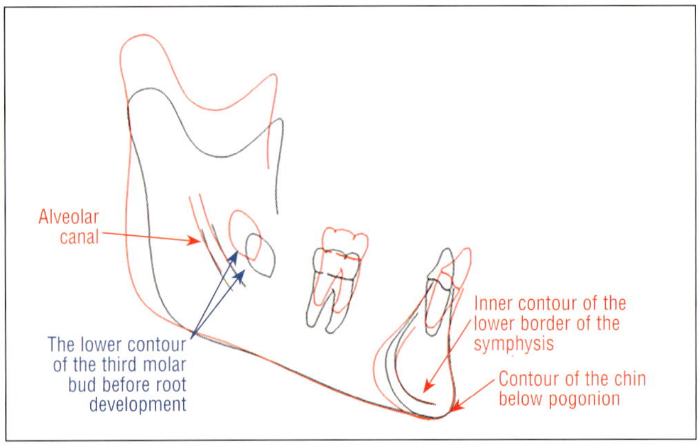

Fig 9-15 2D mandibular regional superimposition using the reference areas recommended by the ABO: the inner contour of the inferior border of the symphysis, the contour of the chin below pogonion, the inferior alveolar canal, and the lower contour of the third molar bud before root development.

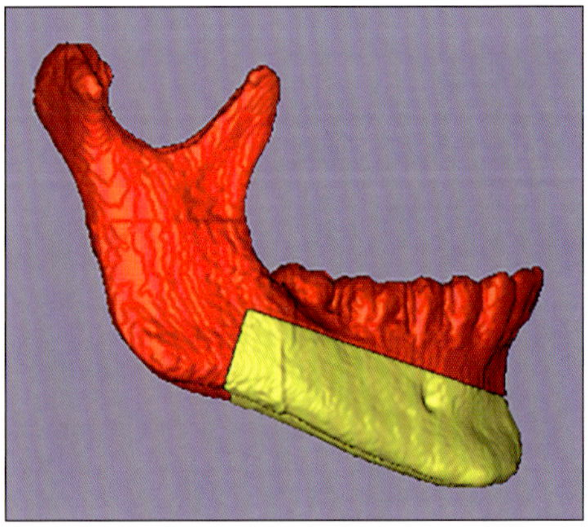

Fig 9-16 3D model of a mandible showing the region of reference *(yellow)* used for mandibular voxel-based registrations as recommended by Ruellas et al.[47] (Courtesy of Dr Antonio Carlos de Oliveira Ruellas, Rio de Janeiro, Brazil.)

transverse dimension. Recently, Ruellas et al described two regions of reference for 3D voxel-based maxillary registration and found that both are very similar with adequate reproducibility[47] (Fig 9-14).

Mandibular superimposition

Similar to maxillary superimposition, the superimposition on stable mandibular structures can be used to evaluate mandibular growth and treatment changes. The structural method of superimposition in 2D cephalometrics was based on the following stable structures of the mandible: *(1)* the anterosuperior contour of the chin, *(2)* the inner cortical structure of the inferior border of the mandibular symphysis, *(3)* the trabecular structure in the symphysis, *(4)* the contour of the mandibular canal, and *(5)* the lower contour of the developing third molar tooth germ before root development begins.[48,49] The ABO recommends the use of the contour of the chin just below pogonion, the inner contour of the cortical plate of the symphysis, and the inferior alveolar canal as primary structures and the lower contour of the third molar bud before root development as a secondary structure[16] (Fig 9-15).

Similar to maxillary superimposition, anatomical structures reported to be stable on 2D radiographs for regional superimpositions may not be reliable for 3D analysis, which involves the transverse dimension.[50] Although 3D studies have supported the fact that the symphysis and the mandibular canals are stable in the sagittal view, as reported by Björk and Skieller, the mandibular canals relocate laterally during growth.[51] Thus, the accuracy and reliability of regions of reference are still controversial for 3D image superimposition.

Ruellas et al tested three different regions for voxel-based registration of the mandible (Björk, modified Björk, and mandibular body mask). They found that the Björk region of reference (or mask) worked properly in only 2 of 16 patients and that the mandibular body mask displayed more consistent results. They concluded that the mandibular body mask (mandible without teeth, alveolar bone, rami, and condyles) is a reliable reference for 3D regional voxel-based registration[52] (Fig 9-16). However, the regional voxel-based superimposition methods

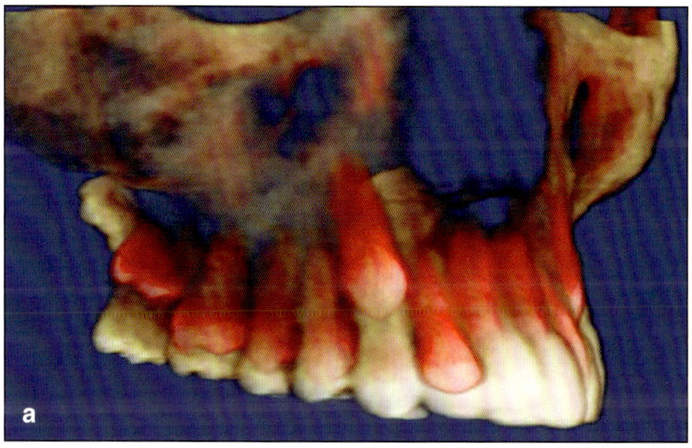

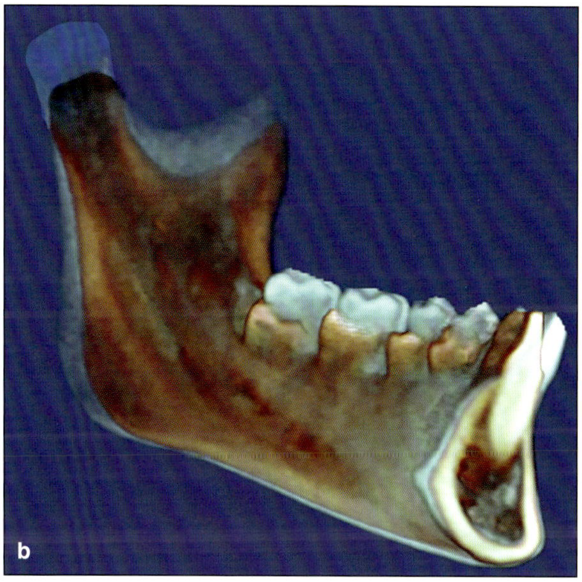

Fig 9-17 *(a)* Semitransparent 3D models after maxillary voxel-based superimposition showing the amount of dental changes due to orthodontic treatment. *Red* is before treatment, and *brown* is after. *(b)* Midsagittal slice of semitransparent 3D models of a growing patient after 3D mandibular voxel-based superimposition showing the amount of mandibular growth and the dental changes due to orthodontic treatment. *Brown* is before treatment, and *blue* is after.

developed by Ruellas et al use different open-source programs and are time-consuming and are therefore not clinically useful.

Some commercially available imaging software programs (Dolphin Imaging, Invivo, and OnDemand3D) recently developed fast and user-friendly algorithms that allow clinicians to do regional superimpositions to evaluate the dental changes in their patients (Fig 9-17). These algorithms still need to be tested for accuracy and reliability.

Conclusion

Outcome assessment is essential for continual improvement and quality control. Radiographic superimposition can provide valuable information regarding growth and development and treatment effects. Most of the anatomical knowledge we have comes from Björk's implant studies, but after a long period of little change in how we do superimposition, a new era of 3D superimposition using millions of points, computerized accuracy, and color-map objective assessment is now available for everyday use.

References

1. Sarnat BG. Growth pattern of the mandible: Some reflections. Am J Orthod Dentofacial Orthop 1986;90:221–233.
2. Björk A. Cranial base development: A follow-up x-ray study of the individual variation in growth occurring between the ages of 12 and 20 years and its relation to brain case and face development. Int J Orthod Dent Chil 1955;41:198–225.
3. Björk A. The use of metallic implants in the study of facial growth in children: Method and application. Am J Phys Anthropol 1968;29:243–254.
4. Melsen B. The cranial base: The postnatal development of the cranial base studied histologically on human autopsy material. Acta Odontol Scand 1974;32(suppl 62):1–126.
5. Arat ZM, Türkkahraman H, English JD, Gallerano RL, Boley JC. Longitudinal growth changes of the cranial base from puberty to adulthood: A comparison of different superimposition methods. Angle Orthod 2010;80:537–544.
6. Afrand M, Ling CP, Khosrotehrani S, Flores-Mir C, Lagravère-Vich MO. Anterior cranial-base time-related changes: A systematic review. Am J Orthod Dentofacial Orthop 2014;146:21–32.
7. Broadbent BH. Measurement of dentofacial changes in relation to the cranium. In: Dewey M, Anderson GM (eds). Practical Orthodontia, ed 5. St Louis: Mosby, 1935:184–204.
8. Steiner CC. Cephalometrics for you and me. Am J Orthod Dentofacial Orthop 1953;39:729–755.
9. Athanasiou AE. Orthodontic Cephalometry. London: Mosby-Wolfe, 1995.
10. Ricketts RM. A foundation for cephalometric communication. Am J Orthod Dentofacial Orthop 1960;46:330–357.
11. Ricketts RM, Bench RW, Gugino CF, Hilgers JJ, Schulhof RJ. Bioprogressive Therapy. Denver: Rocky Mountain Orthodontics, 1979.
12. Baumrind S, Miller D, Molthen R. The reliability of head film measurements: 3. Tracing superimposition. Int J Orthod Dent Chil 1976;70:617–644.
13. Pancherz H, Hansen K. The nasion-sella reference line in cephalometry: A methodology study. Int J Orthod Dent Chil 1984;86:427–434.
14. Ghafari J, Engel FE, Laster LL. Cephalometric superimposition on the cranial base: A review and a comparison of four methods. Am J Orthod Dentofacial Orthop 1987;91:403–413.
15. Arat ZM, Rübendüz M, Akgül AA. The displacement of craniofacial landmarks during puberty: A comparison of three superimposition methods. Angle Orthod 2003;73:374–380.
16. American Board of Orthodontics website. https://www.americanboardortho.com. Accessed 18 May 2017.
17. Harrell WE Jr, Hatcher DC, Bolt RL. In search of anatomic truth: 3-dimensional digital modeling and the future of orthodontics. Am J Orthod Dentofacial Orthop 2002;122:325–330.

18. Baumrind S, Frantz RC. The reliability of head film measurements: 1. Landmark identification. Int J Orthod Dent Chil 1971;60:111–127.
19. Baumrind S, Frantz RC. The reliability of head film measurements: 2. Conventional angular and linear measures. Int J Orthod Dent Chil 1971;60:505–517.
20. Houston WJ, Maher RE, McElroy D, Sherriff M. Sources of error in measurements from cephalometric radiographs. Eur J Orthod 1986;8:149–151.
21. Hägg U, Cooke MS, Chan TC, Tng TT, Lau PY. The reproducibility of cephalometric landmarks: An experimental study on skulls. Aust Orthod J 1998;15:177–185.
22. Gliddon MJ, Xia JJ, Gateno J, et al. The accuracy of cephalometric tracing surperimposition. J Oral Maxillofac Surg 2006;64:194–202.
23. Cooke MS, Wei SH. Cephalometric errors: A comparison between repeat measurements and retaken radiographs. Aust Dent J 1991;36:38–43.
24. Bjerklin K, Ericson S. How a computerized tomography examination changed the treatment plans of 80 children with retained and ectopically positioned maxillary canines. Angle Orthod 2006;76:43–51.
25. Haney E, Gansky SA, Lee JS, et al. Comparative analysis of traditional radiographs and cone-beam computed tomography volumetric images in the diagnosis and treatment planning of maxillary impacted canines. Am J Orthod Dentofacial Orthop 2010;137:590–597.
26. Hodges RJ, Atchison KA, White SC. Impact of cone-beam computed tomography on orthodontic diagnosis and treatment planning. Am J Orthod Dentofacial Orthop 2013;143:665–674.
27. Heymann GC, Cevidanes L, Cornelis M, De Clerck HJ, Tulloch JFC. Three-dimensional analysis of maxillary protraction with intermaxillary elastics to miniplates. Am J Orthod Dentofacial Orthop 2010;137:274–284.
28. Cevidanes LH, Bailey LJ, Tucker GR Jr, et al. Superimposition of 3D cone-beam CT models of orthognathic surgery patients. Dentomaxillofac Radiol 2005;34:369–375.
29. Bookstein F, Schäfer K, Prossinger H, et al. Comparing frontal cranial profiles in archaic and modern homo by morphometric analysis. Anat Rec 1999;257:217–224.
30. Bookstein FL. Morphometric Tools for Landmark Data. Cambridge: Cambridge University, 1991.
31. Ong SC, Khambay BS, McDonald JP, Cross DL, Brocklebank LM, Ju X. The novel use of three-dimensional surface models to quantify and visualize the immediate changes of the mid-facial skeleton following rapid maxillary expansion. Surgeon 2015;13:132–138.
32. Gkantidis N, Schauseil M, Pazera P, Zorkun B, Katsaros C, Ludwig B. Evaluation of 3-dimensional superimposition techniques on various skeletal structures of the head using surface models. PLoS One 2015;10(2):e0118810.
33. Cevidanes LH, Motta A, Proffit WR, Ackerman JL, Styner MA. Cranial base superimposition for 3-dimensional evaluation of soft-tissue changes. Am J Orthod Dentofacial Orthop 2010;137(4 suppl):120S–129S.
34. Cevidanes LH, Styner MA, Proffit WR. Image analysis and superimposition of 3-dimensional cone-beam computed tomography models. Am J Orthod Dentofacial Orthop 2006;129:611–618.
35. Cevidanes LH, Heymann G, Cornelis MA, De Clerck HJ, Tulloch JF. Superimposition of 3-dimensional cone-beam computed tomography models of growing patients. Am J Orthod Dentofacial Orthop 2009;136:94–99.
36. Almukhtar A, Ju X, Khambay B, McDonald J, Ayoub A. Comparison of the accuracy of voxel based registration and surface based registration for 3D assessment of surgical change following orthognathic surgery. PLoS One 2014;9(4):e93402.
37. DCBIA Videos YouTube channel. http://www.youtube.com/user/DCBIA. Accessed 18 September 2016.
38. Gerig G, Jomier M, Chakos M. Valmet: A new validation tool for assessing and improving 3D object segmentation. In: Niessen WJ, Viergever MA (eds). Medical Image Computing and Computer-Assisted Intervention—MICCAI 2001 [Proceedings of the 4th International MICCAI Conference, 14–17 Oct 2001 Utrecht]. Berlin: Springer, 2001:516–528.
39. Lee JH, Kim MJ, Kim SM, Kwon OH, Kim YK. The 3D CT superimposition method using image fusion based on the maximum mutual information algorithm for the assessment of oral and maxillofacial surgery treatment results. Oral Surg Oral Med Oral Pathol Oral Radiol 2012;114:167–174.
40. Nada RM, Maal TJ, Breuning KH, Bergé SJ, Mostafa YA, Kuijpers-Jagtman AM. Accuracy and reproducibility of voxel based superimposition of cone beam computed tomography models on the anterior cranial base and the zygomatic arches. PLoS One 2011;6(2):e16520.
41. Weissheimer A, Menezes LM, Koerich L, Pham J, Cevidanes LH. Fast three-dimensional superimposition of cone beam computed tomography for orthopaedics and orthognathic surgery evaluation. Int J Oral Maxillofac Surg 2015;44:1188–1196.
42. Bazina M, Cevidanes L, Ruellas A, et al. Precision and reliability of Dolphin 3-dimensional voxel-based superimposition. Am J Orthod Dentofacial Orthop 2018;153:599–606.
43. McNamara JA. Influence of respiratory pattern on craniofacial growth. Angle Orthod 1981;51:269–300.
44. Björk A, Skieller V. Growth of the maxilla in three dimensions as revealed radiographically by the implant method. Br J Orthod 1977;4:53–64.
45. Björk A. Sutural growth of the upper face studied by the implant method. Acta Odontol Scand 1966;24:109–127.
46. Nielsen IL. Maxillary superimposition: A comparison of three methods for cephalometric evaluation of growth and treatment change. Am J Orthod Dentofacial Orthop 1989;95:422–431.
47. Ruellas A, Ghislanzoni LT, Gomes M, et al. Comparison and reproducibility of 2 regions of reference for maxillary regional registration with cone-beam computed tomography. Am J Orthod Dentofacial Orthop 2016;149:533–542.
48. Björk A. Prediction of mandibular growth rotation. Int J Orthod Dent Chil 1969;55:585–599.
49. Björk A, Skieller V. Normal and abnormal growth of the mandible: A synthesis of longitudinal cephalometric implant studies over a period of 25 years. Eur J Orthod 1983;5:1–46.
50. Kim I, Oliveira ME, Duncan WJ, Cioffi I, Farella M. 3D assessment of mandibular growth based on image registration: A feasibility study in a rabbit model. Biomed Res Int 2014;2014:276128.
51. Krarup S, Darvann TA, Larsen P, Marsh JL, Kreiborg S. Three-dimensional analysis of mandibular growth and tooth eruption. J Anat 2005;207:669–682.
52. Ruellas A, Yatabe M, Souki B, et al. 3D mandibular superimposition: Comparison of regions of reference for voxel-based registration. PLoS One 2016 23;11(6):e0157625.

10

Growth and Treatment Predictions: Accuracy and Reliability

Achint Utreja, BDS, MS, PhD

The specialty of orthodontics has benefited immensely from the invention of the roentgenographic cephalometer by Dr B. Holly Broadbent.[1] Since its inclusion in mainstream orthodontics, the profession has made great strides, with both clinicians and researchers utilizing cephalometry to elevate the overall level of care provided to patients. The two areas that have received significant attention during the past few decades are *(1)* predicting patterns of craniofacial growth in growing patients and *(2)* forecasting the outcome of orthodontic treatment. The relatively recent adoption by the profession of three-dimensional (3D) imaging techniques, including cone beam computed tomography (CBCT) and facial imaging, have further bolstered efforts to provide the clinician with an opportunity to gaze into the future. However, the accuracy and reliability of most growth and treatment predictions is still open to debate. How close are we to developing and marketing the "orthodontic crystal ball"? This chapter focuses on the evolution and current trends related to forecasting craniofacial growth and orthodontic treatment outcomes.

Craniofacial Growth Studies

The acceptance of cephalometric radiology led to its use in a number of longitudinal studies measuring craniofacial growth over many years. The primary objective of all studies was to identify and analyze craniofacial growth trends in the population. Recently, the American Association of Orthodontists Foundation has done an excellent job of making the data from growth studies available online (http://www.aaoflegacycollection.org/aaof_home.html). Records from 9 out of the 11 documented craniofacial growth studies, collected by researchers over a time span of more than 75 years, are freely available for viewing. The invaluable data collected from these longitudinal growth studies provided a better understanding of craniofacial growth, led to the development of various growth theories, and provided an early method of predicting growth. Additionally, this information has been used over the years as baseline data for later studies.[2]

Table 10-1 **Fishman's skeletal maturity indicators**

	Bone	Stage of maturation
1	Third finger—proximal phalanx	Width of epiphysis equal to diaphysis
2	Third finger—middle phalanx	
3	Fifth finger—middle phalanx	
4	Adductor sesamoid of thumb	Ossification
5	Third finger—distal phalanx	Capping of epiphysis
6	Third finger—middle phalanx	
7	Fifth finger—middle phalanx	
8	Third finger—distal phalanx	Fusion of epiphysis and diaphysis
9	Third finger—proximal phalanx	
10	Third finger—middle phalanx	
11	Radius	

Evolution of Growth-Prediction Methods

Heredity and genetics

Growth and development of the craniofacial structures are interrelated processes influenced by heredity as well as the external environment.[3] Certain traits including the shape and size of the jaws in an individual are predetermined and inherited from both the mother and father. Aberrant craniofacial growth in the young patient who presents for orthodontic treatment usually manifests as a skeletal discrepancy involving the maxilla and/or mandible. The dental malocclusion is often exacerbated by the underlying problem in the skeletal base(s). In such cases, growth predictions are critical as they form the basis of successful treatment outcomes.[4,5]

Initial information regarding the potential for "favorable" growth during and after orthodontic treatment can be obtained by observing both parents when they bring the child to the orthodontist. Because frequently seen problems in the anteroposterior, transverse, and vertical dimensions can have an underlying familial tendency, the observant clinician should note the facial outline of both parents in an effort to ascertain the growth potential of the patient in the dental chair. Identification in either the mother or father of an orthodontic problem similar to that of the child is a strong indicator of future growth potential.[6] This information, combined with the data obtained from cephalometric analyses, can be beneficial during treatment planning to predict the relative stability of various treatment modalities.[7]

Skeletal maturity and the adolescent growth spurt

Prior to the elaborate craniofacial growth studies involving hundreds of subjects, Count Philibert Guéneau de Montbeillard performed one of the first longitudinal studies on his son.[8] He measured his son's height every 6 months from 1759 (at birth) until 1777 (age 18 years) and noticed an accelerated period of growth between 13 and 15 years of age. This adolescent or pubertal growth spurt is the ideal period for orthodontists to attempt growth modification in patients with skeletal Class II or Class III malocclusions because the patient's inherent growth potential can be fully utilized. Tracking changes in height can provide some information regarding skeletal growth; however, peak height velocity is not a good predictor of residual growth in a growing child. As there is significant interindividual variation regarding the initiation and duration of this growth spurt, different methods to estimate the stage of maturation of a growing child have been proposed over the years.

Indicators of skeletal maturity provide the most reliable estimate of elapsed and remaining craniofacial growth potential. However, they do not provide the amount of growth. Over the years, orthodontists have evaluated skeletal maturation at these areas:

- *Frontal sinus:* The morphology of the frontal sinus briefly received attention as an indicator of growth. The greatest advantage was easy visualization of the structure on lateral cephalometric radiographs without exposing patients to additional radiation. Sinus enlargement due to growth was correlated to peak height velocity.[9,10] However, as the onset of the growth spurt is about 2 years before peak height velocity in both girls and boys,[11] this growth estimation technique has limited application in clinical practice.
- *Hand-wrist radiographs:* The ossification sequence of bones in the hand-wrist area is a good predictor of skeletal maturity. Although interindividual variations in the initiation and duration of skeletal growth are seen, the overall sequence of growth correlates well with ossification of bones in the hand and wrist. Greulich and Pyle[12] published an atlas comprised of hand-wrist radiographs taken at 6-month intervals of chronologic age. An orthodontist can compare each bone in a patient's hand-wrist radiograph with corresponding bones in the atlas and estimate the skeletal age. Tanner et al[13] used a different comparison method and assigned weighted scores to individual bones based on data compiled from age- and sex-matched individuals. Besides using averages based on population studies, specific indicators in hand-wrist radiographs can be used to relate skeletal maturation to pubertal growth. Bowden[14] proposed using individual bones including the radius, ulna, carpals, metacarpals, and phalanges to determine the growth curve. Leonard Fishman[15,16] based his analysis on the evaluation of 11 discrete skeletal maturational indicators during adolescent development (Table 10-1). This maturational analysis evaluates in numerical order four ossi-

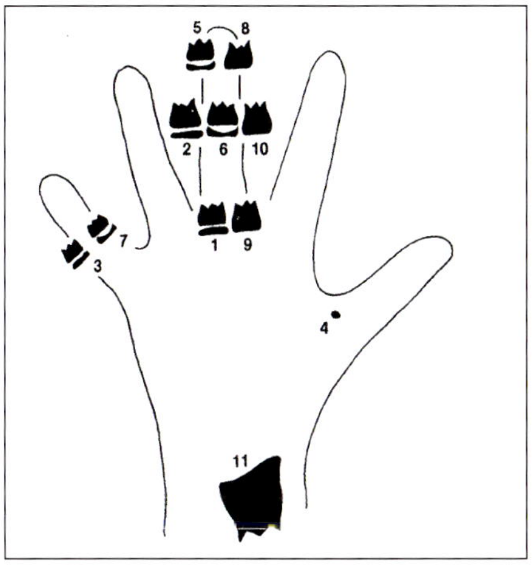

Fig 10-1 Sites of Fishman's 11 skeletal maturity indicators. (Reprinted from Fishman[15] with permission.)

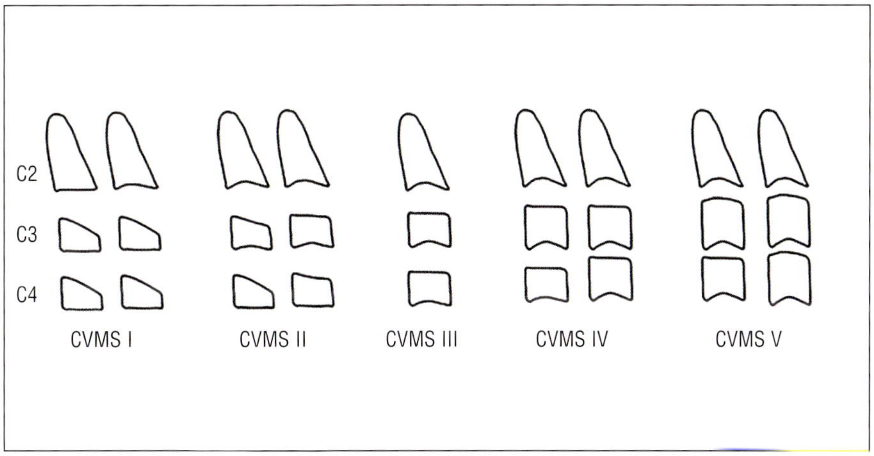

Fig 10-2 The updated CVM method showing representative morphologic changes in the bodies of C2, C3, and C4. CVMS, cervical vertebral maturation stage.

fication stages at six anatomical sites located on the thumb, third finger, fifth finger, and radius (Fig 10-1). He also suggested a quick method of evaluating the ossification stages. Once the sesamoid bone in the thumb (#4) is visible, then the fusion of the distal phalanx of the third finger can be evaluated. If fusion has occurred, then evaluation proceeds to the ninth step of fusion of the proximal phalanx of the third finger.

- *Cervical vertebral maturation:* The greatest advantage of using cervical vertebrae to assess skeletal maturation is the ease with which they can be visualized on lateral cephalometric radiographs. The ventral surfaces of the cervical vertebrae show visual changes in mineralization and growth, changing from flat to concave in a dorsal-ventral order. The second vertebra changes first, followed by the third and then the fourth. While this is occurring, the anterior portion of the vertebra lengthens, changing shape from trapezoid to square. Then both sides of the vertebra lengthen and the ventral surfaces become more concave (see Fig 10-2). Lamparski[17] found a strong correlation between skeletal age assessment based on cervical vertebrae and hand-wrist radiographs. Franchi et al[18] analyzed the validity of the six stages of cervical vertebral maturation (CVM) originally proposed by Lamparski and concluded that the method was useful to predict mandibular skeletal maturity. Subsequently, Baccetti et al[19] studied the morphologic changes in the second through fourth cervical vertebrae and provided an improved CVM staging method for detecting the peak in mandibular growth (Fig 10-2). Based on this method, the peak in mandibular growth of the average patient occurs between CVM stage II and stage III.

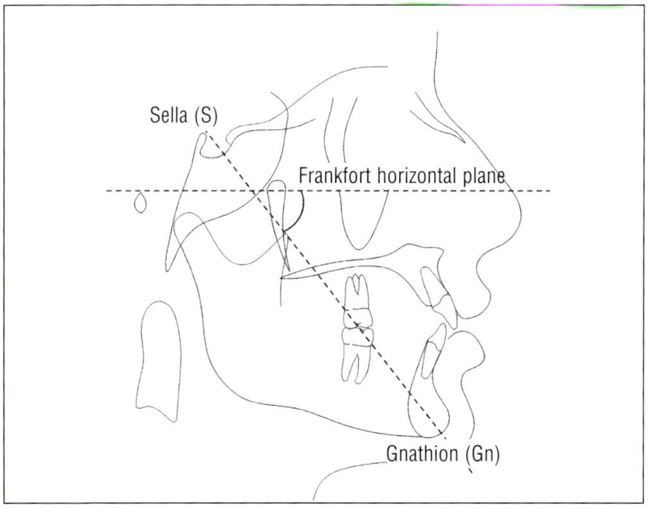

Fig 10-3 The y-axis or growth axis angle is formed at the intersection of the Frankfort horizontal plane and a line joining sella and gnathion.

y-axis

The growth axis or y-axis, a component of the Downs cephalometric analysis, was one of the first attempts at predicting the direction of mandibular growth, and it is still an integral component of various cephalometric analyses. William Downs studied the facial and dental patterns of his patients for 5 years to establish the measurements and norms for his analysis.[20] The tracing technique was subsequently standardized using templates that were placed directly over cephalometric radiographs.

The *y-axis* is defined as the angle between a line connecting sella and gnathion and the Frankfort horizontal plane (Fig 10-3). According to Downs, the mean value of the y-axis is 59 degrees, with a range of 53 to 66 degrees.[20] A large angle indicates vertical growth of the mandible and is common in skeletal Class II malocclusion cases. A small angle suggests horizontal mandibular growth as seen in Class III cases.

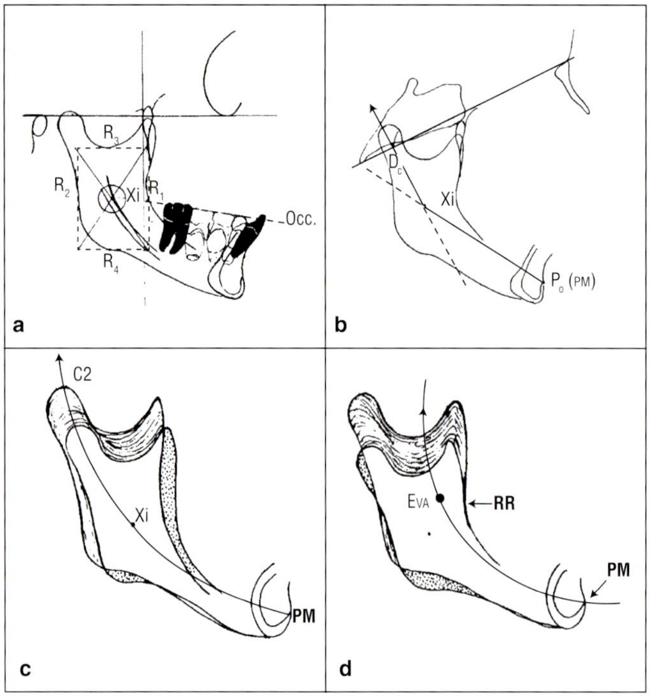

Fig 10-4 Ricketts's concept of arcial growth of the mandible: *(a)* location of Xi point; *(b)* condyle and body axes passing through Xi point; *(c and d)* arcs of mandibular growth. (Reprinted from Ricketts[21] with permission.)

Arcial growth of the mandible

Robert Ricketts was particularly interested in mandibular growth and believed that growth patterns could be predicted based on his research findings. The influx of new information through the work of investigators such as Björk and Moss led to renewed interest in analyzing craniofacial growth trends. Ricketts used radiographic laminography of the mandibular ramus, condyle, and fossa to study growth and enumerated both short- and long-term changes. His research suggested that the mandible grows along an arc (segment of a circle) by superior-anterior (vertical) apposition at the ramus.[21] Because the arcial growth pattern exhibits variation between individuals, he provided a detailed description of the steps involved in determining the radius of the circle comprising the growth arc.

Ricketts first located the center of the mandibular ramus by constructing a rectangle, the sides of which were comprised of tangents to the anterior (R1), posterior (R2), and lower (R3) ramal surfaces and the coronoid notch. Lines connected opposing corners of the rectangle. He called the intersection of the lines the *Xi point* and proposed that the occlusal plane usually passes through it (Fig 10-4a). He then constructed a condyle axis using Xi point as the intersection of the two rays, one bisecting the condyle neck (D_C) and the other forming the body axis passing through pogonion (PM) (Fig 10-4b). These constructed points were used to locate the true arc of mandibular growth (Fig 10-4c). He also added EVA point to the list of constructed landmarks and defined it as the point of concentration of stress lines in the ramus (Fig 10-4d). This method worked well for predicting short-term mandibular growth, although Arne Björk's implant studies showed that the mandibular border resorbed with growth, making it an unreliable landmark.[22]

Subsequently, a 5-year mandibular growth study analyzed lateral and frontal cephalometric radiographs from 40 patients.[21] The interval between the first and second radiographs was based on the development of the dentition. Results suggested that long-range growth forecasting was possible by considering that mandibular growth occurred along arcs passing through mandibular structures and derived cephalometric points. It was also demonstrated that the projected mandible could then be used to forecast the growth of other facial structures.[21] Based on these promising results, both the short- and long-range growth simulations form an essential component of the computerized orthodontic analysis offered by Rocky Mountain Orthodontics Data Services (RMODS) (https://www.rmortho.com/products-services/services/rmods/).

Greenberg and Johnston analyzed the prediction accuracy of RMODS over a 5-year period by comparing initial, final, and predicted lateral cephalogram tracings of random subjects from the Bolton Brush Growth Study Centre.[23] The results suggested that the prediction had limited value, as it was not able to accurately predict all the cephalometric variables that were tested. The additional expense was not justified because a forecasting grid could provide comparable information.

Cephalometric templates

Craniofacial growth is rather complex and varies considerably among individuals. Additionally, because structures comprising the craniofacial complex do not grow at uniform rates, the need for developing baseline standards representative of the growth of component parts was realized. This led to the development of various cephalometric templates and analyses based on these. The primary advantage of template analysis was easy visualization of the imbalance between craniofacial components. Predictions were anticipated to be more reliable because templates permitted comparison of an individual's growth against data interpolated from longitudinal growth studies.

As early as 1952, Baum developed four templates printed on transparencies that could be used with Downs cephalometric analysis.[24] The detailed description provided by the author on the use of this method was intended to encourage its use by orthodontists. Continuing the trend of establishing baseline criteria, Broadbent and Golden constructed templates derived from frontal and lateral cephalograms of 1- to 18-year-old children.[25] Similarly, Popovich and Thompson analyzed records of 120 boys and 90 girls from the Burlington Growth Centre cohort and established craniofacial templates according to the age, sex, and type of growth of an individual.[26] Moorrees developed the mesh diagram to predict growth and treatment changes, taking into account familial resemblance,[27] while Johnston introduced a forecast grid based on longitudinal data from 32 subjects in the Michigan Growth Study.[28] Growth changes in these subjects were measured in units (1 unit/year from 8 to

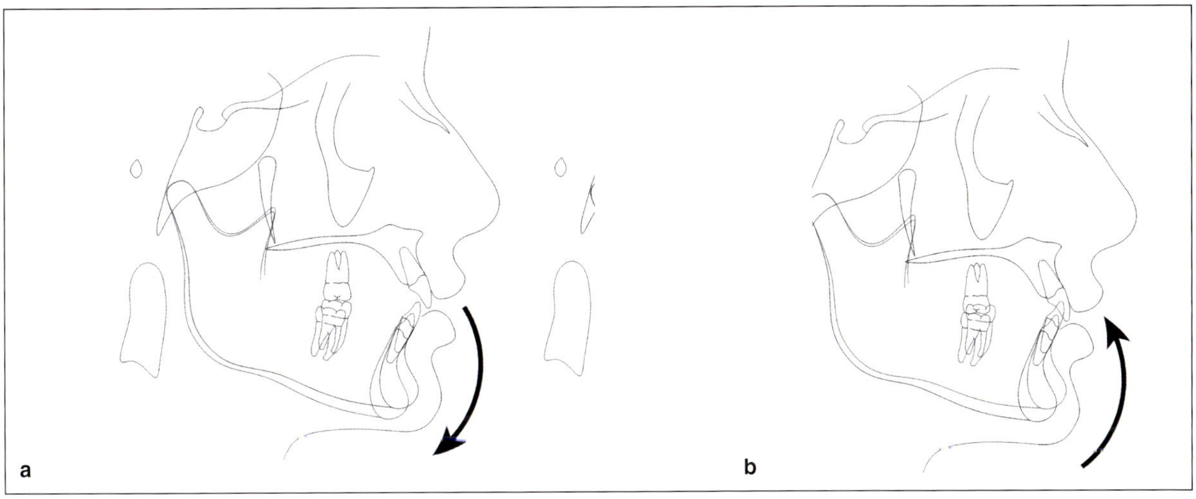

Fig 10-5 *(a)* Clockwise rotation of the mandible, resulting in an open bite. *(b)* Counterclockwise rotation of the mandible, resulting in a deep overbite.

Box 10-1 Seven structural indicators most predictive of significant mandibular rotation during growth according to Björk[30]

1. Inclination of the condylar head
2. Curvature of the mandibular canal
3. Shape of the inferior border of the mandible
4. Inclination of the symphysis
5. Interincisal angle
6. Interpremolar or intermolar angle
7. Lower anterior face height

13 years of age) at the tip of the nose, posterior nasal spine, maxillary first molar, nasion, and points A and B.

Ricketts's short- and long-range forecasting methods were compared with the Johnston forecast grid by Schulhof and Bagha.[29] The final positions of point A, pogonion, the tip of the nose, the mandibular molar, and the center of the ramus were predicted in 50 untreated study subjects from the Michigan Growth Study. Results showed that the Johnston grid was the least accurate growth-prediction method. Ricketts's short-range prediction performed better, with a 10% to 20% improvement over average growth increments related to facial type. The long-range forecast was 21% more accurate than the short-range forecast and 56% more accurate than the grid forecast.

In summary, although Ricketts's prediction method forms the basis of a commercially available service (RMODS), the overall utility of the short- and long-range forecasting methods based on evidence in the scientific literature is still debatable. Correlating the timing and direction of craniofacial growth can be challenging because it can depend on multiple variables.

Predicting rotation during mandibular growth

Simultaneous to the increasing interest in growth prediction in the United States, orthodontic researchers in Europe were equally aware of the individual variation in craniofacial growth and development. The various growth-prediction methods available at that time were categorized as either longitudinal, metric, or structural.[30] Under the category of structural methods, longitudinal data was gathered from landmark research that was performed using metallic implants as fixed references.[22,31–34] The implant studies provided significant insight into craniofacial growth, particularly maxillary and mandibular growth changes. Björk found that the mandible rotates during growth and that its overall shape is maintained by extensive surface remodeling. This rotation was produced by differential anteroposterior mandibular growth and could be in the forward or backward direction, leading to either a deep overbite or an open bite, respectively (Fig 10-5). Schudy used the terms *counterclockwise* and *clockwise* to describe these mandibular rotations.[35] These terms are relative to the American standard of facing the cephalometric profile to the right and not the European custom of facing the profile to the left.

Björk subsequently described seven structural signs that could help predict mandibular rotation during growth[30] (Box 10-1). A six-year evaluation of 44 morphologic variables in 21 subjects led to the identification of four variables that were most predictive of mandibular growth rotation in a growing child[36]: the mandibular inclination, the intermolar angle, the shape of the inferior border of the mandible, and the inclination of the symphysis. Mandibular inclination is a good representation of either forward or backward rotation during growth. The intermolar angle was increased in subjects with forward rotation of the mandible and decreased in cases with backward rotation. The inferior border of the mandible was convex in the anterior region in forward-rotators, whereas it was more straight or convex posteriorly in backward-rotators. The inclination of the symphysis relative to the anterior cranial base also formed a useful indicator of forward and backward growth rotation. The authors recommended early identification of these traits to accurately predict the direction of mandibular growth rotation.[36]

Predictions in skeletal Class II cases

Most clinicians would agree that reliable predictions of the effects of growth and orthodontic treatment could be particularly useful in growing Class II and Class III patients. Based on the research of Björk and Skieller,[22] mandibular growth rotations can be complex and rather challenging to manage clinically, particularly in individuals with a high mandibular plane angle. A retrospective study compared posttreatment lateral cephalograms from 33 high-angle Class II patients with computer-generated visual treatment objectives obtained from the Ricketts computerized growth-prediction system.[37] Comparison of 21 linear and 9 angular measurements showed that half of the computerized predictions were significantly different from the actual treatment values. Inaccuracies in predictions of maxillary length, mandibular rotation, and lower face height (anterior and posterior) were notable.[37]

Predictions of facial growth can be related to both chronologic and skeletal/maturational ages. Two commonly used systems are skeletal maturity indicators from hand-wrist radiographs and the CVM system. A study compared the Fishman maturational analysis (based on hand-wrist radiographs) to the Ricketts and Johnston forecasting methods using serial lateral cephalograms and hand-wrist radiographs of untreated subjects from the Burlington Growth Study.[38] The results suggested that the Fishman analysis was more accurate than the other methods in determining the amount of growth, as it was based on maturational age.

Developing statistical models for prediction

The use of statistical modeling to predict growth changes based on longitudinal data and computer algorithms is an interesting concept in orthodontics. Growth curves have long been plotted on graphs to provide an estimate of an individual's growth status. Chvatal et al[39] used this modified approach to develop complex models for longitudinal growth prediction that would also account for individual variations. Two angular and three linear measurements were selected to compare vertical skeletal changes on serial cephalometric radiographs from 159 girls and 128 boys between 6 and 15 years of age. Horizontal, vertical, and angular changes in the position of menton as well as the mandibular plane angle (measured at the intersection of the sella-nasion and gonion-menton lines) were used to generate the multilevel models. Correlations between actual and predicted values were reasonable, with a direct relation noted between accuracy and measurement change during the prediction period. The authors concluded that 5-year predictions based on the multilevel model were accurate.[39]

The Steiner cephalometric analysis was among the first to be developed for analyzing two-dimensional cephalometric radiographs.[40] The continued interest in growth and treatment prediction led to a study that analyzed the accuracy of Steiner's method by comparing actual and predicted values on posttreatment cephalograms.[41] Results suggested that the analysis was rather inaccurate when predicting treatment changes, probably due to underlying differences in the sample population.

Accuracy of visual treatment objective predictions

Skeletal Class III patients pose a challenge to the clinician, as growth, treatment timing, treatment options, and long-term stability of orthodontic/surgical correction require attention. The visual treatment objective (VTO) tool that is incorporated in most patient-management software offers a forecast of growth and treatment changes and can be useful in these cases. The accuracy of the VTO prediction system in a commonly used imaging software was recently evaluated.[42] This retrospective study examined the records of Class III patients who underwent maxillary advancement and mandibular setback orthognathic surgical procedures. The varying degrees of error for the measurements that were analyzed led the authors to the conclusion that the VTO tool is only useful for gross estimations of treatment outcome and for patient education. Small changes following orthognathic surgery could not be accurately predicted with the VTO software.[42]

3D prediction methods

The underlying principle of 3D imaging techniques is to provide clinicians with adequate information to predict hard tissue, soft tissue, and dental changes in three dimensions over time. As CBCT and stereophotogrammetry are ideally suited to analyze hard and soft tissues, respectively, fusion of these technologies is being explored to allow easy visualization and prediction of hard as well as soft tissue changes related to growth and treatment. Current attempts at combining the data from these two technologies have reported limited success, but the long-term applicability is still debatable.[43] Further research is required and is being conducted in this area.

Future Directions

The desire to foresee the outcome of orthodontic treatment well before the debonding appointment has fueled significant research in this area. Various methodologies developed over the years have been analyzed and compared. The future appears bright with the increasing use of the latest technologic advances such as computer simulations and 3D treatment-planning aids. Moving forward, more concerted efforts are needed to develop the elusive "orthodontic crystal ball" that will enable the clinician to accurately and reliably predict growth and treatment outcomes.

References

1. Broadbent BH. A new x-ray technique and its application to orthodontia. Angle Orthod 1931;1:45–66.
2. Thompson GW, Popovich F. A longitudinal evaluation of the Burlington growth centre data. J Dent Res 1977;56(special issue):C71–C78.
3. Moss ML. Genetics, epigenetics, and causation. Am J Orthod 1981;80:366–375.
4. Mossey PA. The heritability of malocclusion: Part 1—Genetics, principles and terminology. Br J Orthod 1999;26:103–113.
5. Mossey PA. The heritability of malocclusion: Part 2. The influence of genetics in malocclusion. Br J Orthod 1999;26:195–203.
6. Harris JE, Kowalski CJ. All in the family: Use of familial information in orthodontic diagnosis, case assessment, and treatment planning. Am J Orthod 1976;69:493–510.
7. Johannsdottir B, Thorarinsson F, Thordarson A, Magnusson TE. Heritability of craniofacial characteristics between parents and offspring estimated from lateral cephalograms. Am J Orthod Dentofacial Orthop 2005;127:200–207.
8. Hunter CJ. The correlation of facial growth with body height and skeletal maturation at adolescence. Angle Orthod 1966;36:44–54.
9. Ruf S, Pancherz H. Frontal sinus development as an indicator for somatic maturity at puberty? Am J Orthod Dentofacial Orthop 1996;110:476–482.
10. Ruf S, Pancherz H. Development of the frontal sinus in relation to somatic and skeletal maturity. A cephalometric roentgenographic study at puberty. Eur J Orthod 1996;18:491–497.
11. Taranger J, Hägg U. The timing and duration of adolescent growth. Acta Odontol Scand 1980;38:57–67.
12. Greulich WW, Pyle SI. Radiographic Atlas of Skeletal Development of the Hand and Wrist, ed 2. Redwood City, CA: Stanford University, 1959.
13. Tanner JM, Whitehouse RH, Cameron N, Marshall WA, Healy MJR, Goldstein H. Assessment of Skeletal Maturity and Prediction of Adult Height (TW2 Method). Cambridge, MA: Academic, 1983.
14. Bowden BD. Epiphysial changes in the hand/wrist area as indicators of adolescent stage. Aust Orthod J 1976;4:87–104.
15. Fishman LS. Radiographic evaluation of skeletal maturation. A clinically oriented method based on hand-wrist films. Angle Orthod 1982;52:88–112.
16. Fishman LS. Maturational patterns and prediction during adolescence. Angle Orthod 1987;57:178–193.
17. Lamparski DG. Skeletal age assessment utilizing cervical vertebrae. Am J Orthod Dentofacial Orthop 1975;67:458–459.
18. Franchi L, Baccetti T, McNamara JA Jr. Mandibular growth as related to cervical vertebral maturation and body height. Am J Orthod Dentofacial Orthop 2000;118:335–340.
19. Baccetti T, Franchi L, McNamara JA Jr. An improved version of the cervical vertebral maturation (CVM) method for the assessment of mandibular growth. Angle Orthod 2002;72:316–323.
20. Downs WB. Variations in facial relationships: Their significance in treatment and prognosis. Am J Orthod 1948;34:812–840.
21. Ricketts RM. A principle of arcial growth of the mandible. Angle Orthod 1972;42:368–386.
22. Björk A, Skieller V. Normal and abnormal growth of the mandible. A synthesis of longitudinal cephalometric implant studies over a period of 25 years. Eur J Orthod 1983;5:1–46.
23. Greenberg LZ, Johnston LE. Computerized prediction: The accuracy of a contemporary long-range forecast. Am J Orthod 1975;67:243–252.
24. Baum AT. Downs' analysis template transparencies for application directly to cephalometric x-ray films. Angle Orthod 1952;22:217–226.
25. Broadbent BH Sr, Broadbent BH Jr, Golden WH. Bolton Standards of Dentofacial Developmental Growth. St Louis: Mosby, 1975.
26. Popovich F, Thompson GW. Craniofacial templates for orthodontic case analysis. Am J Orthod 1977;71:406–420.
27. Moorrees CFA, Lebret L. The mesh diagram and cephalometrics. Angle Orthod 1962;32:214–231.
28. Johnston LE. A simplified approach to prediction. Am J Orthod 1975;67:253–257.
29. Schulhof RJ, Bagha L. A statistical evaluation of the Ricketts and Johnston growth-forecasting methods. Am J Orthod 1975;67:258–276.
30. Björk A. Prediction of mandibular growth rotation. Am J Orthod 1969;55:585–599.
31. Björk A, Skieller V. Facial development and tooth eruption: An implant study at the age of puberty. Am J Orthod 1972;62:339–383.
32. Björk A, Skieller V. Growth in width of the maxilla studied by the implant method. Scand J Plast Reconstr Surg 1974;8:26–33.
33. Björk A, Skieller V. Growth of the maxilla in three dimensions as revealed radiographically by the implant method. Br J Orthod 1977;4:53–64.
34. Björk A, Skieller V. Contrasting mandibular growth and facial development in long face syndrome, juvenile rheumatoid polyarthritis, and mandibulofacial dysostosis. J Craniofac Genet Dev Biol Suppl 1985;1:127–138.
35. Schudy FF. The rotation of the mandible resulting from growth: Its implications in orthodontic treatment. Angle Orthod 1965;35:36–50.
36. Skieller V, Björk A, Linde-Hansen T. Prediction of mandibular growth rotation evaluated from a longitudinal implant sample. Am J Orthod 1984;86:359–370.
37. Thames TL, Sinclair PM, Alexander RG. The accuracy of computerized growth prediction in Class II high-angle cases. Am J Orthod 1985;87:398–405.
38. Turchetta BJ, Fishman LS, Subtelny JD. Facial growth prediction: A comparison of methodologies. Am J Orthod Dentofacial Orthop 2007;132:439–449.
39. Chvatal BA, Behrents RG, Ceen RF, Buschang PH. Development and testing of multilevel models for longitudinal craniofacial growth prediction. Am J Orthod Dentofacial Orthop 2005;128:45–56.
40. Gottlieb EL. Orthodontics: Dr. Cecil Steiner. J Clin Orthod 1978;12:677.
41. Abdullah RT, Kuijpers MA, Bergé SJ, Katsaros C. Steiner cephalometric analysis: Predicted and actual treatment outcome compared. Orthod Craniofac Res 2006;9:77–83.
42. Peterman RJ, Jiang S, Johe R, Mukherjee PM. Accuracy of Dolphin visual treatment objective (VTO) prediction software on Class III patients treated with maxillary advancement and mandibular setback. Prog Orthod 2016;17:19.
43. Bolandzadeh N, Bischof W, Flores-Mir C, Boulanger P. Multimodal registration of three-dimensional maxillodental cone beam CT and photogrammetry data over time. Dentomaxillofac Radiol 2013;42:22027087.

Measuring Bone with CBCT

Leena Palomo, DDS, MSD
Tarek Elshebiny, BDS, MSD
Ali Z. Syed, BDS, MHA, MS
Juan Martin Palomo, DDS, MSD

Cone beam computed tomography (CBCT) imaging is uniquely suited to dentistry and orthodontics because it has high resolution and significantly lower radiation compared with spiral CT, it provides clear images of highly contrasted structures, and it is extremely useful for evaluating bone.[1,2] While the higher radiation doses for spiral CT allow for better separation of tissues with similar density, the structures we want to see have relatively high differences in density (Fig 11-1). Therefore, the use of CBCT for routine diagnostic purposes in orthodontics is becoming more prevalent.

CBCT was introduced to the dental profession in the United States in the early 2000s with the NewTom 9000 (QR), CB MercuRay (Hitachi), and i-CAT (Imaging Sciences) machines. Initially, the major concern with this technology was the exposure of the patient to increased levels of radiation. However, by changing the parameters of their machines (eg, low settings, pulse technology) and the imaging process (eg, partial rotation around the patient's head), several CBCT manufacturers developed CBCT scanners that are capable of producing similar radiation doses as a conventional panoramic radiograph.[3] Over the last decade, affordable CBCT systems have become commercially available, and several systems are now in use for craniofacial imaging.

CBCT imaging is superior to conventional radiographic techniques including panoramic radiography, full-mouth series, lateral and frontal cephalograms, and occlusal radiographs. With only a single acquisition that can be taken in few seconds, a CBCT can generate reformatted panoramic, cross-sectional, and reconstructed images of the labial and lingual bone plates, which are not apparent in conventional two-dimensional (2D) radiographs due to image superimposition. In addition, views not previously available can be created with CBCT, including axial, coronal, and sagittal views as well as separate views of the right and left sides of the head.

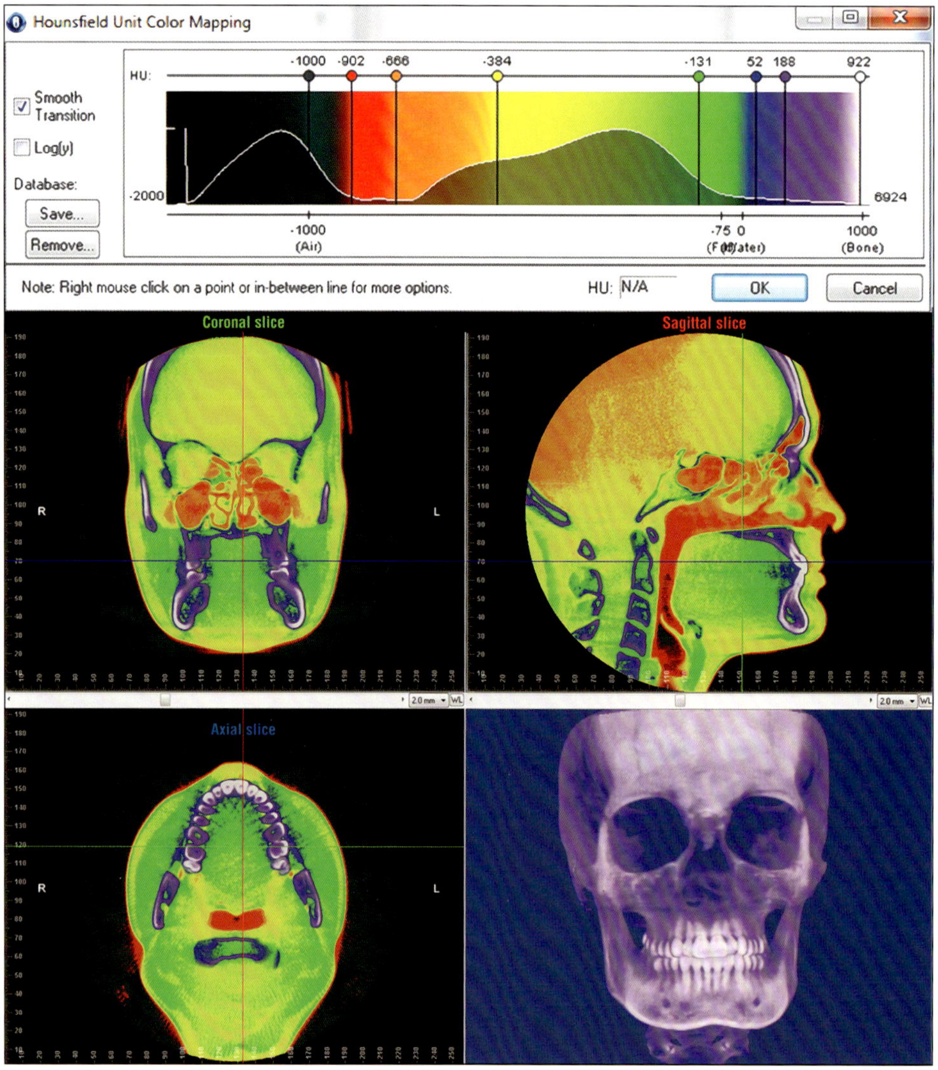

Fig 11-1 Three-dimensional (3D) reconstructed images in different planes of space showing different densities in different tissues in the craniofacial complex with the aid of the Hounsfield Unit Color Mapping tool (Dolphin 3D, Patterson Dental), which helps distinguish between different biologic structures according to their radiolucency measurements. A graph displays the colors as they fall on the Hounsfield scale as a reference, while the image on the screen is colored accordingly.

Accuracy and Spatial Resolution of CBCT

Recently, numerous studies have demonstrated the precision of linear and angular measurements performed on CBCT images. Measurements from synthesized CBCT lateral cephalograms using orthogonal and perspective projections were compared with those from conventional cephalometric radiographs, and it was found that both types of synthesized CBCT projections are similar to conventional cephalograms.[4] Several studies assessing root resorption and localization of impacted teeth using CBCT showed that CBCT provides more accurate assessment than conventional panoramic radiographs.[5,6] The accuracy of linear dental measurements generated on CBCT scans was compared with true anatomical dimensions of the actual teeth, which were used as the gold standard for comparison, and results supported the use of CBCT to analyze the dentition; measurements proved to be reliable and accurate.[7] Several studies have evaluated the accuracy and reliability of CBCT in the diagnosis of naturally occurring fenestrations and bony dehiscences as well as in measuring alveolar bone margins. It was concluded that alveolar bone height can be measured to an accuracy of about 0.6 mm, and root fenestrations can be identified with greater accuracy than dehiscences. The differences between the direct and CBCT methods were most likely due to limitations in spatial resolution.[8]

Spatial resolution takes us to another concept that is always confused with measurement accuracy. The resolution of CBCT imaging is determined by the individual volume elements (voxels) produced from the volumetric data set.[9] The size of a voxel is defined by its height, width, and depth, and CBCT voxels are generally isotropic—equal in three dimensions.[9] The voxel size of a three-dimensional (3D) image is equivalent to the pixel resolution in 2D images.[9] Voxel size is a rational predictor of spatial resolution. *Spatial resolution* is defined as the ability to separate two objects in close proximity in the image, and it depends on the voxel dimension, which is the smallest image unit.[9] A smaller voxel dimension leads to greater image resolution but also a higher dose of radiation.[10]

Few studies related higher accuracy and precision for CBCT with smaller voxel sizes. In one study, images produced by a commercially available CBCT machine (i-CAT model 9140-0035-000C) were evaluated for measurement error and spatial resolution for all settings and in all dimensions.[9] A custom phantom containing 0.3-mm-diameter chromium metal markers approximately 5 mm apart in three planes of space was developed for analyzing distortion and measurement accuracy. This phantom was scanned in the CBCT machine by using all 12 commercially available settings. The distance between the markers was measured three times on the 3D images by using a Digital Imaging and Communications in Medicine (DICOM) viewer and was also measured three times directly on the phantom with a fine-tipped digital caliper. A line-pair phantom was used to evaluate spatial resolution. Thirty evaluators analyzed images and assigned a resolution from 0.2 to 1.6 mm according to the separation of the line pairs. It was found that the voxel size had the greatest effect on resolution.[9]

Molen[11] recommended that smaller voxel sizes should be used with caution if the goal is to assess small variations in bone thickness. Menezes et al[12] evaluated the precision, reproducibility, and accuracy of alveolar crest–level measurements on CBCT images obtained with different voxel sizes. CBCT examinations were performed on 12 dried human mandibles with voxel dimensions of 0.2, 0.3, and 0.4 mm. Bone crest level was measured directly on the mandibles with a digital caliper and on CBCT images. The images with 0.2-mm voxel size showed a decreased number of intra-examiner errors. Compared with the images with larger voxels, a higher accuracy for measurements of bone crest level was observed for all CBCT definitions, except for the mandibular incisors using the 0.4-mm voxel size. It was shown that the mandibular incisor region needs better resolution than that provided by 0.4-mm voxel size for bone crest–level measurements.[12] Patcas et al[13] also evaluated the accuracy of CBCT with different voxel resolutions. CBCT data at two resolutions (0.125- and 0.4-mm voxels) were collected from eight intact cadaver heads. The buccal alveolar bone margin was then determined. Anatomical bony measures were compared with the CBCT measures. It was shown that bony measures obtained with CBCT were accurate and differed only slightly from the physical findings.

These studies show that CBCT renders anatomical measures reliably and is an appropriate tool for linear measurements. However, different voxel size affects the precision of the data. Clinicians and researchers must customize resolution protocol according to the accuracy needed.

Applications of CBCT in Alveolar Bone Assessment

In orthodontics, treatment is most successful when the maximum amount of information on the patient's condition is available to the clinician. That is why the ultimate goal of craniofacial imaging is to answer clinical questions. Clinicians need to consider the appropriate biomechanics according to the patient's bone condition. Assessment of alveolar bone condition in orthodontic patients is a necessity to determine the most appropriate treatment procedures. The quantity and quality of the bone need to be evaluated accurately to avoid periodontal problems as well as to prevent existing problems from worsening during orthodontic treatment. The pretreatment position of teeth in the alveolar boundary could affect diagnosis and treatment-planning decisions. The effect of orthodontic treatment on alveolar bone conditions can be evaluated with CBCT, which is shown to be an accurate and reliable tool when imaging buccal bone morphology and buccal cortical plate thickness.[7,8,13]

Bone coverage and detecting alveolar bone dehiscences and fenestrations

Because the boundaries for orthodontic tooth movement are limited by the bony support of the dentition, the thickness of the alveolar bone of anterior teeth should be considered and measured before and during treatment. According to the definition of Shklar and Carranza,[14] *fenestrations* are isolated areas in which the root is denuded of bone and the root surface is covered only by periosteum and overlying gingiva. *Dehiscences* are bony defects in which the denuded areas involve the alveolar bone margin. The presence of these buccal alveolar bone defects decreases the bony support for the teeth. It is well documented that, under certain conditions, a lack of bony support during orthodontic movement can be detrimental to the health of the teeth and the periodontium.[15–17] In addition, orthodontic tooth movement can create alveolar bone defects.[18–22]

Bony dehiscences and fenestrations cannot be visualized by traditional 2D radiography because of the superimposition of contralateral cortical bony or dental structures. However, studies have shown that CBCT has great diagnostic value for visualization of such defects.[8,23,24] In 2010, one study evaluated the use of CBCT to diagnose naturally occurring bony dehiscences and fenestrations in human skulls. It confirmed that the diagnostic value of CBCT for the detection of buccal defects was high for fenestrations at voxel size of 0.38 mm.[8] In 2012, another study validated the use of 3D surface-rendering images to quantify the height of alveolar dehiscences. Twenty-four dehiscences were created on nine incisors, nine canines, and six premolars in four cadaver skulls. i-CAT CBCTs were taken of each skull at 0.2-mm voxel size, and it was shown that dehiscences can be accurately measured using 3D surface-rendering images.[23] A different study compared the sensitivity of diagnoses of buccal bone coverage in anterior teeth between axial and sagittal reconstructions using CBCT.

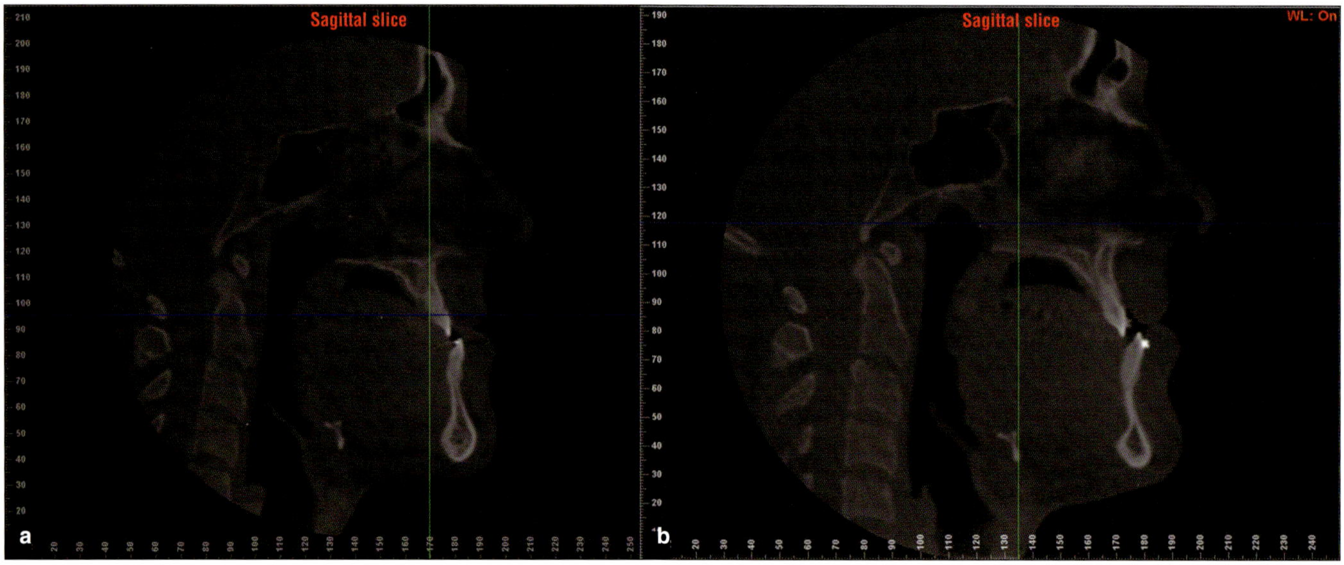

Fig 11-2 *(a)* Clinical example showing the mandibular incisor position in a prognathic mandible before decompensation. *(b)* Mandibular incisors after decompensation. Note the alveolar bone loss in the lingual plate.

Five dry skulls were clinically evaluated to detect bone defects in the anterior maxilla and mandible to establish a gold standard. The skulls were prepared and placed on a Kodak 9000 3D scanner (Trophy) for image acquisition. The images were processed and reconstructed. All bone defects were identified and recorded. It was concluded that CBCT can help in the diagnosis of lack of bone coverage on the buccal surfaces of anterior teeth. There was no difference in the performance of the axial and sagittal reconstructions.[24]

Clinical considerations for alveolar bone thickness

Evangelista et al[25] compared the presence of alveolar defects in patients with Class I and Class II, division 1 malocclusions and different facial types. A total of 79 Class I and 80 Class II patients with no previous orthodontic treatment were evaluated using CBCT. It was found that alveolar defects are a common finding before orthodontic treatment, especially in Class I patients. Another study tested the presence of dehiscence and fenestration among patients with skeletal Class I, Class II, and Class III malocclusions. Results indicated that the Class II group had a greater prevalence of fenestration than the other groups, and no difference was found in the prevalence of dehiscence among the three groups.[26]

Evaluation of the alveolar bone loss around mandibular incisors during surgical-orthodontic treatment in individuals with mandibular prognathism was assessed by comparing CBCT images before treatment, after presurgical orthodontic treatment, and after debonding. The results showed that the vertical alveolar bone level and alveolar bone thickness of the labial and lingual plates of the mandibular central and lateral incisors were reduced after presurgical orthodontic treatment and that special care should be considered in individuals with mandibular prognathism.[27] Another study concluded that special care should be taken to avoid aggravating preexisting alveolar bone loss in the anterior teeth, especially in the mandible, in skeletal Class III patients.[28] Figure 11-2 illustrates a clinical example of mandibular incisor decompensation in a surgical Class III case.

The difference in the alveolar bone thickness, bone loss, or incidence of fenestrations between maxillary and mandibular incisors in skeletal Class I patients with dentoalveolar protrusion before orthodontic treatment was studied by CBCT images. It was shown that incisor periodontal support is poor in these patients and that alveolar bone is minimal even prior to the start of orthodontic treatment.[29] In cases of maxillomandibular protrusion, orthodontic treatment often requires extraction of four premolars with retraction of the anterior teeth. Another study indicated that when maxillary and mandibular incisors are retracted, there is risk for adverse effects, including bone dehiscence.[30] Results showed statistically significant decreases in lingual bone width in both arches after retracting the incisors.

Mandibular anterior alveolar thickness in different skeletal patterns was investigated using CBCT by comparing the mandibular anterior alveolar housing in individuals with low, average, and high mandibular plane angles before and after orthodontic treatment, measuring the alveolar bone loss and root resorption. Total alveolar buccolingual bone thickness at the apex of the mandibular central incisor was larger in the hypodivergent group compared with the normodivergent and hyperdivergent groups.[31]

Another study used CBCT to compare the bone thickness buccal to the teeth in the esthetic zone in four groups: postmenopausal women, premenopausal women, younger men,

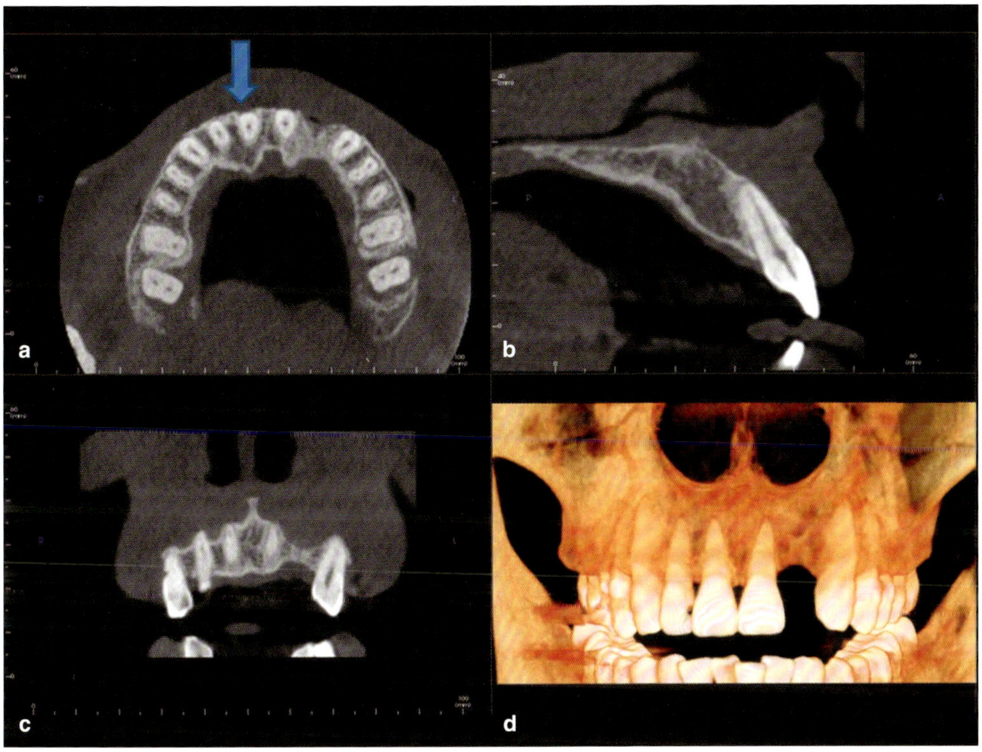

Fig 11-3 Method used to evaluate buccal bone thickness in esthetic areas. Each tooth in the esthetic zone for which buccal bone is to be measured is first identified in all three planes and, for orientation, also in volume-rendering mode. *(a)* The *blue arrow* identifies the buccal bone of the maxillary right central incisor in the axial plane. *(b)* Sagittal view of the maxillary right central incisor. *(c)* Coronal view for orientation. *(d)* Volume-rendering mode for orientation. (Reprinted from Zhang et al[32] with permission.)

and older men (Fig 11-3). The results showed that buccal bone in the esthetic zone is thin in all segments of the population but significantly thinner in postmenopausal women. Strategies to manage the thinner bony housing should be considered before tooth movement.[32]

Orientation and methodology for measuring bone thickness

In order to create different views in a standardized way and to obtain consistent measurements using CBCT images, image orientation should be the first step within the software. The Case Western Reserve University orientation method uses five biologically relevant anatomical structures and one plane[33] (Fig 11-4). After image orientation, the region of interest can be identified in three planes of space (Fig 11-5), and any type of measurement (angular, linear, or creation of paths) can be performed. The buccal or lingual bone thickness from various reference points (cementoenamel junction or alveolar bone crest) or potential dehiscences and fenestrations can be measured for all teeth in the axial, coronal, and sagittal views (Figs 11-6 and 11-7).

Bone Density

Since the discovery of x-radiation in 1895 by Wilhelm Conrad Roentgen,[34] there has been an interest in using radiographs to measure bone density. One early technique was to incorporate a step wedge in the field of exposure to provide a reference to both assess the quality of the radiograph and to estimate bone density.[35–37] Another plain-radiograph technique is radiographic absorptiometry, which uses a phantom with a built-in calibration wedge that can be used to estimate bone density when placed in the field of view (FOV) when taking a radiograph.[38] Dual-energy x-ray absorptiometry (DXA) is a precise method of estimating bone density and is the gold standard for diagnosing osteoporosis.[39,40] More recently, quantitative CT has been used to determine bone density using a spiral CT and has the advantage of 3D and therefore volumetric information.[41] Very recently, magnetic resonance imaging has also been used to estimate bone density by using a standardized phantom made from various hydroxyapatite concentrations in water.[42]

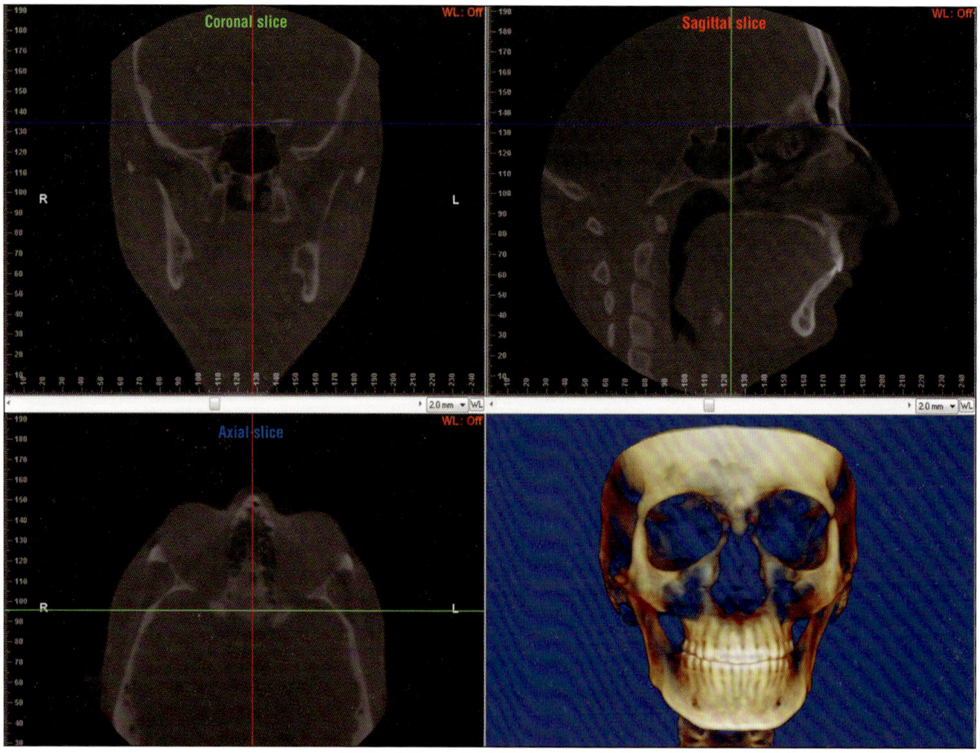

Fig 11-4 Set the axial plane by centering the right and left optical foramina in the coronal view. Set the coronal plane by centering the right and left foramina ovale in the axial view. Set the sagittal plane by viewing foramen cecum in the axial view and placing the axial plane along McRae line (basion to opisthion). Adjust the pitch (clockwise or counterclockwise) to make the palatal plane flush with the axial plane.

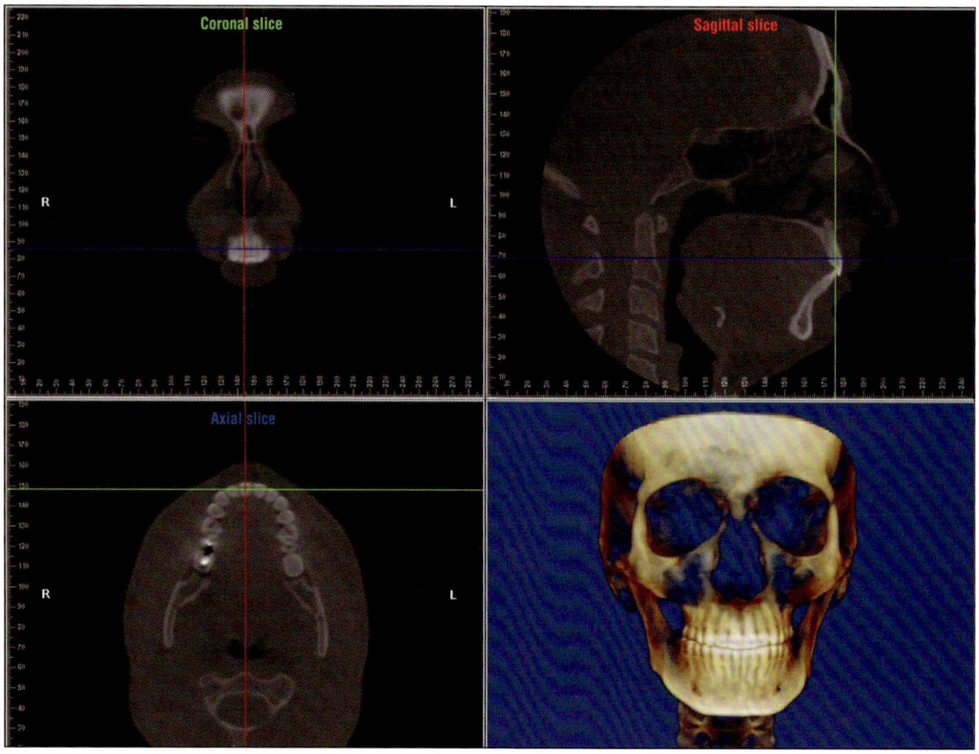

Fig 11-5 Orientation of the region of interest (the maxillary right central incisor).

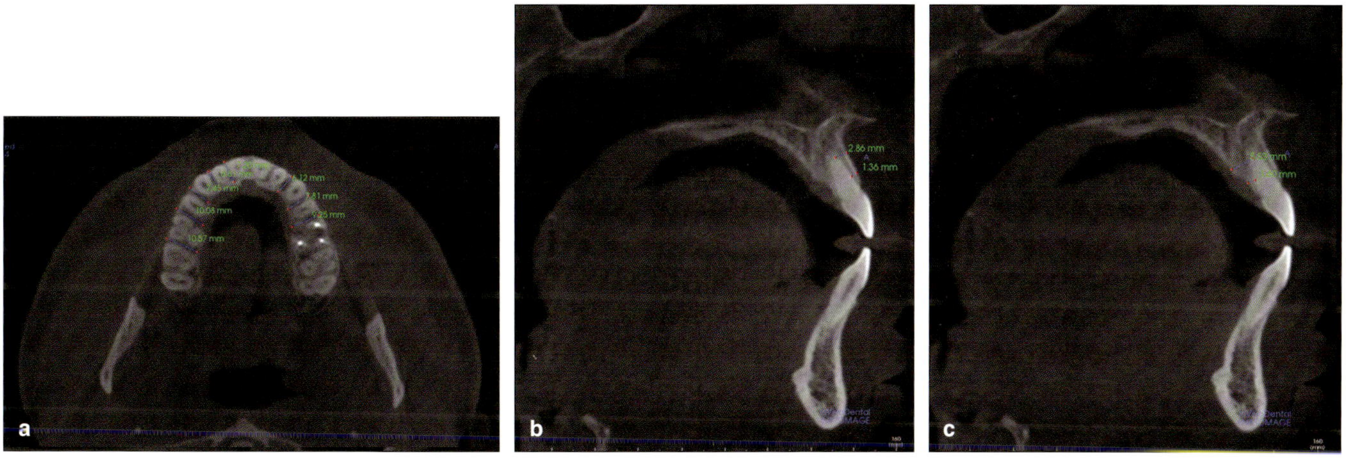

Fig 11-6 *(a)* Alveolar bone thickness measurements performed in an axial slice. *(b)* Buccal bone thickness measurement done at the midroot and root apex in a sagittal view. *(c)* Palatal bone thickness measurement done at the midroot and root apex in a sagittal view.

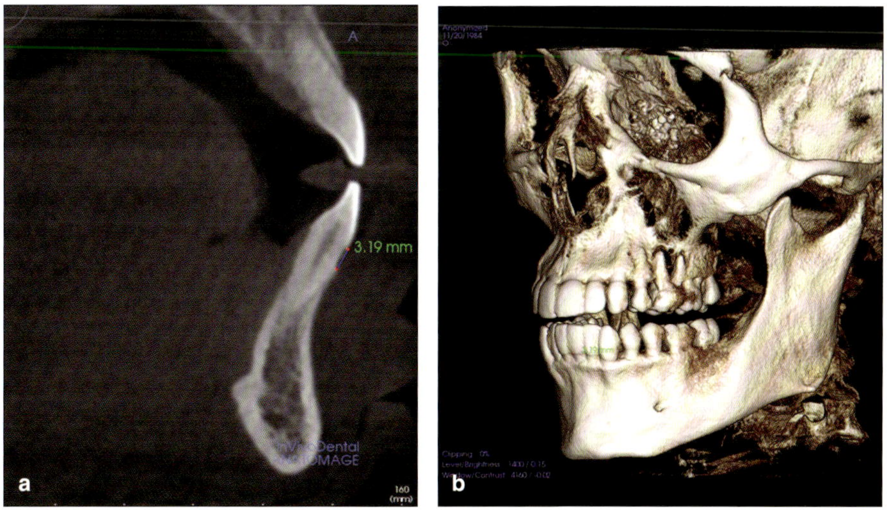

Fig 11-7 *(a)* Sagittal view showing a measurement from the cementoenamel junction to the bone crest as a method of measuring bone dehiscence. *(b)* Volume-rendering presentation for dehiscence measurement.

Spiral CT images acquire information about the radiodensity of various tissues and report the density in Hounsfield units (HU).[43] The formula for deriving Hounsfield units is

$$\text{HU} = 1000 \times \frac{\mu x - \mu water}{\mu water},$$

where μx is the average linear attenuation coefficient of the substance in question and $\mu water$ is the linear attenuation coefficient of water. In spiral CT images, absolute HU values for various types of tissues are calculated using this formula and are standard across machines and across images. While CBCT images also have information about the density of tissues, these values are not absolute and may not be able to be compared across machines or across different images.[44,45] If there were a way to compare these densities, even if they could not be converted to the same scale as spiral CT images, it would be quite advantageous, as the amount of radiation used for a CBCT image is much less than that used for a spiral CT image. If the patient is currently in orthodontic treatment, he or she may have already had a CBCT image taken for diagnostic purposes.

Positive and strong correlation was found between total bone density measured by CBCT and DXA, the gold standard in quantification of bone density in endocrinology and traumatology.[43,44]

Applications of CBCT in measuring bone density

There are many applications for measuring density in the craniofacial region. Beyond the increased visual information a 3D image provides, determining variations in density in the area of pathologic lesions may help to more clearly delineate the borders of the disease, and the amount of tissue to be resected in more serious cases could be more accurately determined. Spiral CT images are already used as a tool for helping to identify lesions, and if CBCT images were able to be used in the same capacity,

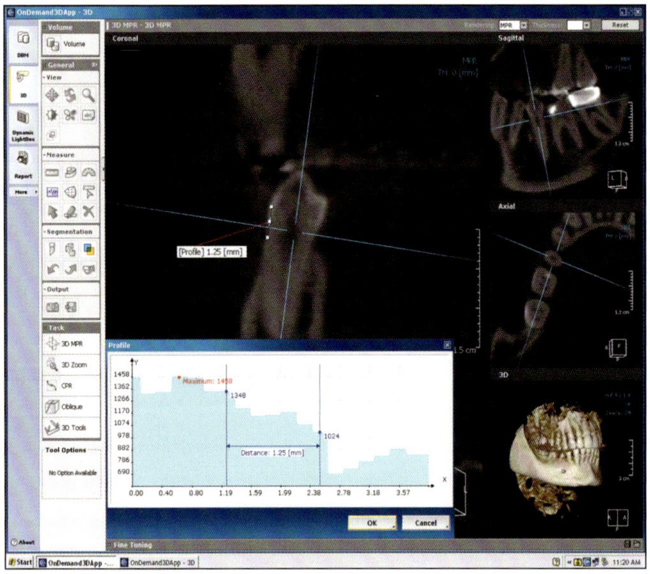

Fig 11-8 A histogram of tissue density showing the different locations of the apical end of enamel as determined by the maximum method (1348) and the half-maximum method (1024). In this instance at the buccal site of a mandibular premolar, the difference between the two methods is 1.25 mm.

the amount of radiation exposure for the patient would be greatly reduced. Asymmetric growth cases could also potentially benefit from knowledge of the density in areas of abnormal growth, as it may shed light on how similar or dissimilar the pathologic site is to its corresponding structure on the opposite side.

Several studies[46–48] have used CBCT technology to evaluate bone density in different regions of the craniofacial complex in attempts to determine the densest sites. This information would be of great significance in treatment planning and could be exploited in orthodontics for the clinical assessment of bone graft quality following alveolar surgery in patients with cleft lip and palate as well as for the use of miniplates and miniscrews. One study investigating relative bone density in the maxilla by means of voxel value measurements found that the mean radiologic density of the vestibular cortical plate was higher than that of the palatal cortical plate; this study confirmed the possibility of using CBCT to measure and evaluate the relative bone density of the dental alveolus with modified grayscale voxel values. Another study[49] showed that the anterior mandible has the highest mean bone density while the posterior maxilla has the lowest mean bone density, confirming that a density scale could help clinicians avoid placing implants into the very poorest-quality bone.

Consideration for using CBCT to assess bone density

CBCT systems offer many advantages over medical CT for dental treatment and planning, including a lower radiation dose to the patient, an affordable cost alternative to medical CT, better resolution, and greater detail.[50–52] One disadvantage associated with CBCT scanners is the inability to display actual HU, the standard scale for measurements of tissue density with medical CT.[53–55] Mah et al[51] reported that values obtained from CBCT are similar to HU from medical CT after using a conversion-factor method to correct for the gray levels from the CBCT. Another study[55] suggested that a pixel value from CBCT machines can be converted into HU values. However, the use of HU in CBCT remains controversial. Different studies reported questionable density values and presented limitations that influence density values using CBCT (such as the scanner, the imaging parameters, and the FOV).[53,55,56] An in vitro study performed to investigate the relationship between computed gray levels in three CBCT scanners and one multislice spiral CT device concluded that caution is essential for evaluation and interpretation of density values, specifically for CBCT images that were not considered reliable for density analysis, because of variations in gray levels among different scanners.[57]

Many available commercial software programs have different tools to measure bone densities in HU or gray value and also to visualize the difference in densities between different types of tissues. A tool available in OnDemand3D software (Cybermed) can be used to estimate the radiologic density of bone; a diagram displays the mean and maximum density values. Figure 11-8 illustrates a histogram of tissue density showing the different locations of the apical end of enamel as determined by the maximum method (1348) and the half-maximum method (1024). In this instance at the buccal site of a mandibular premolar, the difference between the two methods is 1.25 mm. Figure 11-9 illustrates a new feature in Dolphin 3D (Patterson Dental), the Hounsfield Unit Color Mapping tool, which helps distinguish between different biologic structures according to their radiolucency measurements. A graph displays the colors as they fall on the Hounsfield scale as a reference, while the image on the screen is colored accordingly. For instance, in this CBCT scan of a cleft palate patient, the difference in density between the cleft area and the surrounding bone can be visualized. Figure 11-10 shows the mean, maximum, and minimum bone density of the selected area as measured in HU using Invivo software (Anatomage).

Bone Assessment for Placing Temporary Anchorage Devices Using CBCT

Implantologists have long appreciated the third dimension in their clinical work. Conventional CT scans are used routinely to assess bone dimensions, bone quality, alveolar height, and the distance to other anatomical structures such as the mandibular canal or sinus, especially when multiple units are proposed. This has improved the clinical success of these prostheses. CBCT is already being used in implant therapy,[58] and this type of 3D imaging can be just as important when planning to use orthodontic miniscrew implants. Several studies have used CBCT to assess bone quality and quantity to determine the most favorable insertion sites, to report bone thickness in

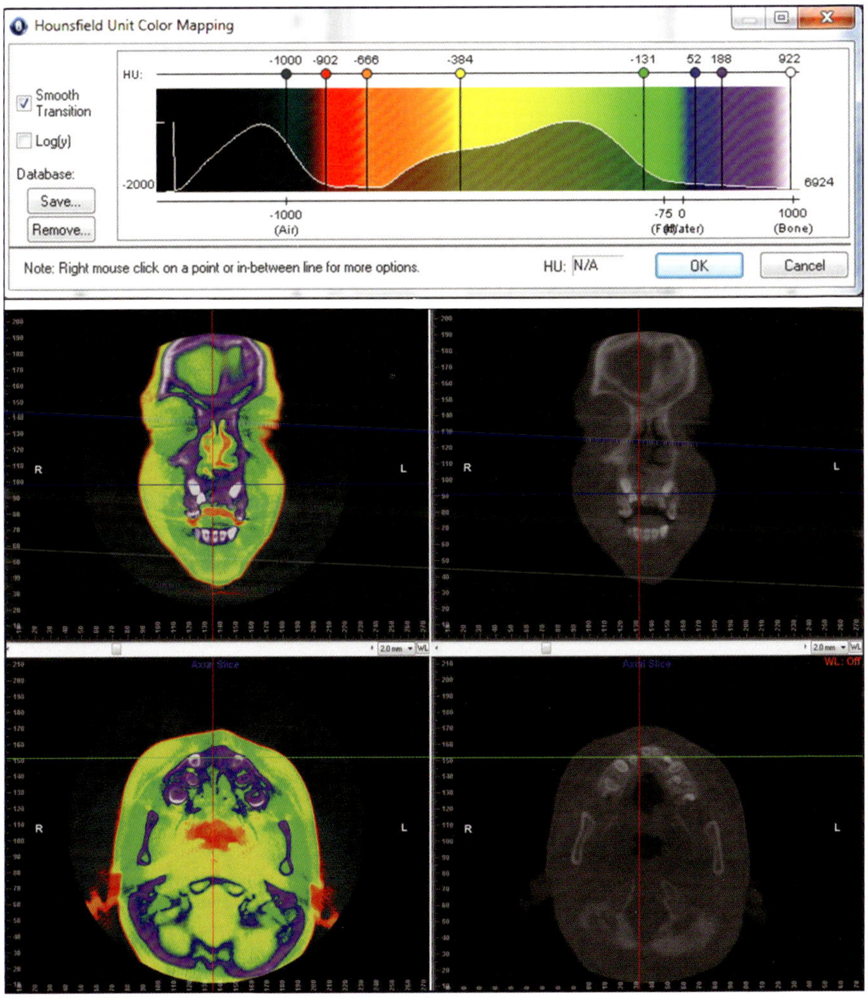

Fig 11-9 Hounsfield Unit Color Mapping tool, which helps distinguish between different biologic structures according to their radiolucency measurements. In this patient with a cleft palate, the difference in density between the cleft area and the surrounding bone can be visualized.

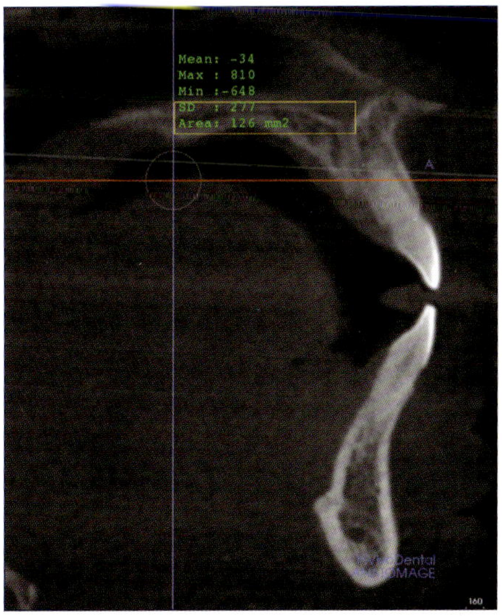

Fig 11-10 The mean, maximum, and minimum bone density of the selected area as measured in HU using Invivo software.

insertion sites commonly used for miniscrew implants, and to evaluate the structures at risk at various insertion sites.[59–61]

Favorable anatomical sites for miniscrew placement

A protocol for safe bicortical placement of miniscrews was proposed by measuring the interradicular spaces of the maxillary teeth and the bone quality. CBCT data were obtained from 50 adults. 3D reconstructions and measurements were made for each interradicular site, and the bone thicknesses and interradicular distances at the planes 1.5, 3.0, 6.0, and 9.0 mm above the cementoenamel junction were measured. It was concluded that bicortical placement would be more stable in the maxilla. For the site between the molars, special care should be taken when inserting miniscrews at a plane higher than 6.0 mm to prevent maxillary sinus penetration. The most favorable interradicular area in the maxilla was between the second premolar and the first molar.[62] Another CBCT study measured the bone thickness in the anterior palate and showed that the lateral anterior palate offers the greatest bone thickness.[63] The authors furthermore recommended a CBCT evaluation if the maximum screw length is to be used.

The thickness of cortical bone is an important factor in mini-implant stability. One study investigated cortical bone thickness and overall bone depth in the palate quantitatively.[59] Thirty dry skulls were imaged with CBCT and showed that bone depth and cortical bone thickness of the palate were most favorable for temporary anchorage device placement at the level of the first and second premolars. In another study, the buccal cortical bone thickness of every interdental area was evaluated as an aid in planning mini-implant placement.[60] Using CBCT scans of 30 dry skulls, the author generated 2D slices through every interdental area. Cortical bone thickness was measured on these slices at 2, 4, and 6 mm from the alveolar crest. Buccal cortical bone thickness was greater in the mandible than in the maxilla. The thickness increased with increasing distance from the alveolar crest in the mandible. Therefore, knowing the

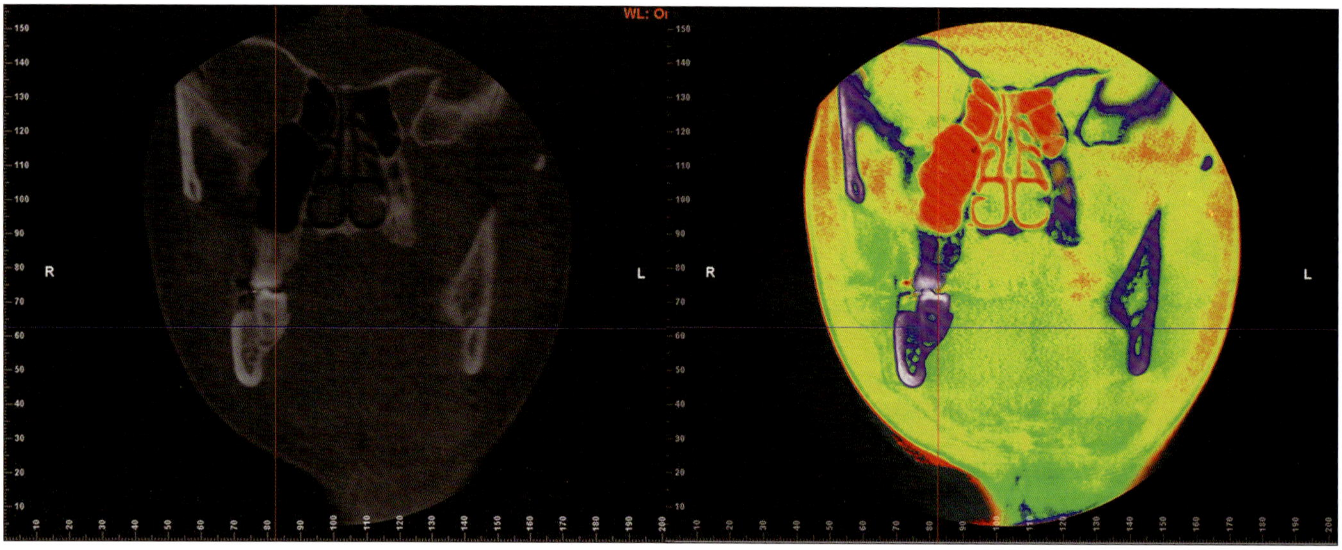

Fig 11-11 Coronal slice representing the mandibular buccal shelf at the distal root of the second molar as an insertion site for miniscrew implant placement.

mean values for thickness can aid clinicians in mini-implant site selection and preparation.

The mandibular buccal shelf has been assessed as a favorable insertion site for orthodontic miniscrews (Fig 11-11). Buccolingual bone width was assessed at three different insertion sites and two height levels at the buccal shelf on CBCT scans of 30 patients (18 female and 12 male, mean age 14.5 ± 2 years).[64] The greatest bone width and insertion depth were found distobuccal to the second molar. It was concluded that the buccal shelf distal to the second molar is the most appropriate site for miniscrew placement.

Bone density effects on miniscrew stability

The effect of bone density on the success rates of orthodontic miniscrews was evaluated with CBCT.[62] Orthodontic miniscrews were placed into the maxillary buccal alveolar bone of 71 patients (53 female, 18 male; mean age, 19.2 years) with malocclusion. The cortical, cancellous, and total bone densities were measured, and the correlations between these measurements and the orthodontic miniscrew success rates were evaluated with CBCT. It was shown that the success rate of orthodontic miniscrews significantly increased with higher cancellous and total bone densities, whereas cortical bone density did not have a significant effect. Another study showed that bone density influences the primary stability of miniscrews.[65] Palatal bone density was evaluated to allow better selection of palatal implant anchorage sites. Bone density was measured in HU. It was suggested that miniscrews for orthodontic anchorage can be effectively placed in most areas with bone density equivalent to that of the palatal area if they are placed at least 3 mm posterior to the incisive foramen.

Anatomical sites at risk during insertion

Root proximity is considered one of the anatomical factors that affect the success of miniscrew implant placement. One study used CBCT images to evaluate the relationship between root proximity and success of miniscrews and concluded that increasing the distance from a miniscrew to the root surface will significantly improve success rates.[66] Another study recommended the use of 3D imaging to prevent damage to the maxillary sinus.[60] The proximity of the inferior alveolar nerve to the miniscrew inserted in the mandibular buccal shelf area was also evaluated.[63] Miniscrews had the greatest proximity to the nerve at the site of the distal root of the second molar. A methodology for nerve tracing is illustrated in Fig 11-12.

A new methodology for virtual miniscrew insertion

Figure 11-13 illustrates a new protocol for virtual placement of miniscrews using CBCT. In order to apply this new method,[67] the insertion area should be scanned with CBCT. A 3D image of the scanned area is constructed and evaluated to determine the best insertion site based on bone thickness and density. STL models of the patient are superimposed on the CBCT volumes to virtually create an outline of the soft tissue contour on the CBCT image (see Fig 11-13a). Commercial software programs allow virtual placement of the miniscrews in the selected insertion sites and selection of the diameter and length of the mini-implants depending on the gathered information from CBCT (see Figs 11-13b and 11-13c).

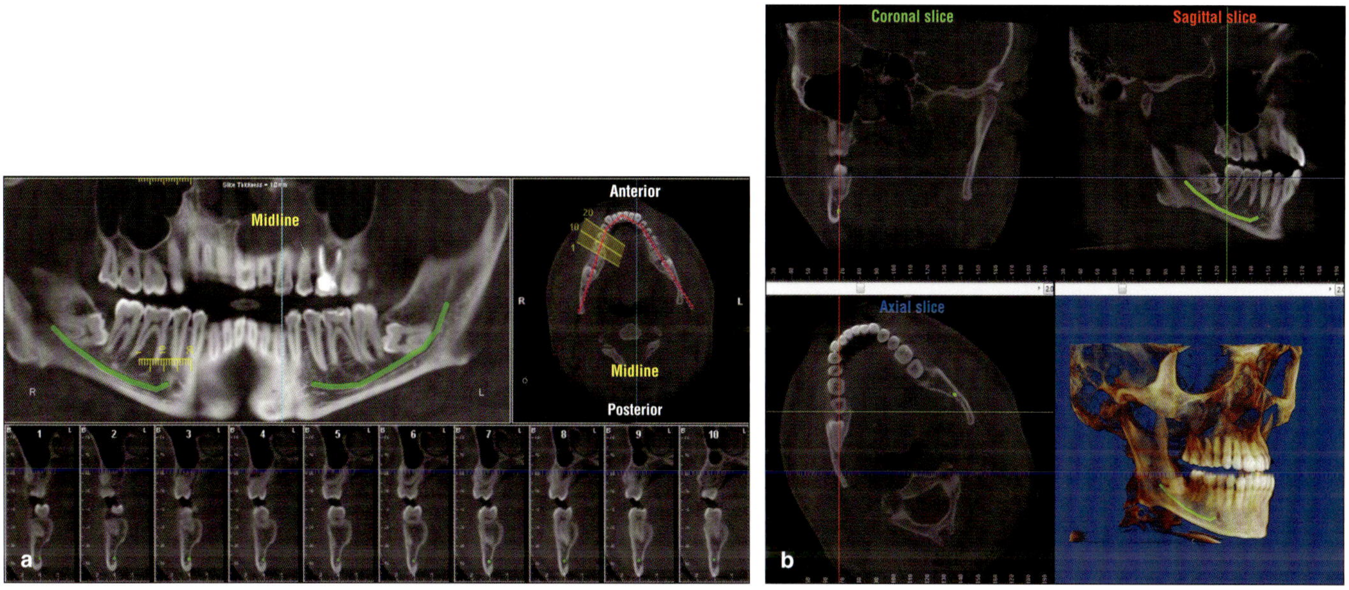

Fig 11-12 *(a)* The inferior alveolar nerve canal can be tracked and traced using the nerve-tracing feature (Dolphin 3D). *(b)* 3D reconstructions of the CBCT images showing the traced nerve canal in different views.

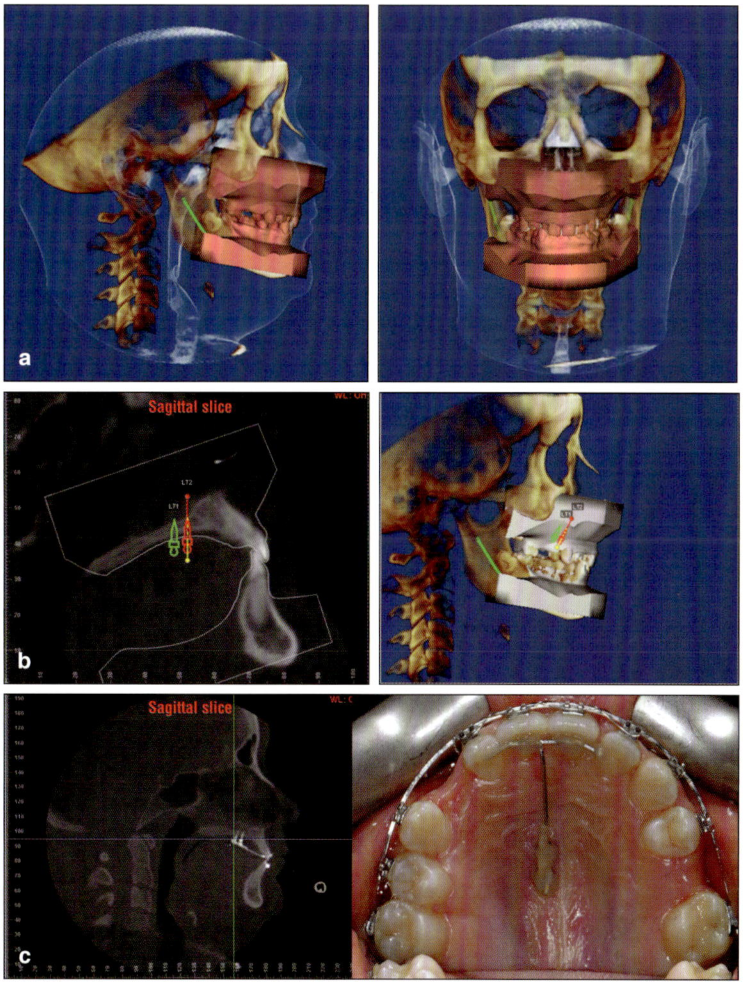

Fig 11-13 *(a)* Maxillary and mandibular STL models superimposed onto the CBCT volume in lateral and frontal views. *(b)* Virtual placement of two miniscrews in the palate. *(c)* CBCT and a clinical photograph showing the outcome of miniscrew placement.

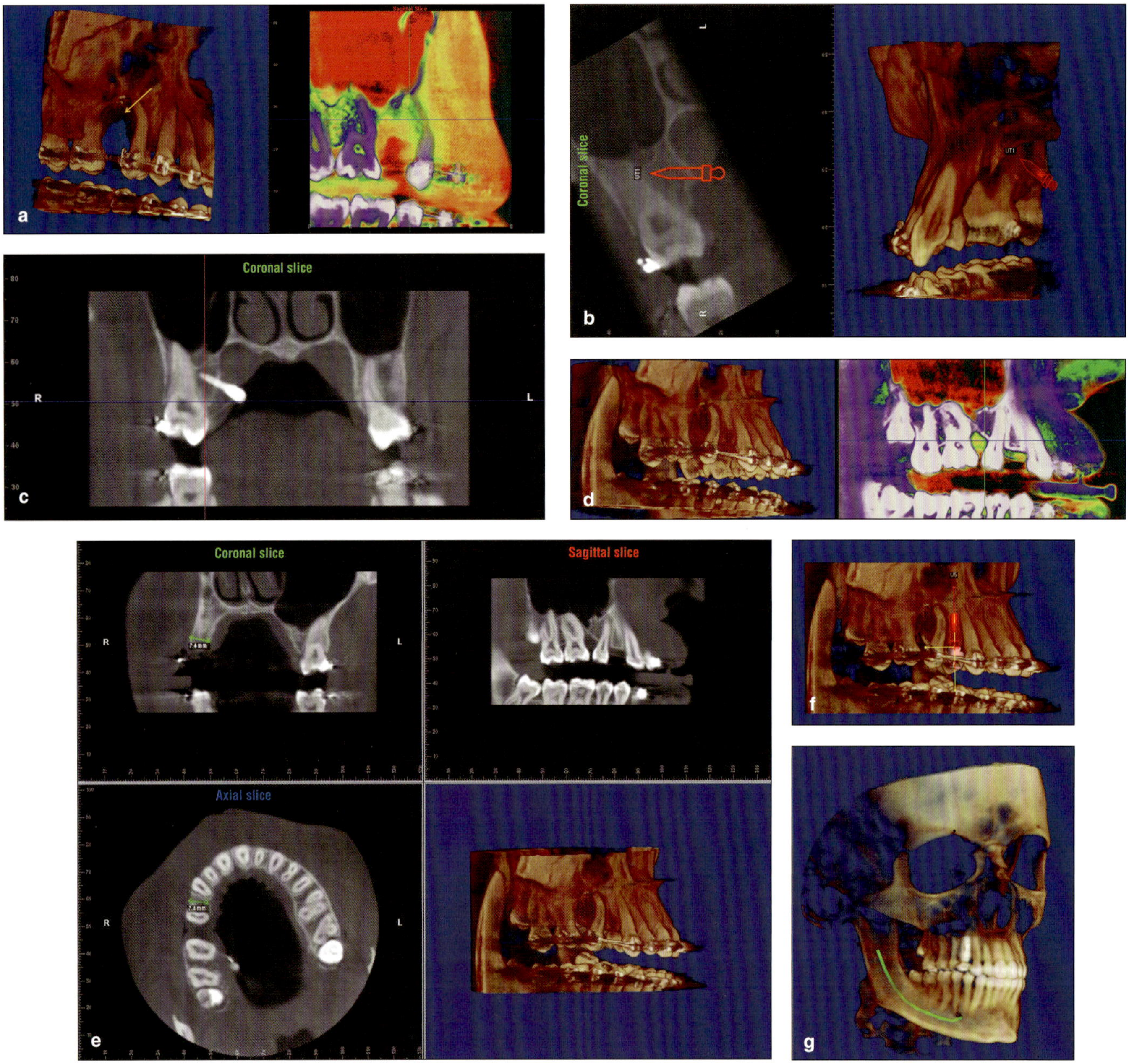

Fig 11-14 *(a)* A small-FOV CBCT showing a bony defect after extraction of an ankylosed maxillary second premolar in a 16-year-old adolescent girl. Note that the bone density in this area is less than that of surrounding bone structures. *(b)* Distalization of the maxillary right first premolar was required to create room for an implant. A miniscrew would need to be placed in the palate to achieve indirect absolute anchorage for this distalization. Miniscrew implant placement was planned with the aid of CBCT virtual placement. *(c)* Clinical outcome of miniscrew implant placement in the posterior palate. *(d)* Small-FOV CBCT showing the progress of distalization. Note the bone formation distal and mesial to the premolar and the increase in bone density according to the HU units in color mapping. *(e)* Small-FOV CBCT was used to aid in placing the dental implant to replace the missing premolar. Bone thickness measurements were performed in the coronal and axial slices. *(f)* Virtual placement of the dental implant after selection of the proper diameter and length. *(g)* Volume rendering showing the final outcome after dental implant placement in the first premolar area.

Clinical Case

Figure 11-14 illustrates a clinical case in which different applications of CBCT were used to assess bone thickness, bone density, and treatment planning for dental implants and miniscrews. A 16-year-old adolescent girl was referred to the clinic at Case Western Reserve University after extraction of her ankylosed maxillary right second premolar (Fig 11-14a). The patient presented after extraction with a bony defect that required precise treatment planning. The treatment plan involved distalization of the maxillary right first premolar to create room for an implant. Absolute anchorage was needed for distalization, so a miniscrew was to be placed in the palate and connected to the first molar as a means of indirect anchorage. The miniscrew implant placement was planned with the aid of CBCT virtual placement (Fig 11-14b). Figure 11-14c shows the outcome of mini-screw placement in the posterior palate, and Fig 11-14d shows bone formation and an increase in bone density achieved with the distalization. A dental implant was then placed to replace the missing premolar (Figs 11-14e and 11-14f). Figure 11-14g shows the final outcome after dental implant placement.

References

1. Farman AG, Scarfe WC. The basics of maxillofacial cone beam computed tomography. Semin Orthod 2009;15:2–13.
2. Kwong JC, Palomo JM, Landers MA, Figueroa A, Hans MG. Image quality produced by different cone-beam computed tomography settings. Am J Orthod Dentofacial Orthop 2008;133:317–327.
3. Ludlow JB, Walker C. Assessment of phantom dosimetry and image quality of i-CAT FLX cone-beam computed tomography. Am J Orthod Dentofacial Orthop 2013;144:802–817.
4. Kumar V, Ludlow J, Soares Cevidanes LH, Mol A. In vivo comparison of conventional and cone beam CT synthesized cephalograms. Angle Orthod 2008;78:873–879.
5. Peck JL, Sameshima GT, Miller A, Worth P, Hatcher DC. Mesiodistal root angulation using panoramic and cone beam CT. Angle Orthod 2007;77:206–213.
6. Van Elslande D, Heo G, Flores-Mir C, Carey J, Major PW. Accuracy of mesiodistal root angulation projected by cone-beam computed tomographic panoramic-like images. Am J Orthod Dentofacial Orthop 2010;137(suppl):S94–S99.
7. Baumgaertel S, Palomo JM, Palomo L, Hans MG. Reliability and accuracy of cone-beam computed tomography dental measurements. Am J Orthod Dentofacial Orthop 2009;136:19–25.
8. Leung CC, Palomo L, Griffith R, Hans MG. Accuracy and reliability of cone beam computed tomography for measuring alveolar bone height and detecting bony dehiscences and fenestrations. Am J Orthod Dentofacial Orthop 2010;137(suppl):S109–S119.
9. Ballrick JW, Palomo JM, Ruch E, Amberman BD, Hans MG. Image distortion and spatial resolution of a commercially available cone-beam computed tomography machine. Am J Orthod Dentofacial Orthop 2008;134:573–582.
10. Davies J, Johnson B, Drage N. Effective doses from cone beam CT investigation of the jaws. Dentomaxillofac Radiol 2012;41:30–36.
11. Molen AD. Considerations in the use of cone-beam computed tomography for buccal bone measurements. Am J Orthod Dentofacial Orthop 2010;137(suppl):S130–S135.
12. Menezes CC, Janson G, Massaro CS, Cambiaghi L, Garib DG. Reproducibility of bone plate thickness measurements with cone-beam computed tomography using different image acquisition protocols. Dent Press J Orthod 2010;15:143–149.
13. Patcas R, Müller L, Ullrich O, Peltomäki T. Accuracy of cone beam computed tomography at different resolutions assessed on the bony covering of the mandibular anterior teeth. Am J Orthod Dentofacial Orthop 2012;141:41–50.
14. Shklar G, Carranza F. The tooth-supporting structures. In: Carranza F, Newman MG, Takei H. Clinical Periodontology, ed 9. Philadephia: Saunders, 2002:68–92.
15. Ericsson I, Thilander B, Lindhe J, Okamoto H. The effect of orthodontic tilting movements on the periodontal tissues of infected and non-infected dentitions in dogs. J Clin Periodontol 1977;4:278–293.
16. Wennström JL, Stokland BL, Nyman S, Thilander B. Periodontal tissue response to orthodontic movement of teeth with infrabony pockets. Am J Orthod Dentofacial Orthop 1993;103:313–319.
17. Artun J, Urbye KS. The effect of orthodontic treatment on periodontal bone support in patients with advanced loss of marginal periodontium. Am J Orthod Dentofacial Orthop 1988;93:143–148.
18. Zachrisson BU, Alnaes L. Periodontal condition in orthodontically treated and untreated individuals. I. Loss of attachment, gingival pocket depth and clinical crown height. Angle Orthod 1973;43:402–411.
19. Wehrbein H, Bauer W, Diedrich P. Mandibular incisors, alveolar bone, and symphysis after orthodontic treatment. A retrospective study. Am J Orthod Dentofacial Orthop 1996;110:239–246.
20. Karring T, Nyman S, Thilander B, Magnusson I. Bone regeneration in orthodontically produced alveolar bone dehiscences. J Periodontal Res 1982;17:309–315.
21. Wainwright WM. Faciolingual tooth movement: Its influence on the root and cortical plate. Int J Orthod Dent Chil 1973;64:278–302.
22. Zachrisson BU, Alnaes L. Periodontal condition in orthodontically treated and untreated individuals. II. Alveolar bone loss: Radiographic findings. Angle Orthod 1974;44:48–55.
23. Ising N, Kim KB, Araujo E, Buschang P. Evaluation of dehiscences using cone beam computed tomography. Angle Orthod 2012;82:122–130.
24. Ferreira PP, Torres M, Campos PS, Vogel CJ, de Araújo TM, Rebello IM. Evaluation of buccal bone coverage in the anterior region by cone-beam computed tomography. Am J Orthod Dentofacial Orthop 2013;144:698–704.
25. Evangelista K, Vasconcelos Kde F, Bumann A, Hirsch E, Nitka M, Silva MA. Dehiscence and fenestration in patients with Class I and Class II division 1 malocclusion assessed with cone-beam computed tomography. Am J Orthod Dentofacial Orthop 2010;138:133.e1–7.
26. Yagci A, Veli I, Uysal T, Ucar FI, Ozer T, Enhos S. Dehiscence and fenestration in skeletal Class I, II, and III malocclusions assessed with cone-beam computed tomography. Angle Orthod 2012;82:67–74.
27. Kim Y, Park JU, Kook YA. Alveolar bone loss around incisors in surgical skeletal Class III patients. Angle Orthod 2009;79:676–682.
28. Sun LY, Wang B, Fang B. The prevalence of dehiscence and fenestration on anterior region of skeletal Class III malocclusions: A cone-beam CT study [in Chinese]. Shanghai Kou Qiang Yi Xue 2013;22:418–422.
29. Nahm KY, Kang JH, Moon SC, et al. Alveolar bone loss around incisors in Class I bidentoalveolar protrusion patients: A retrospective three-dimensional cone beam CT study. Dentomaxillofac Radiol 2012;41:481–488.
30. Sarikaya S, Hayda B, Ciğer S, Ariyürek M. Changes in alveolar bone thickness due to retraction of anterior teeth. Am J Orthod Dentofacial Orthop 2002;122:15–26.
31. Hoang N, Nelson G, Hatcher D, Oberoi N. Evaluation of mandibular anterior alveolus in different skeletal patterns. Progr Orthod 2016;17:22.
32. Zhang CU, DeBaz C, Bhandal G, et al. Buccal bone thickness in the esthetic zone of postmenopausal women: A CBCT analysis. Implant Dent 2016;25:478–484.
33. Wu R, Palomo JM, Landers M, Hans MG. Anatomically Based Cranial Landmarks for Three-Dimensional Superimposition [master's thesis]. Cleveland: Case Western Reserve University, 2012.
34. Discovery of xrays. Br Med J 1945;2:608.
35. Seemann HE, Roth B. New stepped wedges for radiography. Acta Radiol 1960;53:214–226.
36. Bloxom RM, Manson-Hing LR. The accuracy of an x-ray film quality-assurance step-wedge test. Oral Surg Oral Med Oral Pathol 1986;62:449–458.
37. Kribbs PJ, Smith DE, Chesnut CH. Oral findings in osteoporosis. Part I: Measurement of mandibular bone density. J Prosthet Dent 1983;50:576–579.
38. Cutler AM, Whitten S, Wigderowitz C. Measurement of bone mineral density from plain radiographs. J Bone Joint Surg Br 2005;87-B(suppl):229.
39. Nelson DA, Brown EB, Flynn MJ, Cody DD, Schaffer S. Comparison of dual photon and dual energy 11-ray bone densitometers in a clinical setting. Skeletal Radiol 1991;20:591–595.
40. Kanis JA, Glüer CC. An update on the diagnosis and assessment of osteoporosis with densitometry. Committee of Scientific Advisors, International Osteoporosis Foundation. Osteoporos Int 2000;11:192–202.
41. Khoo BCC, Brown K, Cann C, et al. Comparison of QCT-derived and DXA-derived areal bone mineral density and T scores. Osteoporos Int 2009;20:1539–1545.
42. Ho KY, Hu HH, Keyak JH, Colletti PM, Powers CM. Measuring bone mineral density with fat-water MRI: Comparison with computed tomography. J Magn Reson Imaging 2013;37(1):237–242.
43. Brooks RA. A quantitative theory of Hounsfield unit and its application to dual energy scanning. J Comput Assist Tomogr 1977;1:487–493.
44. De Vos W, Casselman J, Swennen GR. Cone-beam computerized tomography (CBCT) imaging of the oral and maxillofacial region: A systematic review of the literature. Int J Oral Maxillofac Surg 2009;38:609–625.
45. Vannier MW. Craniofacial computed tomography scanning: Technology, applications and future trends. Orthod Craniofac Res 2003;6(suppl):23–30.

46. Hamada Y, Kondoh T, Noguchi K, et al. Application of limited cone beam computed tomography to clinical assessment of alveolar bone grafting: A preliminary report. Cleft Palate Craniofac J 2005;42:128–137.
47. Schwarz MS, Rothman SL, Rhodes ML, Chafetz N. Computed tomography: Part I. Preoperative assessment of the mandible for endosseous implant surgery. Int J Oral Maxillofac Implants 1987;2:137–141.
48. Cha JY, Kil JK, Yoon TM, Hwang CJ. Miniscrew stability evaluated with computerized tomography scanning. Am J Orthod Dentofacial Orthop 2010;137:73–79.
49. Attili S, Surapaneni H, Kasina SP, et al. To evaluate the bone mineral density in mandible of edentulous patients using computed toography: An in vivo study. J Int Oral Health 2015;7:22–26.
50. Quereshy FA, Savell TA, Palomo JM. Applications of cone beam computed tomography in the practice of oral and maxillofacial surgery. J Oral Maxillofac Surg 2008;66:791–796.
51. Mah P, Reeves TE, McDavid WD. Deriving Hounsfield units using grey levels in cone beam computed tomography. Dentomaxillofac Radiol 2010;39:323–335.
52. Mah J, Hatcher D. Three-dimensional craniofacial imaging. Am J Orthod Dentofacial Orthop 2004;126:308–309.
53. Spin-Neto R, Marcantonio E Jr, Gotfredsen E, Wenzel A. Exploring CBCT-based DICOM files. A systematic review on the properties of images used to evaluate maxillofacial bone grafts. J Digit Imaging 2011;24:959–966.
54. Katsumata A, Hirukawa A, Okumura S, et al. Effects of image artifacts on gray-value density in limited-volume cone-beam computerized tomography. Oral Surg Oral Med Oral Pathol Oral Radiol Endod 2007;104:829–836.
55. Swennen GJ, Schutyser F. Three-dimensional cephalometry: Spiral multi-slice vs cone-beam computed tomography. Am J Orthod Dentofacial Orthop 2006;130:410–416.
56. Lai RF, Zou H, Kong WD, Lin W. Applied anatomic site study of palatal anchorage implants using cone beam computed tomography. Int J Oral Sci 2010;2:98–104.
57. Azeredo F, de Menezes LM, Enciso R. Computed gray levels in multislice and cone-beam computed tomography. Am J Orthod Dentofacial Orthop 2013;144:147–155.
58. Hatcher DC, Dial C, Mayorga C. Cone beam CT for presurgical assessment of implant sites. J Calif Dent Assoc 2003;31:825–833.
59. Baumgaertel S. Quantitative investigation of palatal bone depth and cortical bone thickness for mini-implant placement in adults. Am J Orthod Dentofacial Orthop 2009;136:104–108.
60. Baumgaertel S. Cortical bone thickness and bone depth of the posterior palatal alveolar process for mini-implant insertion in adults. Am J Orthod Dentofacial Orthop 2011;140:806–811.
61. Baumgaertel S, Hans MG. Buccal cortical bone thickness for mini-implant placement. Am J Orthod Dentofacial Orthop 2009;136:230–235.
62. Lee MY, Park JH, Kim SC, et al. Bone density effects on the success rate of orthodontic microimplants evaluated with cone-beam computed tomography. Am J Orthod Dentofacial Orthop 2016;149:217–224.
63. Yang L, Li F, Cao M, et al. Quantitative evaluation of maxillary interradicular bone with cone-beam computed tomography for bicortical placement of orthodontic mini-implants. Am J Orthod Dentofacial Orthop 2015;147:725–737.
64. Elshebiny T, Palomo JM, Baumgaertel S. Anatomic assessment of the mandibular buccal shelf for miniscrew insertion. Am J Orthod Dentofacial Orthop 2018;153:505–511.
65. Moon SH, Park SH, Lim WH, Chun YC. Palatal bone density in adult subjects: Implications for mini-implant placement. Angle Orthod 2010;80:137–144.
66. Min KI, Kim SC, Kang KH, et al. Root proximity and cortical bone thickness effects on the success rate of orthodontic micro-implants using cone beam computed tomography. Angle Orthod 2012;82:1014–1021.
67. Elshebiny T, Palomo JM, Baumgaertel S. A New Approach for Virtual Miniscrew Placement Using CBCT [master's thesis]. Cleveland: Case Western Reserve University, 2016.

Common Pathologic Findings in Cephalometric Radiology

Paul C. Edwards, DDS, MSc
James Geist, DDS, MS

Cephalometric assessment of the dental and craniofacial skeletal relationships is critical to orthodontic treatment planning. Since the introduction of cone beam computed tomography (CBCT) in the late 1990s, three-dimensional (3D) cephalometric analysis is increasingly used for orthodontic treatment planning in lieu of conventional extraoral lateral cephalometric radiographic analysis. Purported benefits of 3D cephalometric imaging include the ability to obtain distortion-free images of the craniofacial structures with a reduction in magnification and superimposition errors that may complicate interpretation compared with conventional lateral cephalometric imaging. The reader is referred to other chapters in this book for a detailed analysis of the potential benefits and drawbacks of CBCT-derived 3D cephalometric imaging compared with conventional two-dimensional (2D) lateral cephalometric radiographic analysis (see chapters 9 and 13).

Regardless of whether the practicing orthodontist employs conventional or CBCT-derived 3D cephalometric analysis, it is important to recognize that a large number of anatomical structures outside of the dentoalveolar structures fall within the field of view (FOV) covered by both of these modalities. The increasing acceptance of CBCT in orthodontic treatment planning has also significantly increased the practitioner's ability to visualize pathologic entities of the hard tissues of the head and neck. Specifically, because a large-FOV CBCT scan must be acquired to generate the data for a 3D cephalometric reconstruction, the range of pathologies that the interpreting clinician needs to be able to recognize parallels those of the corresponding CBCT scan. Unfortunately, due to the complexities involved in assessing these structures and the limited time available in the postgraduate orthodontic curriculum, few orthodontists graduate with the requisite knowledge or experience needed with respect to head and neck radiographic pathology to comfortably evaluate the complex anatomical structures located beyond the jaws. In fact, studies suggest that orthodontists and orthodontic residents are only able to identify one-third of incidental lesions on CBCT, with false positives approximating 50%. These false-positive findings also contribute to added patient anxiety and health care costs.[1] At the same time, ethical and legal standards of care mandate a thorough assessment of the entire data set obtained in order to identify all deviations from normal anatomy, regardless of the underlying rationale for exposing the patient.[2] Requiring patients to sign a waiver absolving the clinician of the duty to fully assess the entire CBCT data set acquired from which 3D cephalometric reconstruction is generated does not meet legal or professional standards of care.

The importance of conducting a thorough radiographic assessment cannot be overemphasized. Studies have identified upwards of 3.2 incidental findings per scan.[3] Not surprisingly, reported prevalences of incidental findings among studies show significant variations, from 25%[4] to 93%[5] of scans, depending on the original indication for ordering the imaging study, the geographic setting of the study, the FOV employed, and the age range of the patients. The range of incidental findings by type of pathology, as a percentage of scans reviewed, include airway findings (20% to 52%), soft tissue calcifications (20%), bone lesions (15% to 20%), temporomandibular joint lesions (5% to 15%), impacted teeth (22%), endodontic lesions (2% to 11%), condensing osteitis (1%), developmental tooth anomalies (0.7%), and miscellaneous other processes (1% to 3%). While the majority of these incidental findings are of minimal to no clinical significance, important occult pathology nevertheless does occur in the hard tissue structures located outside a dentist's conventional area of expertise but within the FOV of the cephalometric radiograph. Price et al,[3] in reviewing 272 consecutive CBCT scans, found that of the incidental findings they identified, 16% required intervention or referral, and 16% required follow-up monitoring, with the remainder requiring no further treatment.

It is important to note that many retrospective studies fail to adjust their data for anomalies that would have been detected by conventional panoramic, full-mouth intraoral radiographs or conventional cephalometric imaging. Therefore, while it is more than reasonable to anticipate that the improved ability to discriminate normal from abnormal anatomy when interpreting CBCT scans should argue in favor of this modality's ability to better identify pathology that might be missed by conventional imaging, data on the additional "yield" obtained from CBCT compared with properly exposed conventional orthodontic radiographs is lacking.

This chapter focuses on the more common and significant pathologic findings that may be identified in cephalometric radiographs, with the focus on CBCT-based 3D cephalometric reconstructions. Recognizing that a principal limitation of CBCT imaging is that the soft tissue resolution is limited to visualization of the soft tissue profile, the airway, and the higher-density soft tissue structures of the major muscles and salivary glands, the discussion that follows is restricted to hard tissue pathology and intracranial calcifications. Specifically, this chapter reviews some of the more common pathologic findings, grouped as:

- Intracranial
- Paranasal sinuses, nasal cavity, and nasopharynx
- Craniofacial bones including the maxilla and mandible
- Temporomandibular joint
- Cervical spine
- Miscellaneous extracranial soft tissue lesions

Airway changes are discussed in this text in chapter 8. For a detailed review of extracranial soft tissue calcifications (eg, calcifications of the stylohyoid or stylomandibular ligament, calcifications of the lymph nodes, phleboliths, and intradermal calcifications) and lesions involving the external acoustic meatus, the reader is referred to Benavides and Edwards.[6]

Finally, it is important, once again, to emphasize that many of the structures affected by the pathologies discussed in this chapter are best visualized as part of what should be a routine, systematic review of all CBCT data from which 3D cephalometric reconstructions are derived. Many of these pathologic changes are not as easily recognized on conventional 2D cephalometric views alone.

Intracranial

Sella turcica

The sella turcica is the saddle-shaped area on the superior aspect of the body of the sphenoid bone that is bounded anteriorly and posteriorly by the clinoid processes. Changes in sella turcica's anteroposterior dimension or depth, especially when these size differences are greater than two standard deviations of the age-adjusted mean, as well as changes to the shape of this structure should at least raise the possibility of underlying pituitary gland pathology, which may include pituitary adenoma, empty sella syndrome, craniopharyngioma, or intrasellar aneurysm.[7]

Calcifications

Intracranial calcifications are relatively common findings, even in younger patients, on conventional 2D cephalometric radiographs. Tetradis and Kantor[7] noted calcifications of the diaphragma sellae ("bridged sella") in 11%, the falx cerebri in 5% (Fig 12-1), the petroclinoid ligament in 1%, and the pineal gland in 1% of the cephalometric radiographs reviewed. The clear majority of these calcifications are physiologic in nature.[8]

Intracranial internal carotid artery calcifications must be recognized as distinct from the physiologic calcifications noted above. These present as well-defined, single to ringlike densities located on either side of the sella turcica or the sphenoid sinus (Fig 12-2). Risk factors include increased age, a history of smoking, hypercholesterolemia, or cardiac disease.[9] In white individuals over the age of 80 years, the prevalence of intracranial internal carotid artery calcifications exceeds 80%.[10] Their presence is a major risk factor for stroke, contributing to 75% of

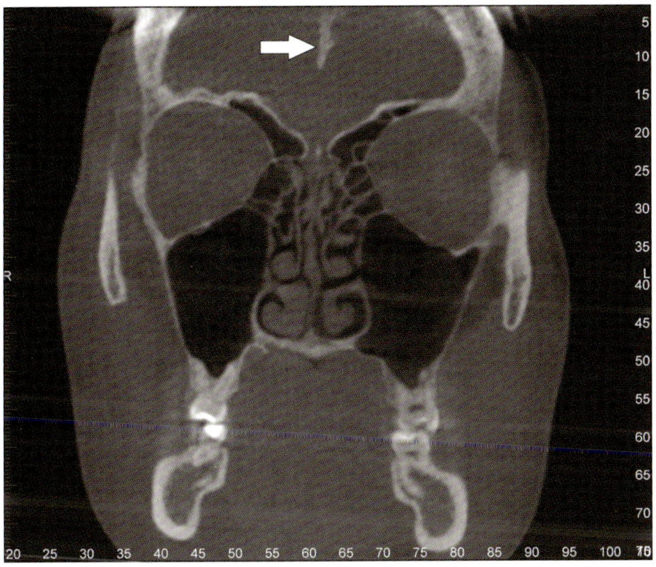

Fig 12-1 Calcified falx cerebri in a 47-year-old woman, indicated by the *arrow* in this coronal CBCT section.

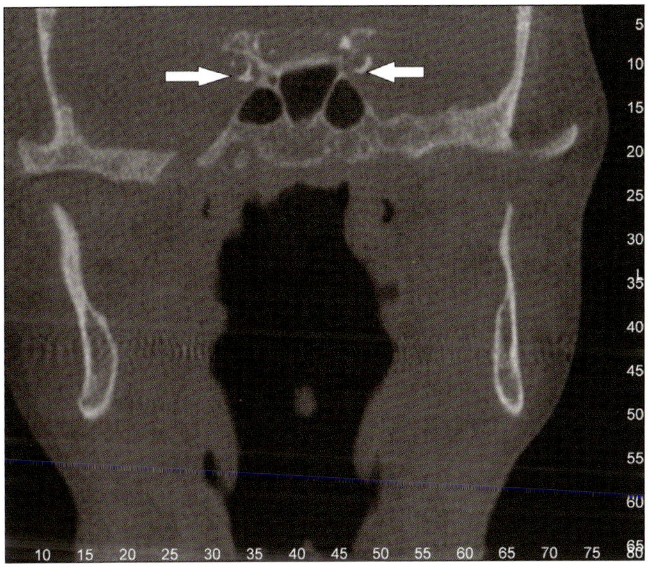

Fig 12-2 Coronal planar CBCT section shows a calcification in the cavernous portion of the intracranial internal carotid artery near the clinoid processes of the sphenoid bone *(arrows)*.

all strokes, compared with only 45% and 25% for calcifications of the aortic arch and extracranial carotid artery, respectively.[11]

Paranasal Sinuses, Nasal Cavity, and Nasopharynx

Inflammatory changes and potentially contributing structural anomalies

Potentially significant pathologic changes are common in the functionally interconnected paranasal sinuses (maxillary, frontal, ethmoid, and sphenoid), nasal cavity, and nasopharyngeal structures. One retrospective study noted potentially significant findings involving the sinonasal complex in 91% of consecutive CBCT scans of the maxillofacial region taken for non-orthodontic assessment, after excluding for findings that would have been evident on intraoral or panoramic radiographic views.[12]

CBCT-evident changes involving the paranasal sinuses are predominantly inflammatory in origin.[13] These primarily involve the maxillary sinuses, with estimated prevalences ranging from 14% to 86%,[14–16] with a trend to higher occurrence on the medial maxillary walls and sinus floor in older men. Radiographically, maxillary sinus change commonly presents as one or more of the following: generalized thickening of the antral mucosal floor, dome-shaped hypodensities (see discussion on antral pseudocysts below), sinus opacification with air-fluid levels and localized thickening of the antral mucosa (suggestive of acute maxillary sinusitis), sinus polyposis, or localized mucosal thickening with opacification of air cells and increased density of the sinus walls (suggestive of chronic sinusitis).

Inflammation of pulpal or periodontal origin is estimated to account for upwards of 10% of cases of chronic maxillary sinusitis[17] and an even greater percentage of cases of generalized or localized mucosal thickening.[18] Not surprisingly, localized mucosal thickening appears to be most closely associated with the presence of periapical lesions, showing a close anatomical relationship between involved teeth and the sinus floor, whereas generalized mucosal thickening is more commonly seen with periodontal bone loss.[14]

As assessed by CBCT, the authors identified chronic sinusitis, defined radiographically by the presence of partial or complete opacification of the sinus with concomitant reactive osseous sclerosis, in 9% of maxillary sinuses, with 8% involving both the ethmoid and sphenoid sinuses, and in 3% of sphenoid sinuses.[19] Fortunately, severe complications resulting from sinusitis, including osteomyelitis, orbital and periorbital cellulitis, intracranial abscesses, and cavernous sinus thrombosis, are rare in adults, with frontal sinus involvement offering the greatest potential hazard.[20]

Obstruction of the openings of the ostiomeatal complex, by interfering with drainage and ventilation between the paranasal sinuses and the nasal cavity, is believed to play a significant role in the pathogenesis of chronic mucosal inflammation. Therefore, factors predisposing to obstruction of these openings, such as acquired or developmental structural abnormalities (eg, concha bullosa, Haller cells, deviated septum, small sinus ostia), and the presence of nasal polyps may predispose to the development of chronic sinusitis.[21]

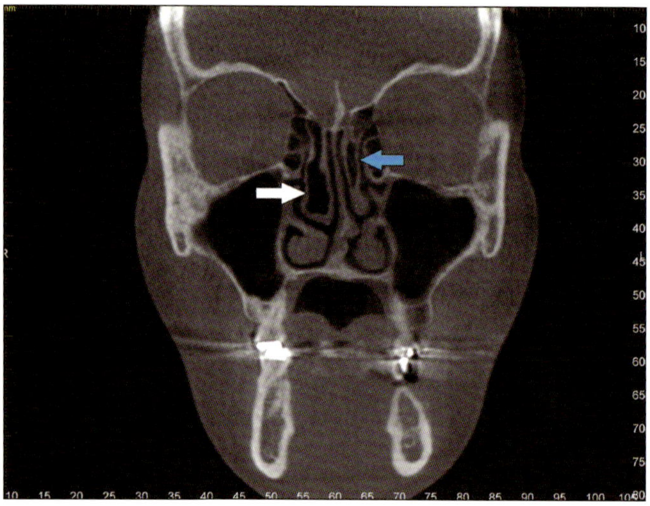

Fig 12-3 Coronal CBCT section reveals an extensive concha bullosa on the right side *(white arrow)* and a smaller lesion confined to the lamellar portion of the turbinate on the left side *(blue arrow)*.

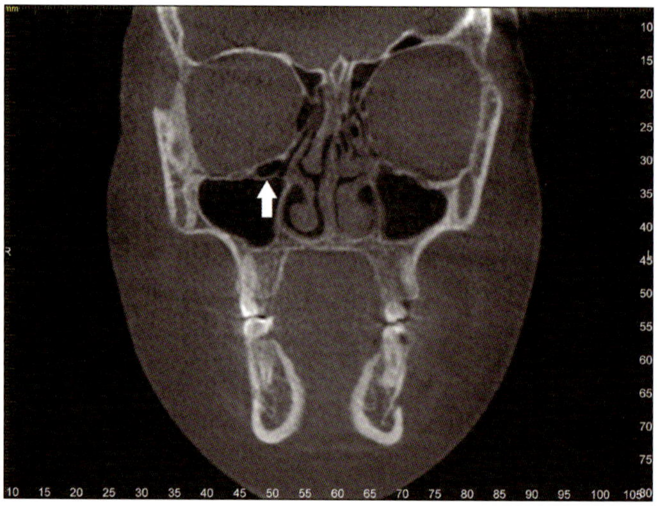

Fig 12-4 Haller cell in the anterior-medial floor of the right orbit *(arrow)* as depicted in the coronal plane.

Three projections from the lateral nasal walls—the superior, middle, and inferior turbinates—overlie the openings to the sphenoid and posterior ethmoid sinuses; the frontal, maxillary, and anterior ethmoid sinuses; and the nasolacrimal ducts, respectively. Pneumatization of the middle turbinate, a condition termed *concha bullosa*, is a common anatomical variant (Fig 12-3), with estimates as high as 53% to 68% of the population.[22,23] Pneumatization may originate in the frontal recess, the anterior ethmoid sinuses, or primarily in the turbinate and may be limited to the lamellar portion of the turbinate or may extensively involve the entire structure. Although some studies have suggested a possible association between the presence of concha bullosa and an increased risk for chronic inflammatory sinonasal disease, the data is contradictory.[24–28]

Haller cells are ethmoidal air cells that extend into the floor of the orbit. These are commonly discovered on CBCT examination (Fig 12-4) and typically have no significance, although some evidence suggests that numerous or large Haller cells may interfere with mucociliary drainage, thereby increasing the risk of maxillary sinusitis.[29]

Sinonasal polyposis is a relatively benign process representing the latter stage of several underlying inflammatory processes involving the sinonasal structures. As noted above, sinonasal polyps predispose to continued obstruction of the ostiomeatal complex. Symptoms, where present, are similar to those of chronic rhinosinusitis: nasal obstruction, postnasal drainage, facial and maxillary tooth pain, sinus pressure, and anosmia.

Nasal polyps present as smooth-surfaced, nodular soft tissue projections from the nasal mucosa, having a propensity to occur in the middle meatus. Polyps may also develop within the paranasal sinuses, with one study[4] noting radiographic findings suggestive of maxillary polyps in 14%, combined ethmoid and sphenoid sinus polyps in 10%, and sphenoid sinus polyps in 8% of scans. Supporting the presumed association with underlying inflammatory processes, sinus polyps were associated with other sinus pathologies in more than two-thirds of affected patients.

Sinonasal polyps appear on CBCT scans as noncorticated, dome-shaped, nodular soft tissue–density lesions. Bone remodeling is uncommon. For smaller polyps, systemic or topically applied corticosteroid therapy may be appropriate. Polyps causing bone remodeling or those that are unresponsive to conservative therapy are best treated by functional endoscopic sinus surgery (removal of the polyps with enlargement of the ostia). The presence of multiple sinonasal polyps in a child should warrant further investigation to rule out cystic fibrosis.

The antral pseudocyst is an extremely common asymptomatic inflammatory lesion, noted in approximately 10% of the population,[30] that is typically discovered incidentally following radiographic examination. The antral pseudocyst represents a nondestructive reactive accumulation of fluid arising in the mucosal lining of the floor of the maxillary sinus that lacks a true epithelial lining. The exact etiology is uncertain, but it is believed to arise as a result of a combination of blockage of seromucinous secretory ducts in the mucoperiosteum, inflammation of the sinus, and odontogenic origin, possibly with an allergic component.

The antral pseudocyst presents radiographically as a single noncorticated, dome-shaped radiopacity overlying the floor of the maxillary sinus that is isodense to soft tissue. It is readily identified on routine panoramic radiographs (Fig 12-5). Early antral pseudocysts may be radiographically indistinguishable from sinus polyps involving the maxillary sinus floor, although the latter tends to be more polypoid in appearance and typically multiple in number. The antral pseudocyst must also be distinguished from sinus mucoceles, destructive and expansile epithelial-lined cysts typically involving the frontal sinuses, and true mucous retention cysts, small mucous-filled cysts that develop secondary to overproduction of mucinous material

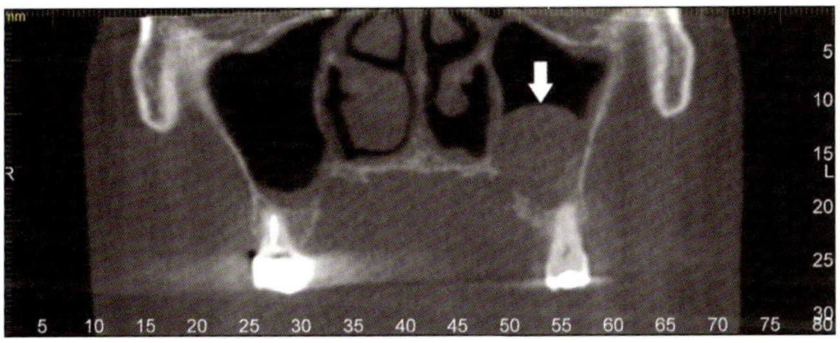

Fig 12-5 Coronal CBCT section reveals an antral pseudocyst in the left maxillary sinus in an 11-year-old girl *(arrow)*. The thickening of the mucosa in the right maxillary sinus is consistent with chronic mucosal inflammatory disease, possibly odontogenic in origin.

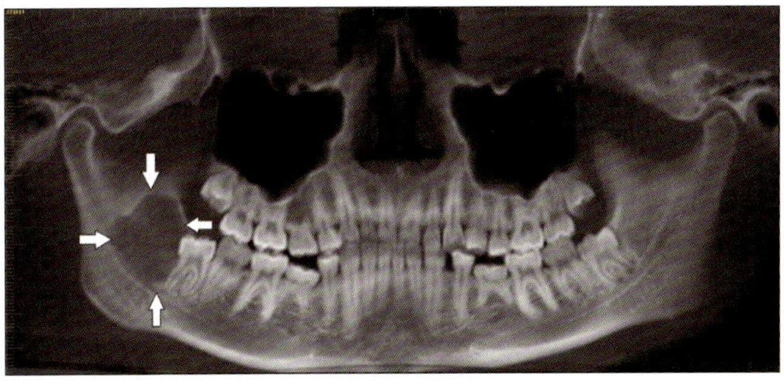

Fig 12-6 Reconstructed pseudo-panoramic view of a CBCT scan that reveals a dentigerous cyst around the right mandibular third molar of a 19-year-old woman *(arrows)*.

by obstructed minor seromucinous glands. As the diagnosis of antral pseudocyst appears to be of minimal clinical significance, treatment is not required once a strong presumptive diagnosis has been rendered.

Postsurgical changes

The oral-antral fistula represents an epithelial-lined pathologic communication between the oral cavity and the maxillary sinus that most commonly follows maxillary molar tooth extraction or other surgical procedures in which a communication is created between these structures.[31] Oral-antral fistulae are responsible for a small number of cases of chronic unilateral maxillary sinusitis. The oral-antral fistula is readily identifiable on CBCT imaging as an osseous defect involving the maxillary bone overlying the sinus with associated inflammatory soft tissue thickening.

Although the more conservative functional endoscopic sinus surgery has largely supplanted the Caldwell-Luc procedure for the treatment of chronic rhinosinusitis, both of these interventions will result in postsurgical changes that may be noted on CBCT imaging.

Finally, the surgical ciliated cyst represents a reactive epithelial-lined cyst that develops following surgical implantation of sinus antral epithelial lining into the maxillary bone, most commonly following a Caldwell-Luc procedure to the area.[32]

Sinus calcifications and foreign material

Antroliths represent calcified concrescences within the maxillary sinus that are assumed to originate secondary to the presence of endogenous (eg, mucus, erythrocytes) or exogenous (eg, gutta-percha) material or fungal organisms that act as a nidus for further calcification.[33] These should generally be readily identifiable on panoramic imaging.

Benign and malignant neoplasms

The sinonasal papillomas represent a group of three pathologically distinct benign neoplastic processes that derive from respiratory mucosa: the exophytic, inverted, and oncocytic papillomas. Sinonasal papillomas are locally destructive lesions with unlimited growth potential. Importantly, inverted papillomas are associated with a 5% to 10% risk of synchronous or metachronous carcinomatous change.[34]

Malignant neoplasms of the paranasal sinuses and nasal cavity are uncommon, accounting for fewer than 1% of all malignancies. Common malignant neoplasms in this site include squamous cell carcinoma, small cell neuroendocrine carcinoma, olfactory neuroblastoma, lymphoepithelial carcinoma, mucosal melanomas, nonkeratinizing carcinoma, sinonasal undifferentiated carcinoma, nasopharyngeal carcinoma, and intestinal type adenocarcinoma. Approximately 60% of sinonasal malignances originate in the maxillary sinus, 30% in the nasal cavity, and 10% in the ethmoid sinuses.[35] Malignant neoplasms of the sphenoid and frontal sinuses are exceedingly rare.

On CBCT, early-stage sinonasal malignancies may be indistinguishable from sinonasal polyps, papillomas, and true sinus mucoceles. As a result, malignant processes involving the maxillary sinus are often initially misdiagnosed as inflammatory odontogenic processes, especially when the characteristic warning signs of dysesthesia are absent or overlooked.[36]

Craniofacial Bones Including the Maxilla and Mandible

Inflammatory and developmental lesions of the jaws

This category includes conditions that are covered extensively in both the predoctoral dental and postgraduate orthodontic curriculum. As a general rule, the practicing orthodontist should be very familiar with this group of lesions. Representative examples include the common inflammatory periradicular lesions (eg, periapical granuloma, apical periodontal cyst, condensing osteitis, external and internal root resorption), developmental odontogenic cysts and tumors (eg, dentigerous cyst [Fig 12-6], odontogenic keratocyst/keratocystic odontogenic tumor, ame-

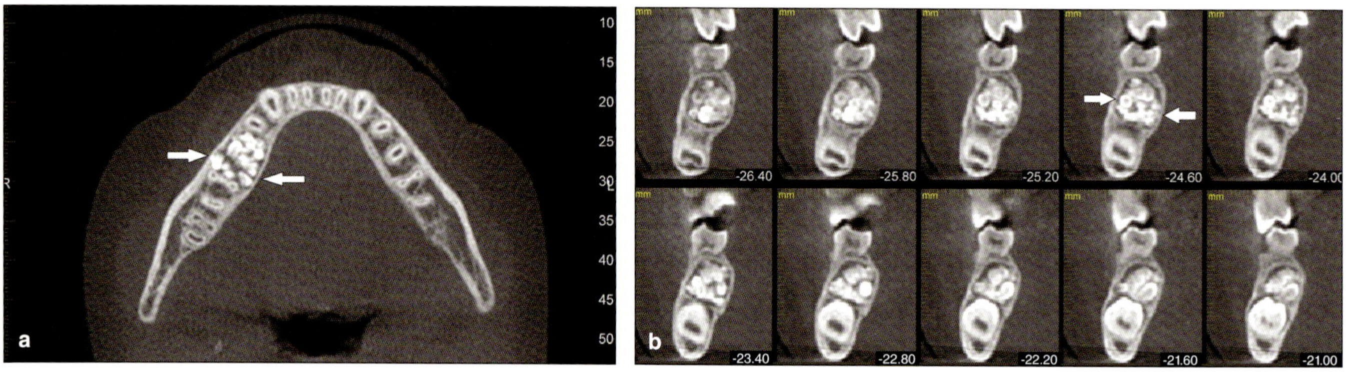

Fig 12-7 This compound odontoma *(arrows)* was discovered in an 11-year-old boy who was being evaluated for orthodontic treatment. *(a)* Axial view. *(b)* Cross-sectional views.

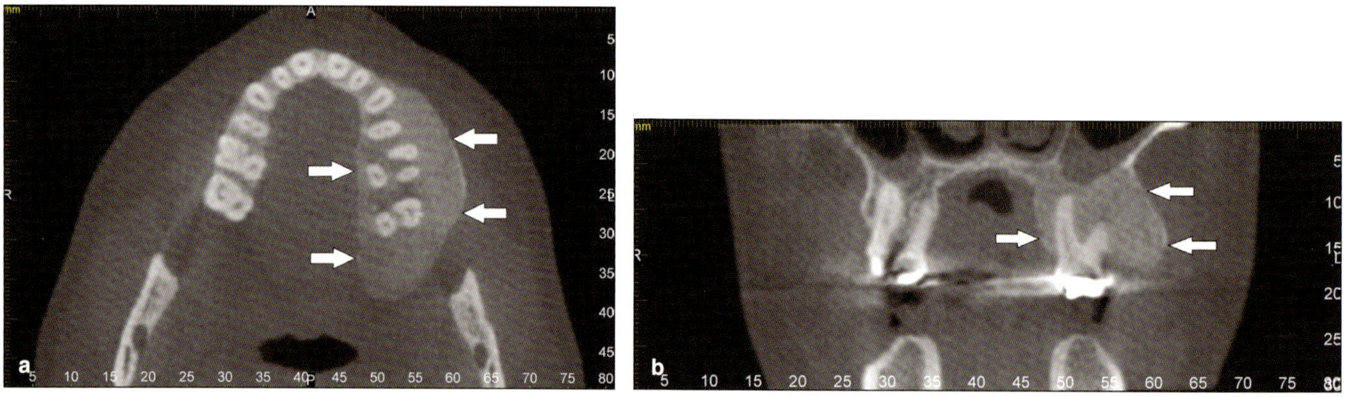

Fig 12-8 A 43-year-old man with fibrous dysplasia of the maxilla *(arrows)*. The patient stated that his jaw began enlarging at 15 years of age. *(a)* Axial section of a CBCT scan through the maxilla. *(b)* Coronal view.

loblastoma), and non-odontogenic developmental lesions (eg, nasopalatine duct cyst, cemento-osseous dysplasias).[37]

The odontoma (Fig 12-7) represents a common hamartomatous process, essentially a tumor-like malformation with limited growth potential comprised of cells and tissues found in areas of the body where that tissue normally occurs. Odontomas produce dental hard and soft tissues, either in the form of small toothlike structures (compound odontoma) or as an amorphous mass of dental tissue (complex odontoma). Odontomas arise during the same time frame as the permanent teeth form, with a tendency for slow growth. Painless expansion of the jaws may occur. Compound odontomas are more commonly located in the anterior maxillary region, while the complex variant is more frequently noted in the posterior segment of the jaws. Many lesions develop around unerupted teeth. Both variants are characterized radiographically by the presence of dental hard tissues surrounded by a thin radiolucency with well-defined borders. These lesions are readily visualized on conventional lateral cephalometric radiographs as well as panoramic and intraoral dental radiographs, so it is an infrequent lesion to be first noted incidentally on CBCT. Nevertheless, CBCT and 3D cephalometric reconstructions may provide valuable additional information on the 3D orientation of these lesions, especially when visualization on plain radiographs is complicated by the superimposition of adjacent structures.

Representative lesions of the craniofacial bones: Fibrous dysplasia and sickle cell anemia

Fibrous dysplasia is a condition associated with a postzygotic mutation involving the *GNAS1* gene in which bone is gradually replaced by delicate fibrous tissue. Abundant, poorly formed, and inadequately mineralized bone trabeculae are produced in affected bone. Fibrous dysplasia usually presents early in life and ceases to progress once the individual reaches skeletal maturity. Affected bones exhibit expansion and have a characteristic homogenous "ground glass" radiopaque pattern. The cortices are attenuated and often become indistinguishable from the medullary bone (Fig 12-8). Most cases involve a single craniofacial bone (monostotic fibrous dysplasia), with the maxilla and mandible being commonly affected sites. Less commonly, multiple craniofacial bones may be affected (polyostotic fibrous dysplasia).

Sickle cell anemia, an inherited mutation in hemoglobin structure, predisposes to a sickling deformity in the erythrocytes under low oxygen tension, leading to erythrocyte destruction in the spleen and potentially to occlusion of small-diameter blood vessels and damage to associated tissues. As a compensatory measure, bone marrow throughout the body becomes hyperplastic as it produces greater numbers of red blood cells.

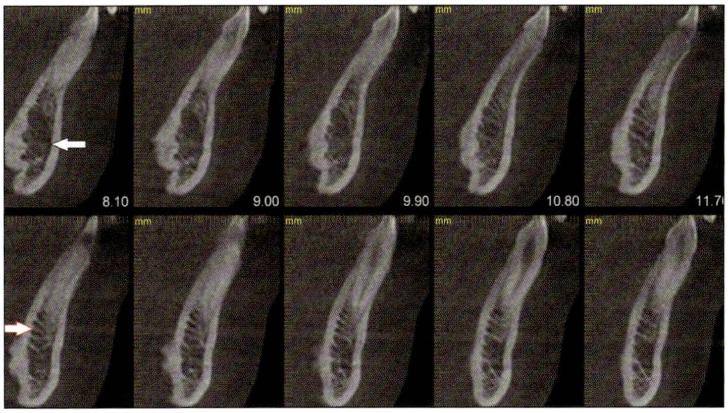

Fig 12-9 Cross-sectional CBCT images of a 19-year-old man with sickle cell anemia. The mandible exhibits reduced numbers of trabeculae with enlarged marrow spaces, producing an osteoporotic appearance *(white arrow at labial surface)*. The trabeculae are often coarse and separated by hyperplastic bone marrow *(white arrow at lingual surface)*.

Radiographs of the skull may reveal thinning of the cortical plates and production of bone at right angles to the cortex, a so-called "hair on end" pattern. The jaws may exhibit reduced numbers of trabecular spaces but an increase in thickness, with enlarged marrow spaces, resulting in an osteoporotic appearance (Fig 12-9).

Temporomandibular Joint

Conditions affecting the temporomandibular joint (TMJ) space range from common degenerative and inflammatory conditions to rare neoplastic processes.

Degenerative joint disease

Degenerative TMJ change represents a common noninflammatory response to supraphysiologic activity on the joint, either from normal forces on a structurally altered joint or excessive parafunctional activity on an otherwise normal joint. Bone or soft tissue remodeling can result in myriad structural changes, ranging from subchondral sclerosis to thinning of the articular cartilaginous surface and flattening of the articular joint curvature. Advanced changes include erosion of the condylar surface, osteophyte formation, subchondral cyst formation, synovial chondromatosis (loose cartilaginous bodies within the synovial membrane), and resorption of the condylar head. Although the anatomy of the articular disc is best assessed by magnetic resonance imaging (MRI), nonspecific late-stage osteoarthritic changes that may be noted on CBCT scans include increased condylar head bone density, subchondral sclerosis, and osteophyte formation.[38,39] Ganglion "cysts," pseudocysts derived from degeneration of the joint capsule, and true synovial cysts of bone represent late findings seen in a wide range of conditions characterized by degeneration of the articular surface.[40]

Inflammatory TMJ conditions

Inflammatory conditions involving the TMJ, including rheumatoid arthritis, infectious arthritis (eg, late-stage Lyme disease), and reactive inflammatory processes resulting from intra-articular crystalline deposits (eg, gout and pseudogout secondary to monosodium urate and calcium pyrophosphate crystal deposits, respectively) tend to present with overlapping radiographic features similar to what is noted in non-inflammatory degenerative TMJ disease.

Neoplastic conditions

Malignant neoplasms of the TMJ are extremely rare, with metastatic lesions being more common than primary malignancies.[41,42] The initial radiographic presentation has a tendency to mimic the more common degenerative or inflammatory TMJ conditions. More advanced disease will present on CBCT as unilateral destructive lesions with irregular margins. Due to the underlying neoplastic soft tissue component, additional MRI imaging is recommended.

Developmental and traumatically acquired anomalies

CBCT provides valuable treatment-planning data in orthodontic patients presenting with obvious facial asymmetry or a limited range of mandibular movement that characterizes the myriad possible developmental osseous disorders that may involve the TMJ structures. Examples include morphologic changes, condylar hypoplasia, condylar hyperplasia, coronoid hyperplasia, and repaired condylar fractures with residual joint deformities.

The bifid condyle, a rare anomaly characterized by duplication of the condylar head (Fig 12-10), usually presents unilaterally, although extremely rare bilateral cases have been reported.[43] Although the cause of bifid condyle is unknown, it has been suggested that the persistence of a fibrous septum within the cartilaginous condylar head early in its formation may lead to altered condylar head development. Alternatively, trauma to the condylar area during development may play a role.

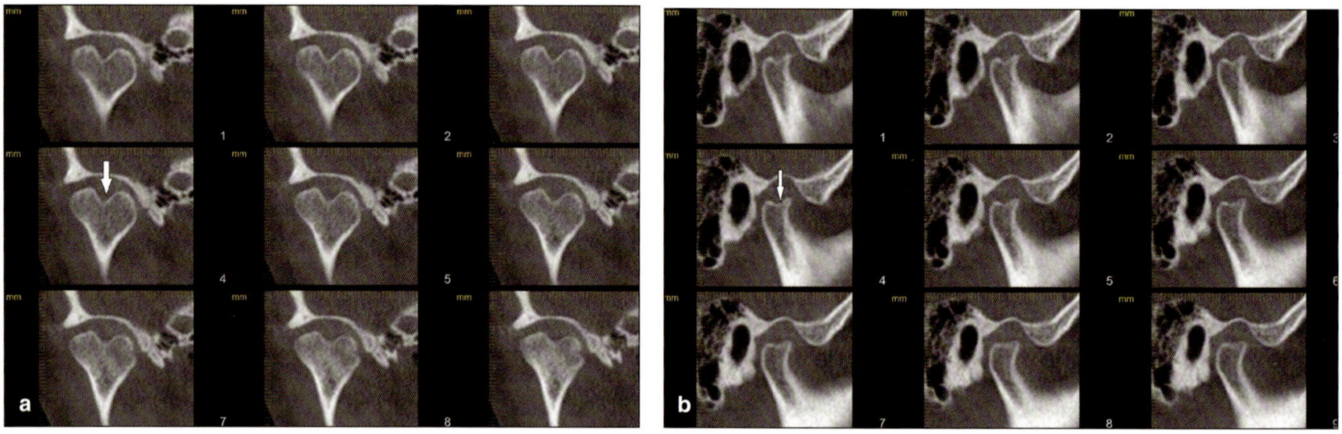

Fig 12-10 Bifid condylar head *(arrow)*. *(a)* Coronal view. *(b)* Sagittal view. The CBCT sections are corrected along the long axis of the condylar head.

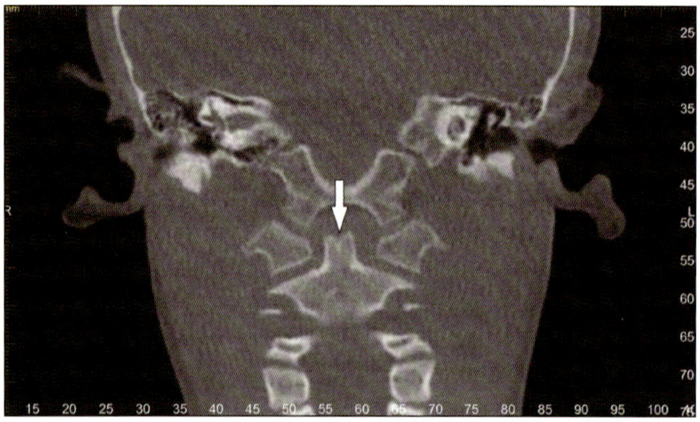

Fig 12-11 Dens bicornis *(arrow)* as shown on a coronal planar CBCT section through the cervical vertebrae.

Cervical Spine

Surface remodeling and changes in bone density

Extended-FOV CBCT scans may be used to assess peak mandibular growth via analysis of cervical vertebrae maturation.[44] Particularly in older patients, these extended-FOV scans will frequently demonstrate remodeling changes of the cervical spine, including flattening, exostosis formation, osteophytes (compensatory outgrowths of bone that form around damaged joints, more commonly known as *bone spurs*), and changes in bone density (both osteopenia and osteosclerosis).

Metastatic lesions to the cervical spine

Malignancies of the cervical spine are relatively uncommon. However, overall the spine is the third most common site for distant cancer metastasis, with the cervical spine involved in 8% to 20% of cases.[45] Malignant neoplasms with a propensity to metastasize to bone include prostate, breast, and colon primaries. These are more common in older adults. Multiple myeloma and lymphomas are relatively common hematogenous malignancies involving bone.

Structural anomalies: Dens bicornis, ponticulus posticus, and ponticulus lateralis

In dens bicornis, the superior aspect of the dens (odontoid process of C2) remains bicornuate. The proatlas is formed from the caudal aspect of the fourth occipital sclerotome and the cranial portion of the first cervical sclerotome (Fig 12-11). The caudal portion of the proatlas gives rise to the apical aspect of the odontoid process, or dens, of C2. The apical portion separates from the basiocciput to join with the basal aspect of the dens, which arises from the first cervical sclerotome. Two ossification centers develop on each side of the basal dental process in utero and normally fuse around the time of birth. Dens bicornis results when the fusion does not occur at the time of ossification of the apical portion of the dens, which is usually between age 3 and 5 years.[46] Fortunately, there are no associated abnormalities in function.

Ponticulus posticus is an abnormality in the atlas consisting of a calcification that completely or partially bridges the vertebral groove of the posterior arch (Fig 12-12). It can form in the first decade of life but appears to be more common after puberty.[47] Lesions can be unilateral or bilateral. Evidence suggests that partial ponticuli tend to progress to complete lesions with age. The prevalence of ponticulus posticus has been reported to range between 1% and 45%.[48] Ponticulus posticus has been related to vertebrobasilar insufficiency syndrome as well as headache, alterations in vision, and difficulty in speaking and swallowing.

Ponticulus lateralis consists of a bridge of bone that extends from the lateral aspect of the superior articular process in an inferior direction to the lateral process of C1 (Fig 12-13). It is less common than ponticulus posticus but may be associated with similar problems.[47]

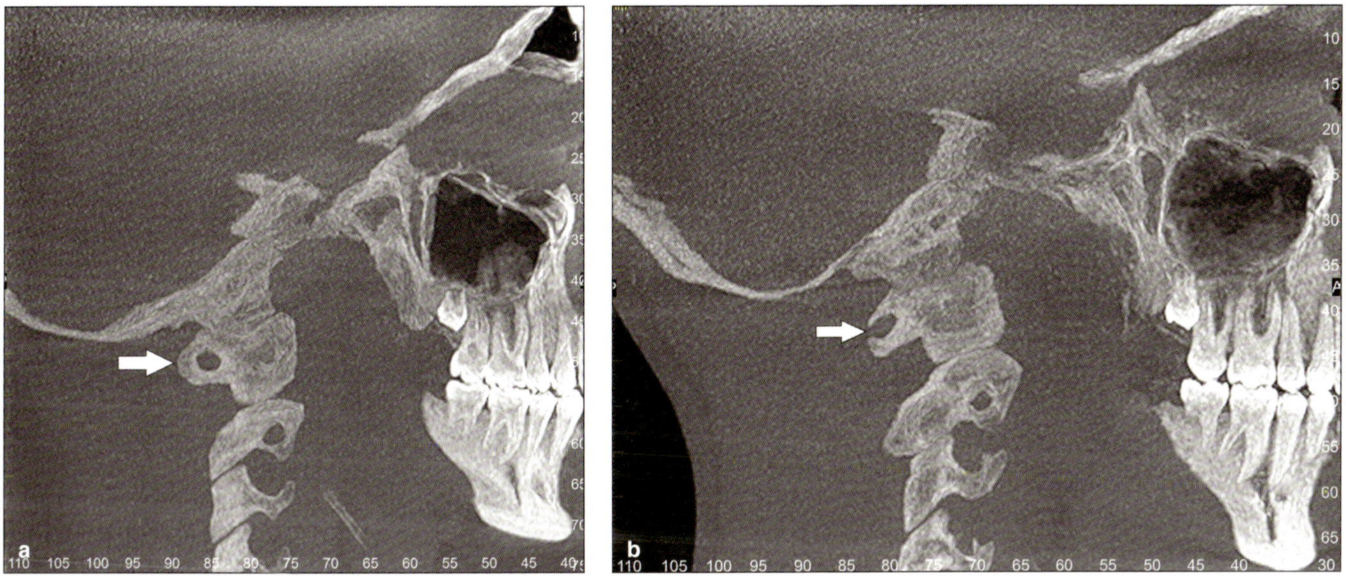

Fig 12-12 Ponticulus posticus *(arrows)* as revealed in sagittal CBCT sections. *(a)* Complete ponticulus posticus in an 11-year-old girl. *(b)* Partial ponticulus posticus in a 17-year-old adolescent boy.

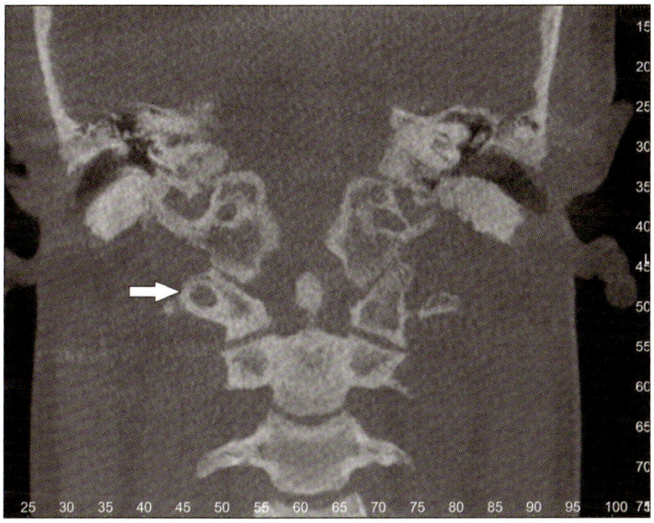

Fig 12-13 Complete ponticulus lateralis *(arrow)* as depicted in a coronal CBCT section.

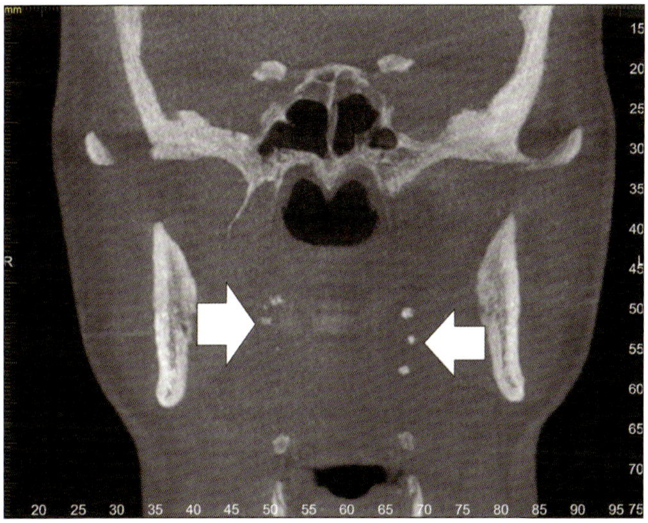

Fig 12-14 Tonsillar calcifications: multiple small bilateral calcifications in the tonsils in the coronal plane *(arrows)*.

Miscellaneous Extracranial Soft Tissue Lesions

Tonsillar calcifications

Tonsilloliths, or tonsillar calcifications, are commonly discovered on CBCT scans (Fig 12-14). These represent a form of dystrophic calcification of entrapped debris, sometimes in association with microorganisms, involving the tonsillar crypts. Recurrent tonsillitis can lead to fibrosis and subsequent dystrophic calcification. Tonsilloliths are commonly asymptomatic, although these can be associated with oral malodor and discomfort involving the throat.[49]

Calcification of carotid artery atheromas

Atherosclerosis is a common disease of adulthood, characterized by deposition of atheromas below the tunica intima of arteries, including the carotid artery. Atheromas, which consist of deposits of lipids containing a mixture of macrophages, fibroblasts, and cell debris, cause narrowing of the artery walls. These lesions can undergo dystrophic calcification, especially

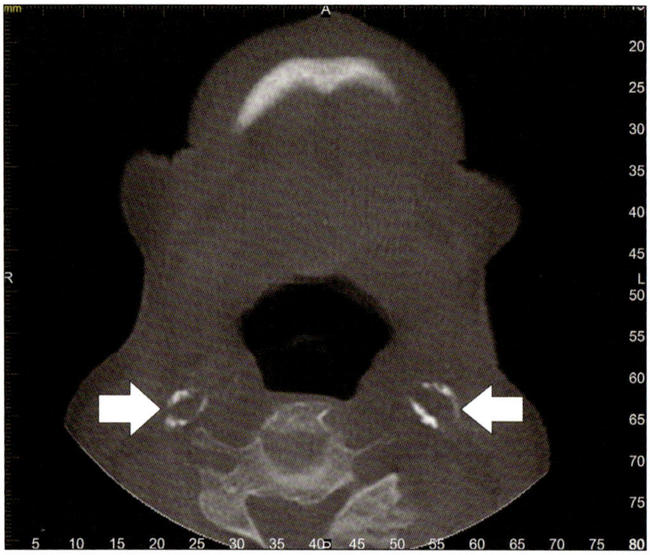

Fig 12-15 Calcified carotid artery atheromas at the bifurcation of the internal and external carotid arteries *(arrows)* as observed in an axial CBCT section.

at sites of shearing force of blood flow such as the bifurcation of the internal and external carotid artery. In the external carotid artery, calcified atheromas appear as curved or linear radiopacities posterolateral to the pharyngeal air space and anterolateral to the anterior tubercle of the transverse process of C3 or C4 when viewed in the axial plane[50] (Fig 12-15).

Cosmetic implants involving the chin, cheek, and other soft tissue structures are identified in CBCT scans as foreign bodies of varying size, shape, and density.

Conclusion

The increasing use of CBCT in orthodontic treatment planning has also heightened the need for practitioners to be able to identify and knowledgeably assess the full spectrum of pathologic entities and anatomical variants that may be seen within the extended CBCT FOV that is acquired when generating data for 3D cephalometric reconstruction. This chapter has briefly reviewed several representative pathologies, but the examples provided are not intended to cover the full spectrum of pathologies that may be encountered.

References

1. Ahmed F, Brooks SL, Kapila SD. Efficacy of identifying maxillofacial lesions in cone-beam computed tomographs by orthodontists and orthodontic residents with third-party software. Am J Orthod Dentofacial Orthop 2012;141:451–459.
2. Zinman EJ, White SC, Tetradis S. Legal considerations in the use of cone beam computer tomography imaging. J Calif Dent Assoc 2010;38:49–56.
3. Price JB, Thaw KL, Tyndall DA, Ludlow JB, Padilla RJ. Incidental findings from cone beam computed tomography of the maxillofacial region: A descriptive retrospective study. Clin Oral Implants Res 2012;23:1261–1268.
4. Cha JY, Mah J, Sinclair P. Incidental findings in the maxillofacial area with 3-dimensional cone-beam imaging. Am J Orthod Dentofacial Orthop 2007;132:7–14.
5. Cağlayan F, Tozoğlu U. Incidental findings in the maxillofacial region detected by cone beam CT. Diagn Interv Radiol 2012;18:159–163.
6. Benavides E, Edwards PC. Detection and diagnosis of incidental findings in CBCT imaging and their clinical implications. In: Kapila S (ed). Cone Beam Computed Tomography in Orthodontics: Indications, Insights, and Innovations. Ames, IA:Wiley-Blackwell, 2014:185–219.
7. Tetradis S, Kantor ML. Prevalence of skeletal and dental anomalies and normal variants seen in cephalometric and other radiographs of orthodontic patients. Am J Orthod Dentofacial Orthop 1999;116:572–577.
8. Sedghizadeh PP, Nguyen M, Enciso R. Intracranial physiological calcifications evaluated with cone beam CT. Dentomaxillofac Radiol 2012;41:675–678.
9. de Weert TT, Cakir H, Rozie S, et al. Intracranial internal carotid artery calcifications: Association with vascular risk factors and ischemic cerebrovascular disease. AJNR Am J Neuroradiol 2009;30(1):177–184.
10. Bos D, van der Rijk MJ, Geeraedts TE, et al. Intracranial carotid artery atherosclerosis: Prevalence and risk factors in the general population. Stroke 2012;43:1878–1884.
11. Bos D, Portegies ML, van der Lugt A, et al. Intracranial carotid artery atherosclerosis and the risk of stroke in whites: The Rotterdam Study. JAMA Neurol 2014;71:405–411.
12. Edwards PC, Scanlon C, Norton N, Saini T. Review of extragnathic pathology noted during routine volumetric computed tomography [Abstract from the AAOMP annual conference, 7–8 May 2007, Kansas City, MO]. Oral Surg Oral Med Oral Pathol Oral Radiol Endod 2007;103(suppl 1).
13. Scanlon C, Saini T, Norton N, Edwards PC. Systematic protocol for cone beam computed tomography interpretation. J Dent Res 2007;86(special issue A):466.
14. Vogiatzi T, Kloukos D, Scarfe WC, Bornstein MM. Incidence of anatomical variations and disease of the maxillary sinuses as identified by cone beam computed tomography: A systematic review. Int J Oral Maxillofac Implants 2014;29:1301–1314.
15. Ritter L, Lutz J, Neugebauer J, et al. Prevalence of pathologic findings in the maxillary sinus in cone-beam computerized tomography. Oral Surg Oral Med Oral Pathol Oral Radiol Endod 2011;111:634–640.
16. Nascimento EH, Pontual ML, Pontual AA, Freitas DQ, Perez DE, Ramos-Perez FM. Association between odontogenic conditions and maxillary sinus disease: A study using cone-beam computed tomography. J Endod 2016;42:1509–1515.
17. Mehra P, Jeong D. Maxillary sinusitis of odontogenic origin. Curr Allergy Asthma Rep 2009;9:238–243.
18. Shanbhag S, Karnik P, Shirke P, Shanbhag V. Association between periapical lesions and maxillary sinus mucosal thickening: A retrospective cone-beam computed tomographic study. J Endod 2013;39:853–857.
19. Bourek H, Saini TS, Edwards PC, et al. Incidental recognition of sphenoid sinus pathosis during routine cone beam computed tomography of dental patients. J Dent Res 2008;87(special issue A):240.
20. Rosenfeld RM, Andes D, Bhattacharyya N, et al. Clinical practice guideline: Adult sinusitis. Otolaryngol Head Neck Surg 2007;137(suppl):S1–S31.
21. Hamilos DL. Chronic rhinosinusitis: Epidemiology and medical management. J Allergy Clin Immunol 2011;128:693–707.
22. Zinreich SJ, Mattox DE, Kennedy DW, Chisholm HL, Diffley DM, Rosenbaum AE. Concha bullosa: CT evaluation. J Comput Assist Tomogr 1988;12:778–784.
23. Smith KD, Lanphier TF, Edwards PC, et al. Using cone beam computed tomography (CBCT) imaging to study the incidence of concha bullosa in the nasal cavity. Clin Anat 2010;23:490.
24. Smith KD, Edwards PC, Saini TS, Norton NS. The prevalence of concha bullosa and nasal septal deviation and their relationship to maxillary sinusitis by volumetric tomography. Int J Dent 2010;2010:404982.
25. Bolger WE, Butzin CA, Parsons DS. Paranasal sinus bony anatomic variations and mucosal abnormalities: CT analysis for endoscopic sinus surgery. Laryngoscope 1991;101:56–64.
26. Stallman JS, Lobo JN, Som PM. The incidence of concha bullosa and its relationship to nasal septal deviation and paranasal sinus disease. AJNR Am J Neuroradiol 2004;25:1613–1618.

27. Subramanian S, Lekhraj Rampal GR, Wong EF, Mastura S, Razi A. Concha bullosa in chronic sinusitis. Med J Malaysia 2005;60:535–539.
28. Lam WW, Liang EY, Woo JK, Van Hasselt A, Metreweli C. The etiological role of concha bullosa in chronic sinusitis. Eur Radiol 1996;6:550–552.
29. Goncalves FG, Jovem CL, de Oliveira Moura L. Computed tomography of intra- and extramural ethmoid cells: Iconographic essay. Radiol Bras 2011;44:321–326.
30. Carter LC, Calamel A, Haller A, Aguirre A. Seasonal variation in maxillary antral pseudocysts in a general clinic population. Dentomaxillofac Radiol 1998;27:22–24.
31. Franco-Carro B, Barona-Dorado C, Martínez-González MJ, Rubio-Alonso LJ, Martínez-González JM. Meta-analytic study on the frequency and treatment of oral antral communications. Med Oral Patol Oral Cir Bucal 2011;16:e682–687.
32. Leung YY, Wong WY, Cheung LK. Surgical ciliated cysts may mimic radicular cysts or residual cysts of maxilla: Report of 3 cases. J Oral Maxillofac Surg 2012;70:e264–e269.
33. Güneri P, Kaya A, Calişkan MK. Antroliths: Survey of the literature and report of a case. Oral Surg Oral Med Oral Pathol Oral Radiol Endod 2005;99:517–521.
34. Karligkiotis A, Lepera D, Volpi L, et al. Survival outcomes after endoscopic resection for sinonasal squamous cell carcinoma arising on inverted papilloma. Head Neck 2016;38:1604–1614.
35. Franchi A, Miligi L, Palomba A, et al. Sinonasal carcinomas: Recent advances in molecular and phenotypic characterization and their clinical implications. Crit Rev Oncol Hematol 2011;79:265–277.
36. Edwards PC, Hess SJ, Saini T. Sinonasal undifferentiated carcinoma of the maxillary sinus. J Can Dent Assoc 2006;72:163–167.
37. Edwards PC. Pathology of the hard tissues of the jaws. In: Rosen CJ (ed), American Society for Bone and Mineral Research. Primer on the Metabolic Bone Diseases and Disorders of Mineral Metabolism, ed 8. Ames, IA: Wiley-Blackwell, 2013:922–927.
38. Wasserburger M, Dendinger EJ, Edwards PC, et al. Assessing bone density changes in condyles using cone beam CT. J Dent Res 2007;86(special issue A):461.
39. Wasserburger M, Edwards PC, Saini TS, Norton NS. A comparison of dental iCAT scans and routine histological slides in observing osteoarthritic changes in the mandibular condyles of cadavers. Fed Am Soc Exp Biol J 2007;21:623–624.
40. Sano T, Yamamoto M, Okano T, Gokan T, Westesson PL. Common abnormalities in temporomandibular joint imaging. Curr Probl Diagn Radiol 2004;33:16–24.
41. dos Santos DT, Cavalcanti MG. Osteosarcoma of the temporomandibular joint: Report of 2 cases. Oral Surg Oral Med Oral Pathol Oral Radiol Endod 2002;94:641–647.
42. Kruse AL, Luebbers HT, Obwegeser JA, Edelmann L, Graetz KW. Temporomandibular disorders associated with metastases to the temporomandibular joint: A review of the literature and 3 additional cases. Oral Surg Oral Med Oral Pathol Oral Radiol Endod 2010;110:e21–e28.
43. Gunduz K, Avsever H, Karacayli U. Bilateral bifid condylar process. Int J Morphol 2010;28:941–944.
44. Baccetti T, Franchi L, McNamara JA Jr. An improved version of the cervical vertebral maturation (CVM) method for the assessment of mandibular growth. Angle Orthod 2002;72:316–323.
45. Molina CA, Gokaslan ZL, Sciubba DM. Diagnosis and management of metastatic cervical spine tumors. Orthop Clin North Am 2012;43:75–87.
46. Pang D, Thompson DN. Embryology and bony malformations of the craniovertebral junction. Childs Nerv Syst 2011;27:523–564.
47. Geist JR, Geist SM, Lin LM. A cone beam CT investigation of ponticulus posticus and lateralis in children and adolescents. Dentomaxillofac Radiol 2014;43:20130451.
48. Sekerci AE, Soylu E, Arikan MP, Ozcan G, Amuk M, Kocoglu F. Prevalence and morphologic characteristics of ponticulus posticus: Analysis using cone-beam computed tomography. J Chiropr Med 2015;14:153–161.
49. Chan J, Rashid M, Karagama Y. An unusual case of a tonsillolith. Case Rep Med 2012;2012:587503.
50. MacDonald D, Chan A, Harris A, Vertinsky T, Farman AG, Scarfe WC. Diagnosis and management of calcified carotid artery atheroma: Dental perspectives. Oral Surg Oral Med Oral Pathol Oral Radiol 2012;114:533–547.

13

The Cost of 2D Versus 3D Radiology

Eric Dellinger, DDS, MSD

"Risk comes from not knowing what you're doing."

— Warren Buffett

Though many academic journals have promoted the additional information and efficacy of three-dimensional (3D) scans relative to panoramic-cephalometric machines, usage and cost considerations of this technology are also important. Even if we could know exactly what treatment outcomes are best based on radiology, a $25,000 radiographic scan would be prohibitively expensive at a time when average orthodontic fees are in the $6,000 to $9,000 range. The cost of radiology must also be assessed relative to usage. Information used on a daily basis may have much more clinical value than information that is only used once a month.

With this in mind, I reviewed my practice usage of our in-office LED Dental 3D machine (Fig 13-1) relative to the use of two-dimensional (2D) panoramic-cephalometric images. Cost and training were also reviewed, and the information below reflects this data based on 2016 costs. This exercise is just one example of the decision-making necessary in acquiring new technology for a private orthodontic office.

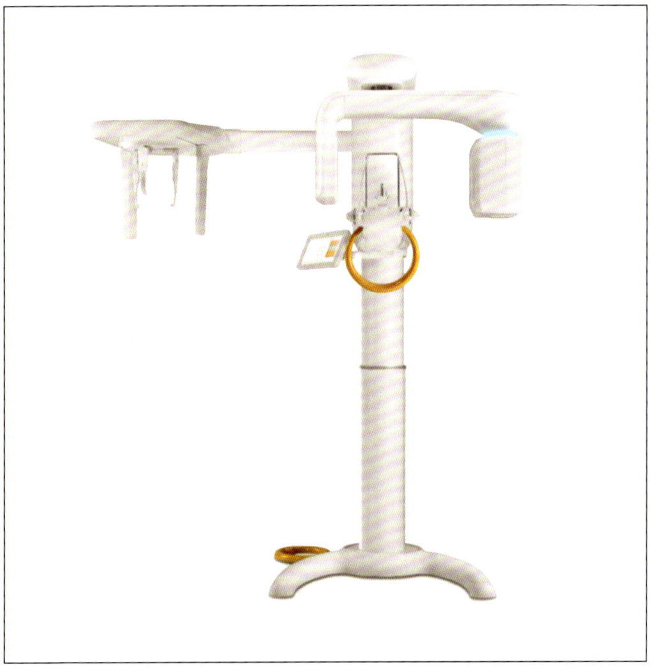

Fig 13-1 LED Dental 3D imaging machine used in the author's practice.

Table 13-1 2016 costs of panoramic and cone beam machines

Manufacturer	2D cost[a]	3D cost[b]	Software cost
Encompass/Panoramic	$37,000 to $43,000	NA	NA
Sirona 3D Orthophos	NA	$145,000	NA
LED Dental	$41,000	$85,000	$1,795
Carestream/Orthotrac	$37,999	$79,999	$1,495
Planmeca	$56,000	$121,000 to $131,000	NA
Soredex	$43,000	NA	NA

NA, not applicable.
[a] Digital panoramic-cephalometric machine.
[b] Cone beam system.

Overall Relative Cost of 2D Versus 3D Digital Imaging

In my review of costs, I found a $42,000 to $44,000 increase in cost for a 3D machine relative to a traditional panoramic-cephalometric machine. This is significantly reduced from the difference of $100,000 or more that was the norm a few years ago. Nonetheless, this cost is a twofold increase in the normal cost for digital x-ray equipment, and thus this expense must be covered by supplemental treatment fees. In addition to the extra expense of the hardware, the 3D software costs another $2,000.

On average, our office has used our 3D scanner eight times per month since we purchased it. On an annual basis, therefore, we use it 96 times per year (8 × 12 = 96). The machine cost $85,000 (compared with $41,000 for the 2D panoramic-cephalometric machine), which means in the first year each 3D scan cost us an average of $458 (the difference in machine cost, $44,000, divided by 96). Assuming the increased cost is amortized over a 3-year period, the average cost per scan would decrease to about $153, but then there is also the increased cost of financing. At 5% interest, the difference in expenditure in the first year would be approximately $2,200 financing costs per year on $44,000.

Given this significant expense, the question becomes "is this worth the cost"? The ability to refine diagnosis for patients with clefts, impacted canines, or craniofacial dysostosis might be a rarity in some offices. Within my own office, each year we see about 12 patients with clefts, 100 patients with impacted teeth, and 24 patients presenting for clear aligner treatment. Thus, in my practice we see only 136 patients per year who can potentially benefit from the 3D scan. Again, this is relative to my own practice, and a review of your own numbers involving clear retainers, clefts, and impactions would be wise before engaging in the cost analysis of the 3D machine.

Another cost involves staff training. Under the assumption that the average staff member costs about $20 per hour, and my staff required training over 8 hours for 10 people, our training costs approximated $1,600. Assuming some extra phone calls involved with follow-up questions, it is not unreasonable to anticipate around $2,000 in training costs.

With all of these extra charges, the final cost of the machine over a 3-year period is $2,000 training + $85,000 machine cost + finance costs of $6,711 (if the total of $85,000 is financed at 5% over 3 years) + sales tax (7% in Indiana) $5,950 = $99,661. Thus, much like automobile purchases, the total cost of the machine can be deceptively higher than the reduced sticker price may appear. As always, when approaching a significant expense for your practice, professional advice from your accountant may be very helpful in avoiding unpleasant surprises. The choice of charging more for 3D scans and submitting this charge to medical insurance is also an option to defray costs, but development of this reimbursement technique is beyond the scope of this book.

Additional costs for shipping and warranties may also be involved with the purchase of a new machine. We found the highest cost for shipping and warranties to be $2,300 and $5,000, respectively, and both of these highest charges involved a specific brand of unit. Additional costs may be incurred as a result of difficulties with proper function and training of use of these machines. In discussions with my staff, they expressed concerns about poor customer service, product function, and training with our previous hardware, and this directly affected my personal decision to purchase our 3D unit. I would not advise purchase of any unit, regardless of price or features, if the company has failed to provide you with excellent customer service.

So what is a reasonable monthly expenditure for a 3D machine? If we assume a $100,000 cost divided over a 3-year amortization period, this comes to $2,778 per month. Assuming 20 uses per month, this leaves a cost of $138 per usage of the machine. By the same token, a 2D panoramic-cephalometric machine used 40 times a month at an initial cost of $45,000 (including some financing and training fees as well) comes to a price of only $62.50 per usage. Allowing these rough estimates, we see that the cost of 3D digital radiology will be about twice the cost of panoramic radiology. While the advantages of surgical evaluation of sinus structure and bone support can be invaluable in situations of cleft repair and impacted canines and third molars, and although this information is useful to the orthodontist, the cost may exceed that of a referral to a radiology clinic for a magnetic resonance imaging (MRI) or 3D scan for evaluation of the patient, particularly in offices with fewer patients (Table 13-1).

Conclusion

Despite the additional monetary costs involved with 3D imaging, I find the personal reassurance of knowing the exact location of impactions and clefts to be of significant value. The confidence and reassurance of knowing the precise positions of anatomy can lead to a much happier and confident clinician as well as a better treatment result for our patients. The cost of the 3D scan can thus produce several psychologic benefits, and these benefits can easily justify the additional cost for many clinicians. Given the advantages of 3D technology, it seems likely that we will continue to see improvements in this technology as well as increases in its use within dentistry and specifically within the practice of orthodontics.

14

Clinical Cases

Ahmed Ghoneima, BDS, PhD, MSD
Katherine Kula, MS, DMD, MS

Authors' note: Please see Table 3-1 for descriptions and definitions of all landmarks not otherwise defined in this chapter.

Case 1

Initial medical history

A 9-year-old Caucasian boy was referred from the Cleft and Craniofacial Team with a diagnosis of cleft lip and no other significant medical history.

Photographic and clinical evaluation

The profile showed slight protrusion of the lips (Fig 14-1a). Frontal views at rest and smiling showed scarring of the right upper lip and an anterior crossbite with noncoincident midlines (Figs 14-1b and 14-1c). The nose and smile were asymmetric, with the right ear more prominent. Intraoral photographs showed a Class I molar relationship, noncoincident midlines, an anterior crossbite, small maxillary lateral incisors, and crowding in both arches (Figs 14-1d to 14-1h). The gingival tissue distal to the maxillary right central incisor was erythemic, and an unusually thick white frenum was present between the right central and lateral incisors. The maxillary occlusal view showed unusual erythema and a palatal indentation from the area of the right lateral incisor to the midpalatal raphae, but no fistula (see Fig 14-1g). Generalized erythema, gingival swelling, and plaque were noted.

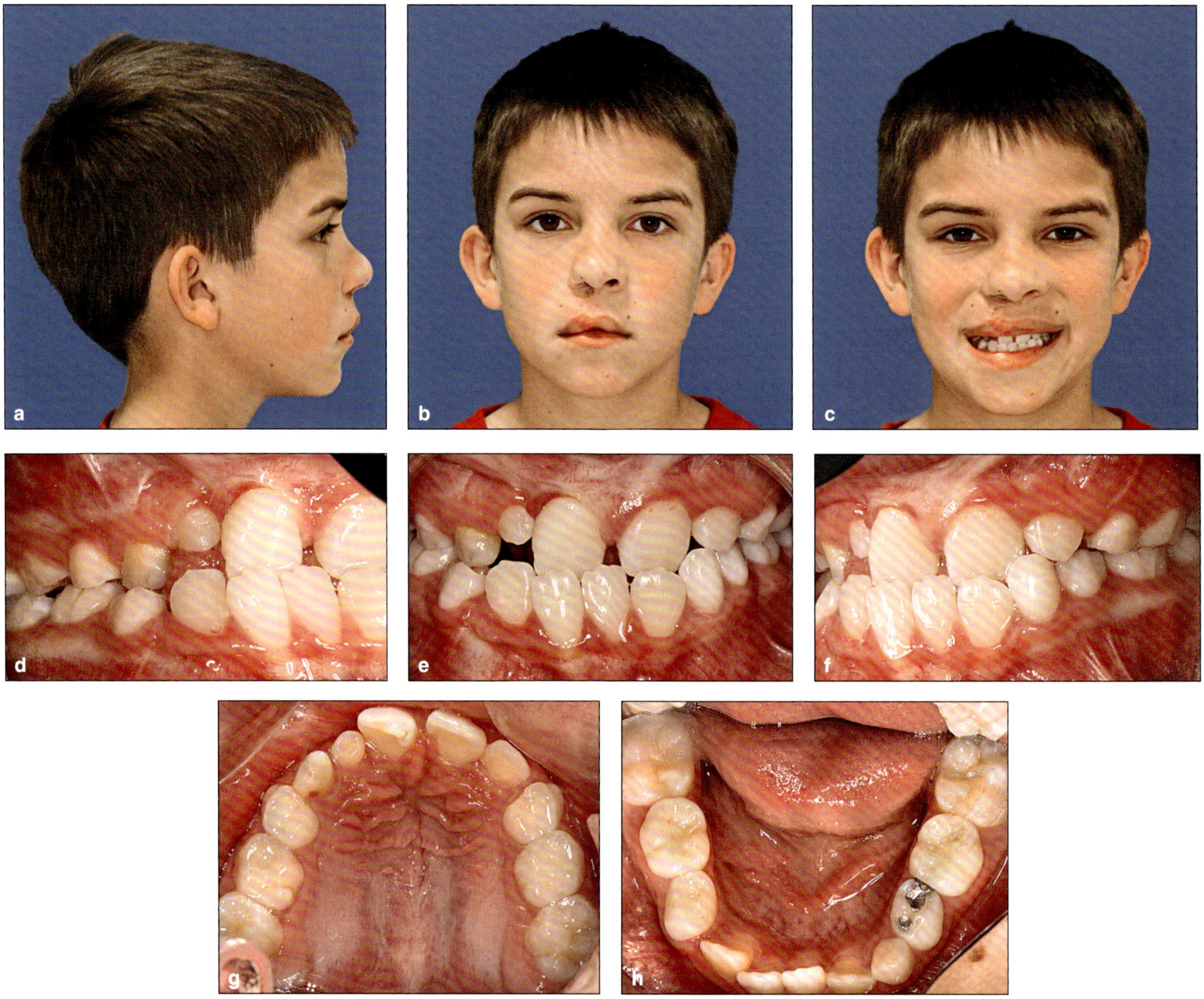

Fig 14-1 *(a to h)* Pretreatment extraoral and intraoral photographs.

Cephalometric evaluation

The measures for the maxilla were contradictory (Fig 14-1i and Table 14-1). Compared with the cranial base, the maxilla was within normal limits (SNA), but it was short according to ANS-PNS. The maxilla was protrusive according to A-N perp. Some of the discrepancy was probably due to the interference of the upright maxillary incisors with A-point identification. The occlusal plane to SN was steeper than normal, although the palatal plane to SN was within the normal range. This was probably due to the overeruption and retroclination of the maxillary incisors.

The mandible was recessive compared with the cranial base (SNB, SNPg, B-N perp, Pg-N perp, mandibular length) but expected to grow with age. The Frankfort mandibular angle (FMA) was within normal limits, but the cranial base to mandibular plane (SN-MP) was excessive. The differential between the

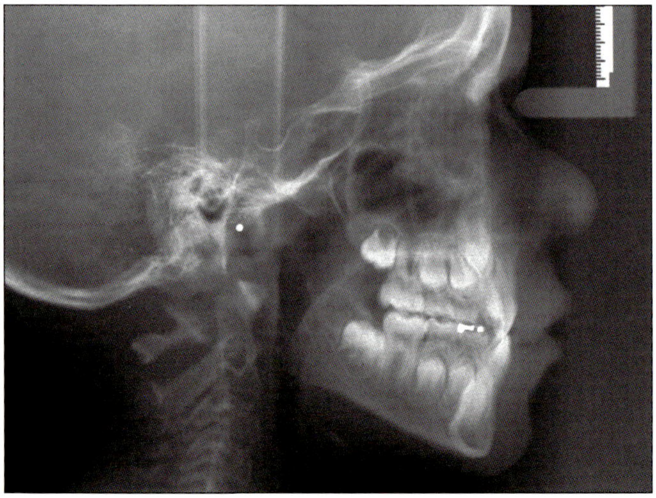

Fig 14-1i Pretreatment lateral cephalogram.

Table 14-1 Case 1 pretreatment cephalometric values

Group/measurement	Value	Norm	SD	Dev norm
Maxilla to cranial base				
SNA (degrees)	79.8	82.0	3.5	–0.6
SN-PP (degrees)	10.0	8.0	3.0	0.7
SN-OP (degrees)	28.3	14.4	2.5	5.5*****
A-N perp (mm)	2.6	0.0	2.0	1.3*
Mandible to cranial base				
SNB (degrees)	73.7	80.9	3.4	–2.1**
SNPg (degrees)	73.5	80.0	3.5	–1.9*
FMA (MP-FH) (degrees)	28.1	25.6	4.5	0.5
SN-MP (degrees)	38.5	32.9	5.2	1.1*
MP-OP (degrees)	11.9	15.3	5.0	–0.7
B-N perp (mm)	–5.3	–6.0	8.0	0.1
Pg-N perp (mm)	–6.0	–5.0	4.0	–0.3
y-axis (SGnSN) (degrees)	70.9	67.0	5.5	0.7
Maxilla to mandible				
ANB (degrees)	6.1	1.6	1.5	3.0***
PP-MP (degrees)	30.2	25.0	6.0	0.9
Wits appraisal (mm)	–2.0	–1.0	1.0	–1.0*
Maxillary length (ANS-PNS) (mm)	41.9	51.6	4.3	–2.3**
Mandibular length (CoGn) (mm)	96.0	111.6	4.0	–3.9***
Cranial base				
BaSN (degrees)	127.5	130.0	5.0	–0.5
Upper incisors to maxilla				
U1-SN (degrees)	72.9	102.3	5.5	–5.3*****
U1-NA (degrees)	–6.8	22.8	5.7	–5.2*****
U1-NA (mm)	–5.3	4.3	2.7	–3.5***
U1-PP (degrees)	83.0	110.0	5.0	–5.4*****
Lower incisors to mandible				
L1-MP (degrees)	87.6	95.0	7.0	–1.1*
L1-NB (degrees)	22.3	25.3	6.0	–0.5
L1-NB (mm)	4.0	4.0	1.8	0.0
L1 protrusion (L1-APg) (mm)	0.6	1.0	2.3	–0.2
Incisors to each other				
Interincisal angle (U1-L1) (degrees)	158.4	130.0	6.0	4.7****
Soft tissue				
Upper lip to E-plane (mm)	1.2	–3.0	2.0	2.1**
Lower lip to E-plane (mm)	1.9	–2.5	2.5	1.8*
ILG (HP) (mm)	1.1	2.0	2.0	–0.4
Nasolabial angle (CoLSnUL) (degrees)	95.3	102.0	8.0	–0.8
H-angle (Pg′UL-Pg′N′) (degrees)	21.4	10.0	4.0	2.9**
LFH (Sn′Me′) (mm)	66.5	63.0	3.0	1.2*

(cont)

Table 14-1 (cont) **Case 1 pretreatment cephalometric values**

Group/measurement	Value	Norm	SD	Dev norm
Facial proportions (hard tissue)				
UFH (N-ANS) (mm)	45.4	50.0	2.5	–1.8*
LFH (ANS-Me) (mm)	60.9	60.0	4.5	0.2
UFH (N-ANS/[N-ANS+ANS-Me]) (%)	42.8	45.0	5.0	–0.4
LFH (ANS-Me/[N-ANS+ANS-Me]) (%)	57.2	57.0	5.0	0.0
Posterior face height (ArGo) (mm)	28.9	40.5	4.5	–2.6**
PFH:AFH (CoGo:NMe) (%)	46.0	60.0	1.0	–14.0******
Profile				
Convexity (NA-APg) (degrees)	13.7	9.2	3.0	1.5*
Facial angle (FH-NPg) (degrees)	86.5	86.9	3.0	–0.1

Dev norm, deviation from the norm; PP, palatal plane; OP, occlusal plane; MP, mandibular plane; U1, maxillary incisor; L1, mandibular incisor; ILG (HP), interlabial gap (horizontal plane); CoL, condylion lateral; UL, upper lip; UFH, upper face height; LFH, lower face height; PFH:AFH, posterior face height to anterior face height.
*Each asterisk represents a standard deviation (SD).

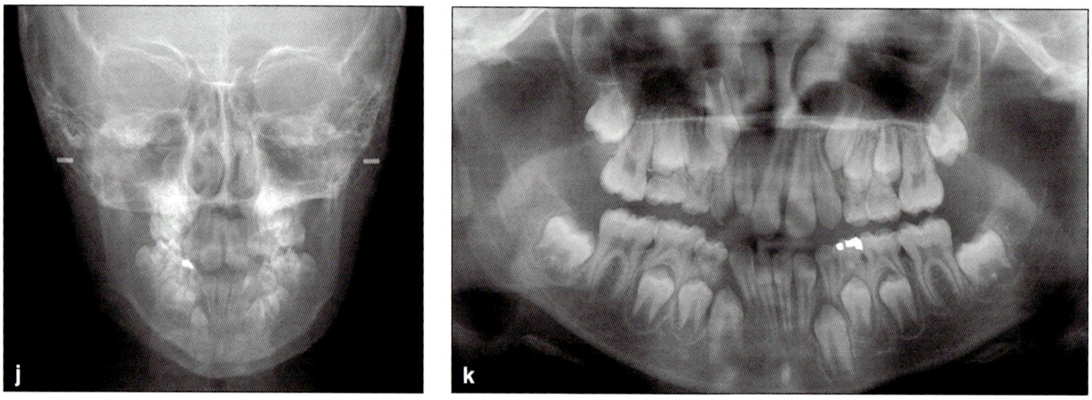

Fig 14-1 *(cont)* *(j)* Pretreatment frontal cephalogram. *(k)* Pretreatment panoramic radiograph.

maxilla and the mandible (ANB, Wits appraisal) was greater than the norm, indicating a Class II skeletal pattern.

The maxillary incisors were retroclined (U1-SN, U1-NA, U1-PP) and retrusive (U1-NA in mm). The mandibular incisors were retroclined to the mandibular plane (L1-MP) but within the normal range for the facial profile (L1-NB), and they were within the normal range for protrusion (L1-NB in mm, L1-APg). The interincisal angle exceeded the normal range, confirming upright incisors. The overjet and overbite were smaller than the normal range.

Both lips were protrusive (upper lip to E-plane and lower lip to E-plane), and facial proportion measurements indicated that the upper face height (NaMe, G′Sn′) was shorter than the norm, while the lower face height (Sn′Me′) was greater than the norm. The posterior face height was shorter than the norm and probably confirmed the increased mandibular plane to cranial base angle.

The profile (NA-APg) was more convex than the norm, confirming the mandibular retrusion, whereas the facial angle (FH-NPg) indicated that the profile was within normal limits. The cervical vertebral maturation (CVM) stage was 1 to 2, indicating growth potential.

An initial frontal cephalogram (Fig 14-1j) showed some asymmetry but no obvious clefting.

Panoramic evaluation

The panoramic radiograph showed probable impaction of the maxillary right canine and an indentation of the alveolar bone in the area between a microdont lateral incisor and the right central incisor (Fig 14-1k). The indentation appeared to continue toward the alveolar crest.

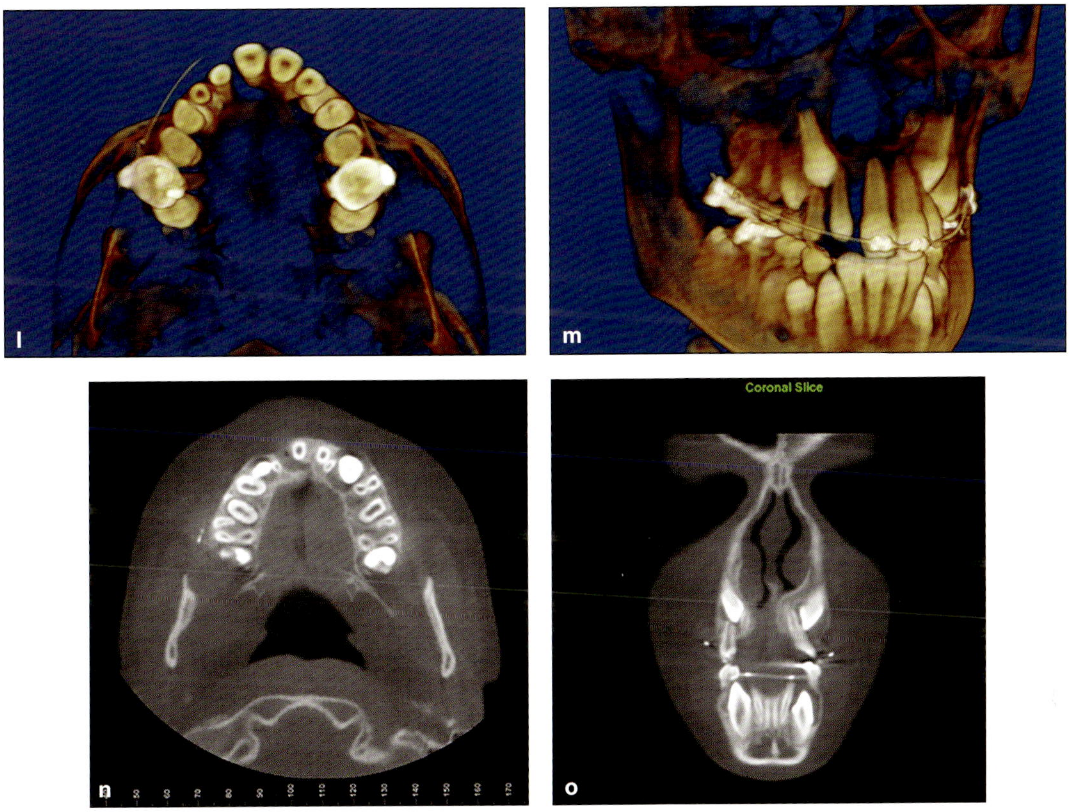

Fig 14-1 *(cont)* *(l and m)* Progress 3D CBCT reconstructions showing the cleft from an axial view and a semilateral view. *(n)* Axial CBCT section showing the cleft with lack of alveolar continuity between the right lateral and central incisors. *(o)* Coronal CBCT section showing the position of the maxillary canines relative to the lateral incisor roots.

CBCT evaluation

The case was started based on the lateral and frontal cephalograms and panoramic radiograph, and the patient was not scheduled for an alveolar graft or extractions. During re-evaluation of the case, the decision was made to take a three-dimensional (3D) cone beam computed tomography (CBCT) scan based on the appearance of the anterior maxillary arch, the frenum, the nasal asymmetry, and the grooving in the panoramic radiograph (see Fig 14-1k). Review of the 3D CBCT reconstruction showed obvious clefting from the frontal view (Fig 14-1l), and an axial cut at the level of the alveolar crest revealed a cleft between the right central and lateral incisors (Figs 14-1m and 14-1n) that was masked in the panoramic radiograph by two overlapping pieces of alveolar bone. The alveolar bone anterior to the maxillary and mandibular incisors was minimal. The alveolar bone palatal to the maxillary right central incisor was also minimal.

Classification

This case was classified as a Class I molar, Class II skeletal malocclusion with alveolar clefting, possible impaction of the right canine (Fig 14-1o), crowding, and minimal alveolar bone.

Treatment plan

Re-evaluation of the case resulted in a two-phase treatment. The objectives of phase I were to correct the anterior crossbite, achieve coincident midlines pending grafting of the cleft, obtain alveolar continuity via surgical grafting in the anterior right maxilla, relieve crowding via extraction of the maxillary lateral incisors and mandibular first premolars and primary first molars and maintain the spaces until the maxillary canines erupted, and improve the gingival health and level of oral hygiene. The distal and lingual movement of the maxillary right central incisor needed to be minimized until after alveolar grafting to prevent the root from entering the cleft.

The objectives of phase II were to maintain the Class I molar relationships, perform canine substitution for the maxillary lateral incisors, and coordinate the arches.

Final evaluation

The final photographs reveal a straight facial profile with a relatively well-balanced face (Figs 14-1p to 14-1w). The midlines are coincident, the canines are anatomically reasonable substitutes for the lateral incisors, and the molars are in Class I relationships but need to settle. The arches are coordinated with Class I molar relationships (Fig 14-1x). The tissue is slightly erythematous in the area of the former cleft.

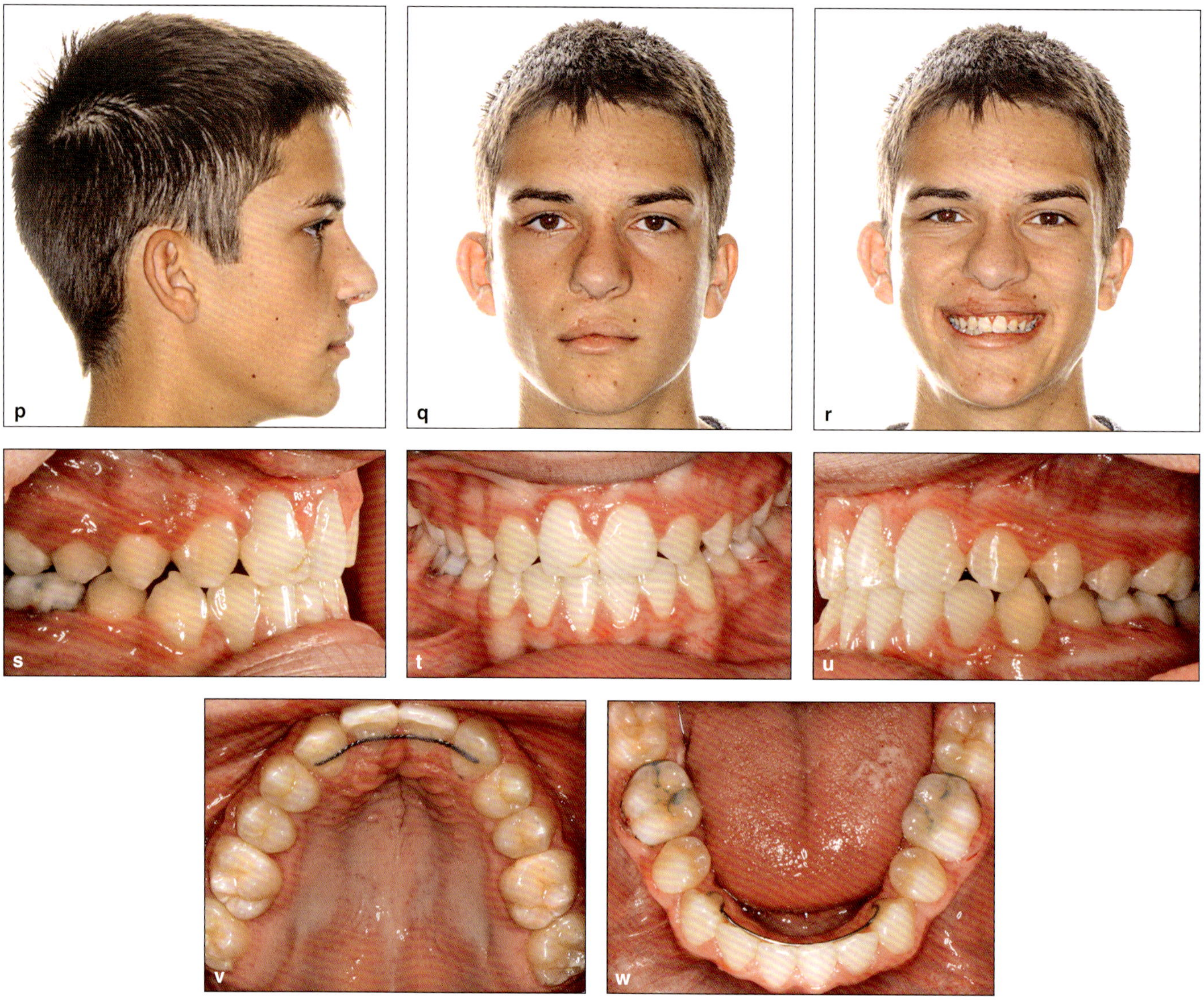

Fig 14-1 *(cont)* *(p to w)* Posttreatment extraoral and intraoral photographs.

Cephalometric analysis

The differential between the maxilla and mandible decreased appreciably (SNB, SNPg, B-N perp, and Pg-N perp increased, and ANB decreased) (Fig 14-1y). The maxilla appeared to grow smaller, the difference probably affected by the change in A-point, which was misidentified in the initial radiograph due to the upright maxillary incisors. The palatal plane to mandibular plane angle decreased considerably, as did SN-OP. The maxillary incisor became more proclined (U1-SN, U1-NA, and U1-PP) and more protrusive (U1-NA in mm). The mandibular incisor reclined more (L1-MP, L1-NB) and was more retrusive (L1-NB in mm), although L1-APg was still within the normal range. The interincisal angle became smaller, confirming the proclination of the maxillary incisors. Table 14-2 shows all of the posttreatment cephalometric values.

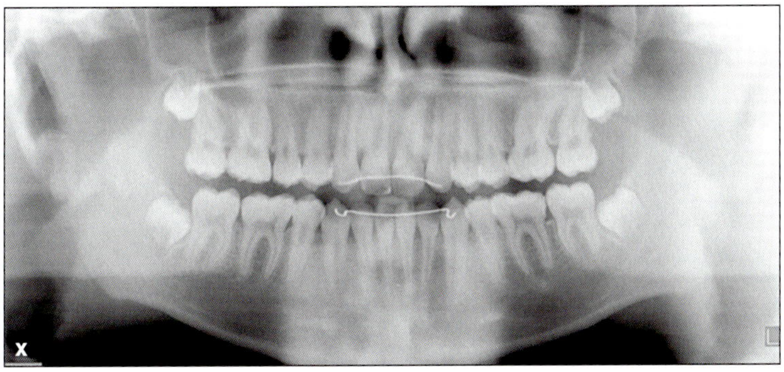

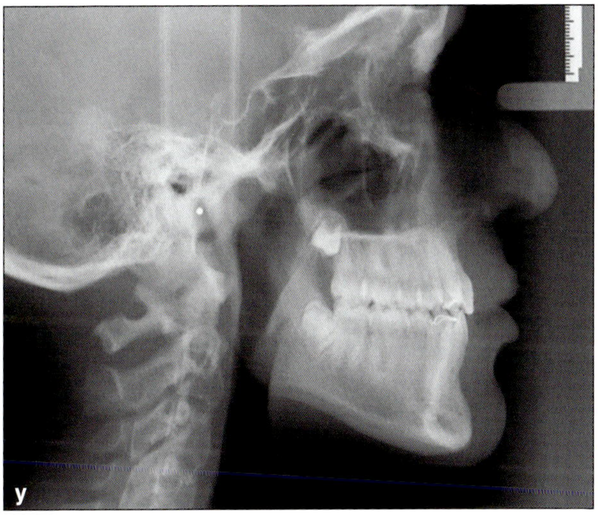

Fig 14-1 *(cont)* *(x)* Posttreatment panoramic radiograph. *(y)* Posttreatment lateral cephalogram.

Table 14-2 **Case 1 posttreatment cephalometric values**

Group/measurement	Value	Norm	SD	Dev norm
Maxilla to cranial base				
SNA (degrees)	75.4	82.0	3.5	–1.9*
SN-PP (degrees)	9.0	8.0	3.0	0.3
SN-OP (degrees)	22.0	14.4	2.5	3.0***
A-N perp (mm)	–1.0	0.0	2.0	–0.5
Mandible to cranial base				
SNB (degrees)	74.6	80.9	3.4	–1.9*
SNPg (degrees)	76.2	80.0	3.5	–1.1*
FMA (MP-FH) (degrees)	23.5	23.6	4.5	0.0
SN-MP (degrees)	34.5	32.9	5.2	0.3
MP-OP (degrees)	12.5	17.7	5.0	–1.0*
B-N perp (mm)	–3.0	–6.0	8.0	0.4
Pg-N perp (mm)	–0.3	2.0	4.0	–0.6
y-axis (SGnSN) (degrees)	70.4	67.0	5.5	0.6
Maxilla to mandible				
ANB (degrees)	0.8	1.6	1.5	–0.6
PP-MP (degrees)	25.5	25.0	6.0	0.1
Wits appraisal (mm)	–3.7	–1.0	1.0	–2.7**
Maxillary length (ANS-PNS) (mm)	44.1	51.6	4.3	–1.7*
Mandibular length (CoGn) (mm)	114.4	123.8	4.0	–2.3**
Cranial base				
BaSN (degrees)	129.6	130.0	5.0	–0.1
Upper incisors to maxilla				
U1-SN (degrees)	96.1	102.9	5.5	–1.2*
U1-NA (degrees)	20.7	22.8	5.7	–0.4
U1-NA (mm)	3.4	4.3	2.7	–0.3
U1-PP (degrees)	105.1	110.0	5.0	–1.0*

(cont)

Table 14-2 (cont) Case 1 posttreatment cephalometric values

Group/measurement	Value	Norm	SD	Dev norm
Lower incisors to mandible				
L1-MP (degrees)	80.8	95.0	7.0	–2.0**
L1-NB (degrees)	12.6	25.3	6.0	–2.1**
L1-NB (mm)	2.0	4.0	1.8	–1.1*
L1 protrusion (L1-APg) (mm)	0.2	1.0	2.3	–0.3
Incisors to each other				
Interincisal angle (U1-L1) (degrees)	146.0	130.0	6.0	2.7**
Soft tissue				
Upper lip to E-plane (mm)	–5.3	–3.0	2.0	–1.1*
Lower lip to E-plane (mm)	–1.7	–2.5	2.5	0.3
ILG (HP) (mm)	–1.0	2.0	2.0	–1.5*
Nasolabial angle (CoLSnUL) (degrees)	93.5	102.0	8.0	–1.1*
H-angle (Pg′UL-Pg′N′) (degrees)	13.3	10.0	4.0	0.8
LFH (Sn′Me′) (mm)	69.4	63.0	3.0	2.1**
Facial proportions (hard tissue)				
UFH (N-ANS) (mm)	51.8	50.0	2.5	0.7
LFH (ANS-Me) (mm)	68.6	60.0	4.5	1.9*
UFH (N-ANS/[N-ANS+ANS-Me]) (%)	43.0	45.0	5.0	–0.4
LFH (ANS-Me/[N-ANS+ANS-Me]) (%)	57.0	57.0	5.0	0.0
Posterior face height (ArGo) (mm)	49.7	49.6	4.5	0.0
PFH:AFH (CoGo:NMe) (%)	54.8	60.0	1.0	–5.2*****
Profile				
Convexity (NA-APg) (degrees)	–1.9	4.3	3.0	–2.1**
Facial angle (FH-NPg) (degrees)	89.9	88.9	3.0	0.3

Dev norm, deviation from the norm; PP, palatal plane; OP, occlusal plane; MP, mandibular plane; U1, maxillary incisor; L1, mandibular incisor; ILG (HP), interlabial gap (horizontal plane); CoL, condylion lateral; UL, upper lip; UFH, upper face height; LFH, lower face height; PFH:AFH, posterior face height to anterior face height.
*Each asterisk represents a standard deviation (SD).

Cephalometric superimposition

The upper and lower lip became more retrusive, and the nose and chin both became more prominent. The nasolabial angle increased slightly, probably due to the increase in nasal growth. Both the upper and the lower face grew, and the proportions approached normal measures. The facial profile became straight to slightly convex, and the facial angle stayed within the normal range (Fig 14-1z).

Posttreatment CBCT evaluation

The CBCT showed that the right maxillary central incisor root was more protrusive than the left. The alveolar graft had made the alveolus continuous, although there was a slight radiolucency in the alveolar bone lingual to the maxillary right central incisor (Figs 14-1aa and 14-1bb).

The patient maintained poor oral hygiene throughout treatment despite frequent hygiene instruction. However, the par-

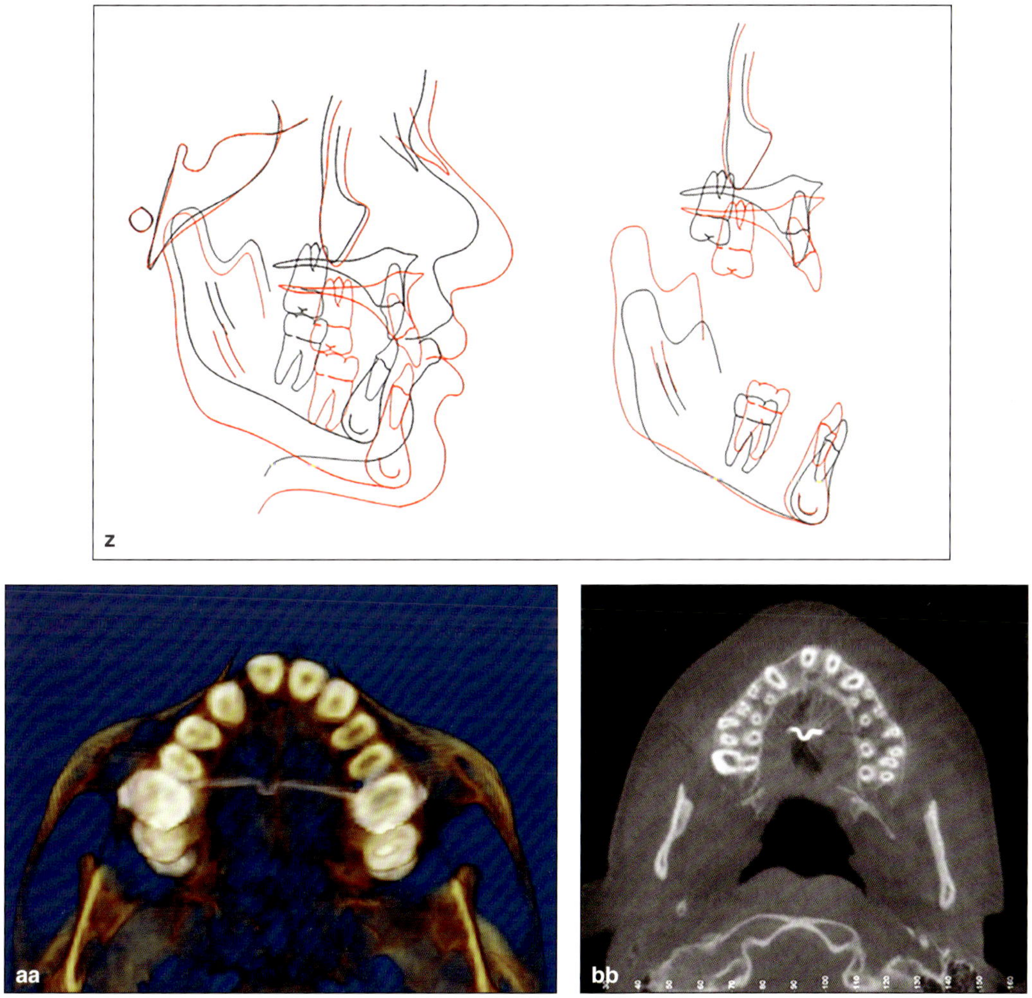

Fig 14-1 *(cont)* *(z)* Superimposition of pretreatment and posttreatment cephalometric tracings. *(aa and bb)* Posttreatment 3D CBCT reconstruction and axial section showing the maxillary dentition and fixed transpalatal bar for retention.

ents were satisfied with treatment. If a 3D CBCT had been taken initially, the cleft would have been recognized, resulting in a shorter treatment time for phase I and fewer radiographs. If a 3D CBCT had not been taken at all, the cleft would have gone unrecognized, and the movement of incisors in the area might have resulted in loss of these incisors. Subsequent placement of a dental implant to replace any extracted teeth in the area of the cleft might have resulted in loss of the implant.

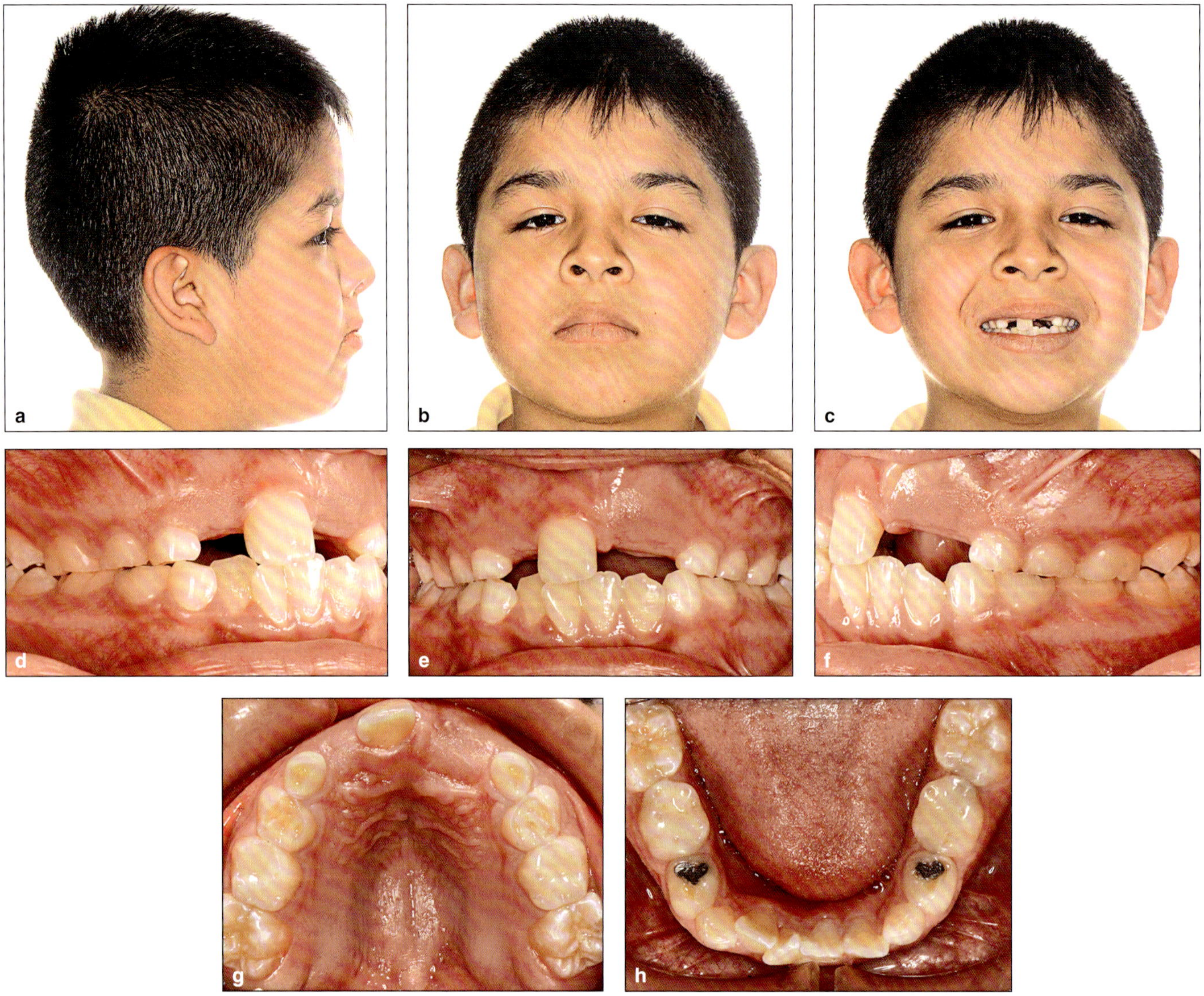
Fig 14-2 *(a to h)* Pretreatment extraoral and intraoral photographs.

Case 2

Initial medical history

A 7-year-old Hispanic boy with a noncontributory medical history was referred from private practice because of his impacted left central and lateral incisors. His dental history was sketchy because his parents did not speak English well.

Chief complaint

The patient's chief complaint was that only one permanent maxillary central incisor had erupted.

Photographic and clinical evaluation

The patient's profile was slightly convex (Fig 14-2a). Frontal extraoral photographs showed that the left side of the face was wider than the right side, and the left ear was more prominent than the right ear (Figs 14-2b and 14-2c). The left eye had slight ptosis (see Fig 14-2b). The extraoral smile view showed multiple missing maxillary incisors (see Fig 14-2c).

Slight gingival erythema and swelling was present. The molars and primary canines were in Class I relationships (Figs 14-2d to 14-2f). The midlines were noncoincident, and there was moderate (6 mm) mandibular crowding. The maxillary right and left lateral incisors and left central incisors had not erupted, and the arch forms were broad (Figs 14-2g and 14-2h). Occlusal amalgams were present in the mandibular primary first molars.

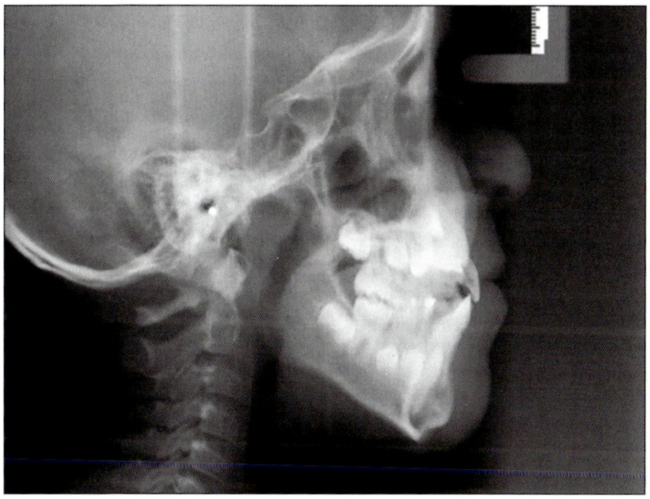

Fig 14-2i Pretreatment lateral cephalogram.

Table 14-3 Case 2 pretreatment cephalometric values

Group/measurement	Value	Norm	SD	Dev norm
Maxilla to cranial base				
SNA (degrees)	84.0	82.0	3.5	0.6
SN-PP (degrees)	13.2	8.0	3.0	1.7*
SN-OP (degrees)	18.0	14.4	2.5	1.4*
A-N perp (mm)	3.4	0.0	2.0	1.7*
Mandible to cranial base				
SNB (degrees)	76.4	80.9	3.4	–1.3*
SNPg (degrees)	77.0	80.0	3.5	–0.9
FMA (MP-FH) (degrees)	39.8	26.0	4.5	3.1***
SN-MP (degrees)	42.4	32.9	5.2	1.8*
MP-OP (degrees)	31.4	14.7	5.0	3.3***
B-N perp (mm)	–4.8	–6.0	8.0	0.1
Pg-N perp (mm)	–4.3	–5.0	4.0	0.2
y-axis (SGnSN) (degrees)	74.6	67.0	5.5	1.4
Maxilla to mandible				
ANB (degrees)	7.6	1.6	1.5	4.0****
PP-MP (degrees)	36.2	25.0	6.0	1.9*
Wits appraisal (mm)	3.1	–1.0	1.0	4.1****
Maxillary length (ANS-PNS) (mm)	46.5	51.6	4.3	–1.2*
Mandibular length (CoGn) (mm)	103.0	108.8	4.0	–1.4*

(cont)

Cephalometric evaluation

The maxillary position (SNA) was at the higher end of normal limits but was protrusive based on A-N perp (Fig 14-2i and Table 14-3). The measures for the mandible were controversial. SNB indicated that the mandible was retrusive, but SNPg, B-N perp, and Pg-N perp were within normal limits. The y-axis indicated a downward grower. The mandibular plane angle was steep (SN-MP, FMA).

The differential between the maxilla and mandible measures (ANB) indicated a Class II skeletal relationship, although the Wits analysis indicated a Class III. Both maxillary and mandibular lengths were short, which was probably a factor of age.

Table 14-3 (cont) Case 2 pretreatment cephalometric values

Group/measurement	Value	Norm	SD	Dev norm
Cranial base				
BaSN (degrees)	127.7	130.0	5.0	–0.5
Upper incisors to maxilla				
U1-SN (degrees)	94.5	102.1	5.5	–1.4*
U1-NA (degrees)	10.5	22.8	5.7	–2.2**
U1-NA (mm)	0.1	4.3	2.7	–1.6*
U1-PP (degrees)	107.7	110.0	5.0	–0.5
Lower incisors to mandible				
L1-MP (degrees)	86.3	95.0	7.0	–1.2*
L1-NB (degrees)	32.8	25.3	6.0	1.2*
L1-NB (mm)	7.1	4.0	1.8	1.7*
L1 protrusion (L1-APg) (mm)	3.3	1.0	2.3	1.0*
Incisors to each other				
Interincisal angle (U1-L1) (degrees)	129.1	130.0	6.0	–0.1
Soft tissue				
Upper lip to E-plane (mm)	–2.4	–3.0	2.0	0.3
Lower lip to E-plane (mm)	0.7	–2.5	2.5	1.3*
ILG (HP) (mm)	0.0	2.0	2.0	–1.0*
Nasolabial angle (CoLSnUL) (degrees)	104.2	102.0	8.0	0.3
H-angle (Pg'UL-Pg'N') (degrees)	14.5	10.0	4.0	1.1*
LFH (Sn'Me') (mm)	75.5	63.0	3.0	4.2****
Facial proportions (hard tissue)				
UFH (N-ANS) (mm)	42.4	50.0	2.5	–3.1***
LFH (ANS-Me) (mm)	69.9	60.0	4.5	2.2**
UFH (N-ANS/[N-ANS+ANS-Me]) (%)	37.7	45.0	5.0	–1.5*
LFH (ANS-Me/[N-ANS+ANS-Me]) (%)	62.3	57.0	5.0	1.1*
Posterior face height (ArGo) (mm)	31.6	38.4	4.5	–1.5*
PFH:AFH (CoGo:NMe) (%)	36.6	60.0	1.0	–23.4******
Profile				
Convexity (NA-APg) (degrees)	13.7	10.3	3.0	1.1*
Facial angle (FH-NPg) (degrees)	87.3	86.5	3.0	0.3

Dev norm, deviation from the norm; PP, palatal plane; OP, occlusal plane; MP, mandibular plane; U1, maxillary incisor; L1, mandibular incisor; ILG (HP), interlabial gap (horizontal plane); CoL, condylion lateral; UL, upper lip; UFH, upper face height; LFH, lower face height; PFH:AFH, posterior face height to anterior face height.
*Each asterisk represents a standard deviation (SD).

The maxillary incisors were upright (U1-SN, U1-NA in degrees) and retruded (U1-NA in mm). The mandibular incisors were upright to the steep mandibular plane (L1-MP) but proclined (L1-NB in degrees) and protrusive (L1-NB in mm) to the face.

Proportionately, the lower face height (LFH) was longer than normal, and the upper face height (UFH) was shorter than normal. The ratio of the posterior face height to the anterior face height indicated a shorter posterior face height.

An indentation was noted on the bony chin that was not noted in later radiographs. The face was convex (NA-APg), and the CVM stage was 1, indicating the potential for growth.

Panoramic evaluation

The maxillary lateral incisors and left central incisor were present but not erupting (Fig 14-2j). The lack of eruption of the lateral incisors could have been due to age, but the left lateral

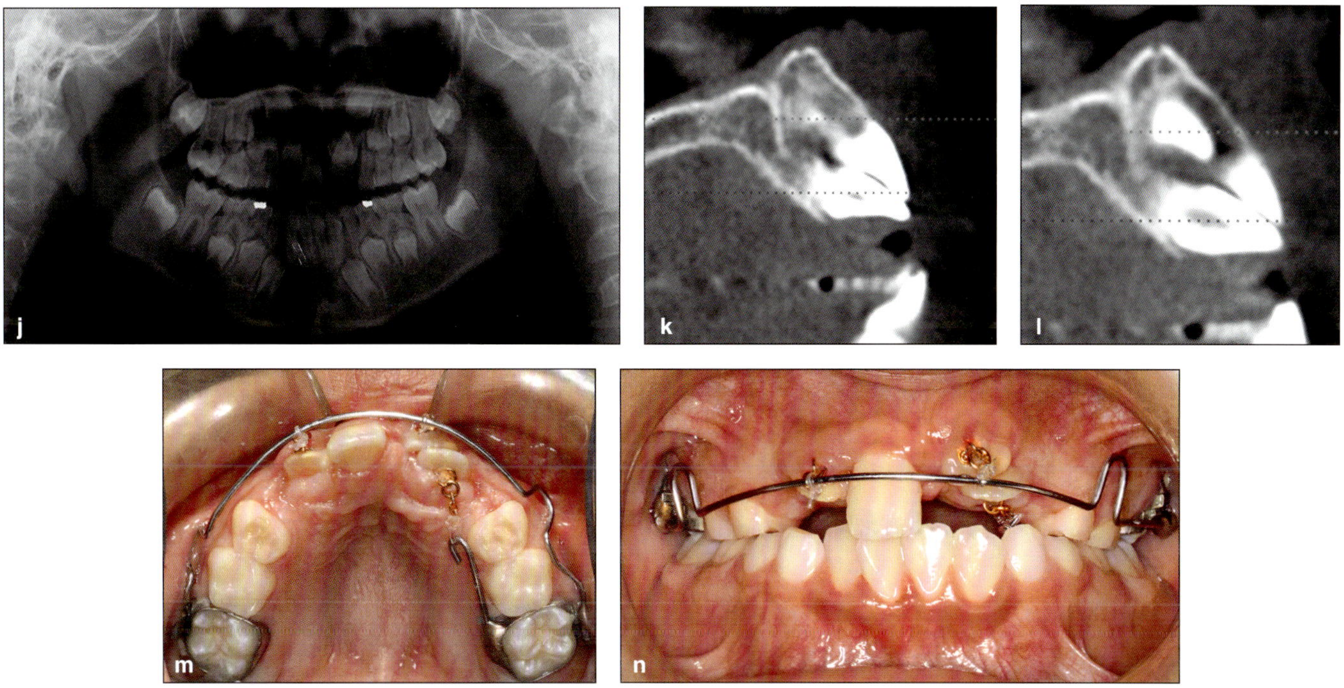

Fig 14-2 *(cont)* *(j)* Pretreatment panoramic radiograph. *(k and l)* CBCT implant views showing that the position of the maxillary left lateral incisor crown is directly ventral and palatal to the central incisor crown *(k)* and the position of the permanent left canine crown is superior and labial to the distal portion of the lateral incisor crown *(l)*. The distal of the central incisor crown is also labial to the lateral incisor crown. *(m and n)* Views of the appliance used to apply a distal erupting force to the right lateral incisor and erupting forces to the hypomineralized left lateral and central incisors.

and central incisors appeared to be crossed. The third molars were not apparent yet.

CBCT evaluation

Evaluation of the CBCT showed the left lateral incisor crown distal to and touching the left central incisor crown (Fig 14-2k). The position of the permanent left canine was mesial and would interfere with the root of the lateral incisor if the lateral incisor was properly positioned (Fig 14-2l).

Classification

The case was classified as a Class I molar and Class II skeletal malocclusion with impactions and moderate to severe crowding.

Treatment plan

Two-phase treatment was planned with the objectives of erupting the maxillary incisors following surgical exposure and extraction of the primary maxillary canines. The first premolars were planned for serial extraction when the primary first molars were exfoliating, and the premolar roots were longer. An appliance was designed incorporating a soldered labial bow and a lingual hook soldered to the molar band from which eruptive forces could be applied using elastomeric threads (Figs 14-2m and 14-2n). Following eruption of all the incisors, the left lateral incisor crown was brought from its erupted position in the palate into the arch using a thread tied to the lingual arch but in a distobuccal direction. The incisors were bracketed, and round wires were then used to align and level the incisor crowns but not the roots.

End of phase I evaluation

Figures 14-2o to 14-2v show reasonable alignment of the maxillary incisors. The roots of the lateral incisors were intentionally kept palatally to minimize contact with the maxillary canines. These will be properly positioned during phase II. The maxillary arch maintained its shape, and adequate overbite and overjet were achieved for phase I.

Cephalometric analysis

During the observation phase between phases I and II, the first premolars were extracted to allow the permanent canines room for eruption and distalization. The maxillary position appears more retruded (SNA), and the maxilla-to-mandible relationship is better (ANB). The mandibular plane (FMA, SN-MP) and incisor positions are also more normal (Fig 14-2w and Table 14-4). The indentation on the chin is no longer apparent.

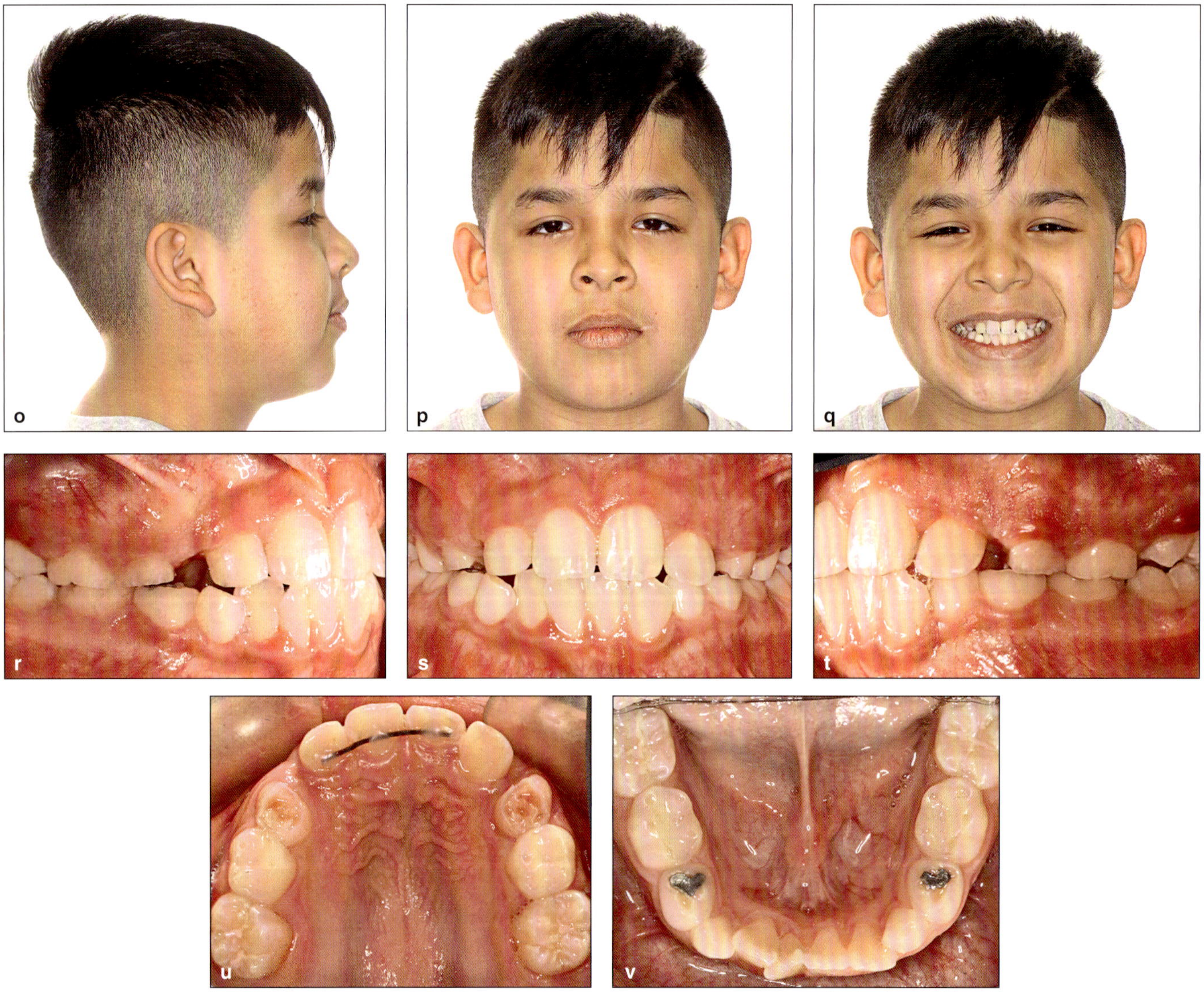

Fig 14-2 *(cont)* *(o to v)* Extraoral and intraoral photographs at the end of phase I showing a lingual fixed retainer for the maxillary incisors.

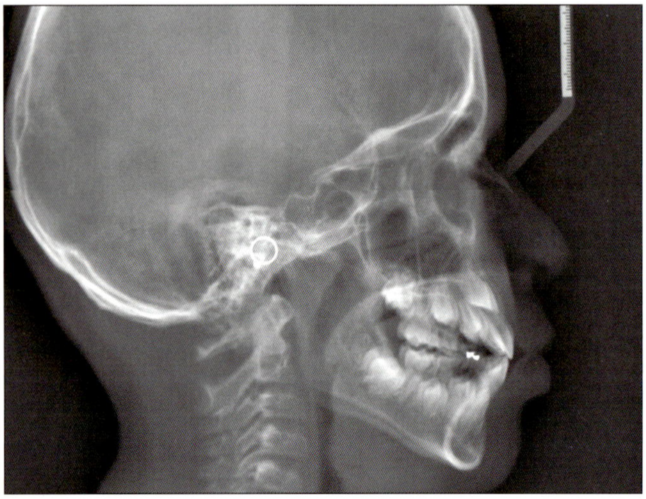

Fig 14-2w Pre–phase II cephalogram.

Panoramic analysis

The first premolars were extracted to allow the permanent canines room for eruption and distalization. The left canine will need to be re-evaluated for surgical exposure. The third molars are now showing formation (Fig 14-2x).

Cephalometric superimposition

Superimposition shows downward growth of the maxilla and mandible (Fig 14-2y). There was considerable increase in the size of the nose and soft tissue. Even though the mandibular teeth were not included in phase I treatment, the computer superimposition shows the mandibular incisors coming forward. The mandibular molars also came forward, possibly as a result of the first premolar extractions.

Table 14-4 Case 2 pre–phase II cephalometric values

Group/measurement	Value	Norm	SD	Dev norm
Maxilla to cranial base				
SNA (degrees)	80.9	82.0	3.5	–0.3
SN-PP (degrees)	7.2	8.0	3.0	–0.3
SN-OP (degrees)	23.1	14.4	2.5	3.5***
A-N perp (mm)	8.6	0.0	2.0	4.3****
Mandible to cranial base				
SNB (degrees)	75.4	80.9	3.4	–1.6*
SNPg (degrees)	75.4	80.0	3.5	–1.3*
FMA (MP-FH) (degrees)	22.2	25.7	4.5	–0.8
SN-MP (degrees)	38.1	32.9	5.2	1.0*
MP-OP (degrees)	17.8	15.2	5.0	0.5
B-N perp (mm)	6.4	–6.0	8.0	1.5*
Pg-N perp (mm)	7.1	–5.0	4.0	3.0***
y-axis (SGnSN) (degrees)	72.6	67.0	5.5	1.0*
Maxilla to mandible				
ANB (degrees)	5.5	1.6	1.5	2.6**
PP-MP (degrees)	33.6	25.0	6.0	1.4*
Wits appraisal (mm)	–0.9	–1.0	1.0	0.1
Maxillary length (ANS-PNS) (mm)	39.3	51.6	4.3	–2.9**
Mandibular length (CoGn) (mm)	99.6	111.4	4.0	–3.0***
Cranial base				
BaSN (degrees)	128.2	130.0	5.0	–0.4
Upper incisors to maxilla				
U1-SN (degrees)	98.6	102.3	5.5	–0.7
U1-NA (degrees)	17.7	22.8	5.7	–0.9
U1-NA (mm)	2.4	4.3	2.7	–0.7
U1-PP (degrees)	105.8	110.0	5.0	–0.8
Lower incisors to mandible				
L1-MP (degrees)	96.5	95.0	7.0	0.2
L1-NB (degrees)	32.8	25.3	6.0	1.2*
L1-NB (mm)	7.8	4.0	1.8	2.1**
L1 protrusion (L1-APg) (mm)	4.7	1.0	2.3	1.6*
Incisors to each other				
Interincisal angle (U1-L1) (degrees)	124.1	130.0	6.0	–1.0*
Soft tissue				
Upper lip to E-plane (mm)	1.6	–3.0	2.0	2.3**
Lower lip to E-plane (mm)	3.9	–2.5	2.5	2.6**
ILG (HP) (mm)	0.2	2.0	2.0	–0.9
Nasolabial angle (CoLSnUL) (degrees)	107.4	102.0	8.0	0.7
H-angle (Pg'UL-Pg'N') (degrees)	20.7	10.0	4.0	2.7**
LFH (Sn'Me') (mm)	69.6	63.0	3.0	2.2**

(cont)

Table 14-4 (cont) Case 2 pre–phase II cephalometric values

Group/measurement	Value	Norm	SD	Dev norm
Facial proportions (hard tissue)				
UFH (N-ANS) (mm)	44.5	50.0	2.5	−2.2**
LFH (ANS-Me) (mm)	64.3	60.0	4.5	1.0*
UFH (N-ANS/[N-ANS+ANS-Me]) (%)	40.9	45.0	5.0	−0.8
LFH (ANS-Me/[N-ANS+ANS-Me]) (%)	59.1	57.0	5.0	0.4
Posterior face height (ArGo) (mm)	43.3	40.4	4.5	0.6
PFH:AFH (CoGo:NMe) (%)	42.1	60.0	1.0	−17.9******
Profile				
Convexity (NA-APg) (degrees)	11.2	9.2	3.0	0.7
Facial angle (FH-NPg) (degrees)	94.0	86.8	3.0	2.4**

Dev norm, deviation from the norm; PP, palatal plane; OP, occlusal plane; MP, mandibular plane; U1, maxillary incisor; L1, mandibular incisor; ILG (HP), interlabial gap (horizontal plane); CoL, condylion lateral; UL, upper lip; UFH, upper face height; LFH, lower face height; PFH:AFH, posterior face height to anterior face height.
*Each asterisk represents a standard deviation (SD).

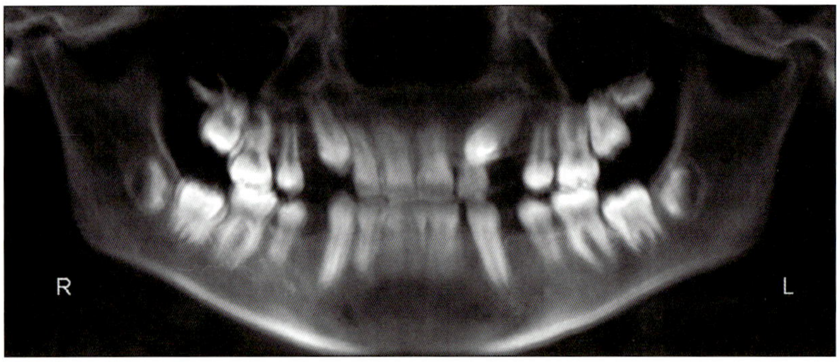

Fig 14-2x Pre–phase II panoramic radiograph.

Treatment analysis

The parents and patient were happy with the results. The anterior teeth were reasonably aligned for phase I, facial esthetics and occlusal function were improved, and the arch width was maintained despite the multiple forces applied to the left molar. The roots of the incisors did not appear to be affected by the eruption process. The patient was well prepared for phase II treatment.

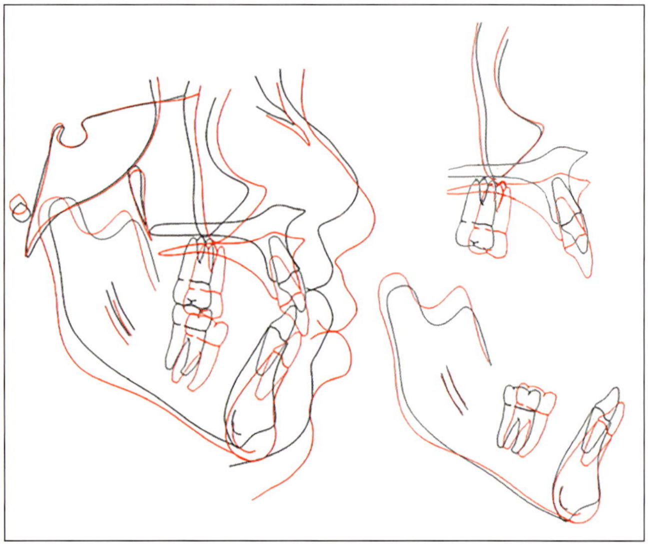

Fig 14-2y Superimposition of pretreatment and pre–phase II treatment cephalometric tracings.

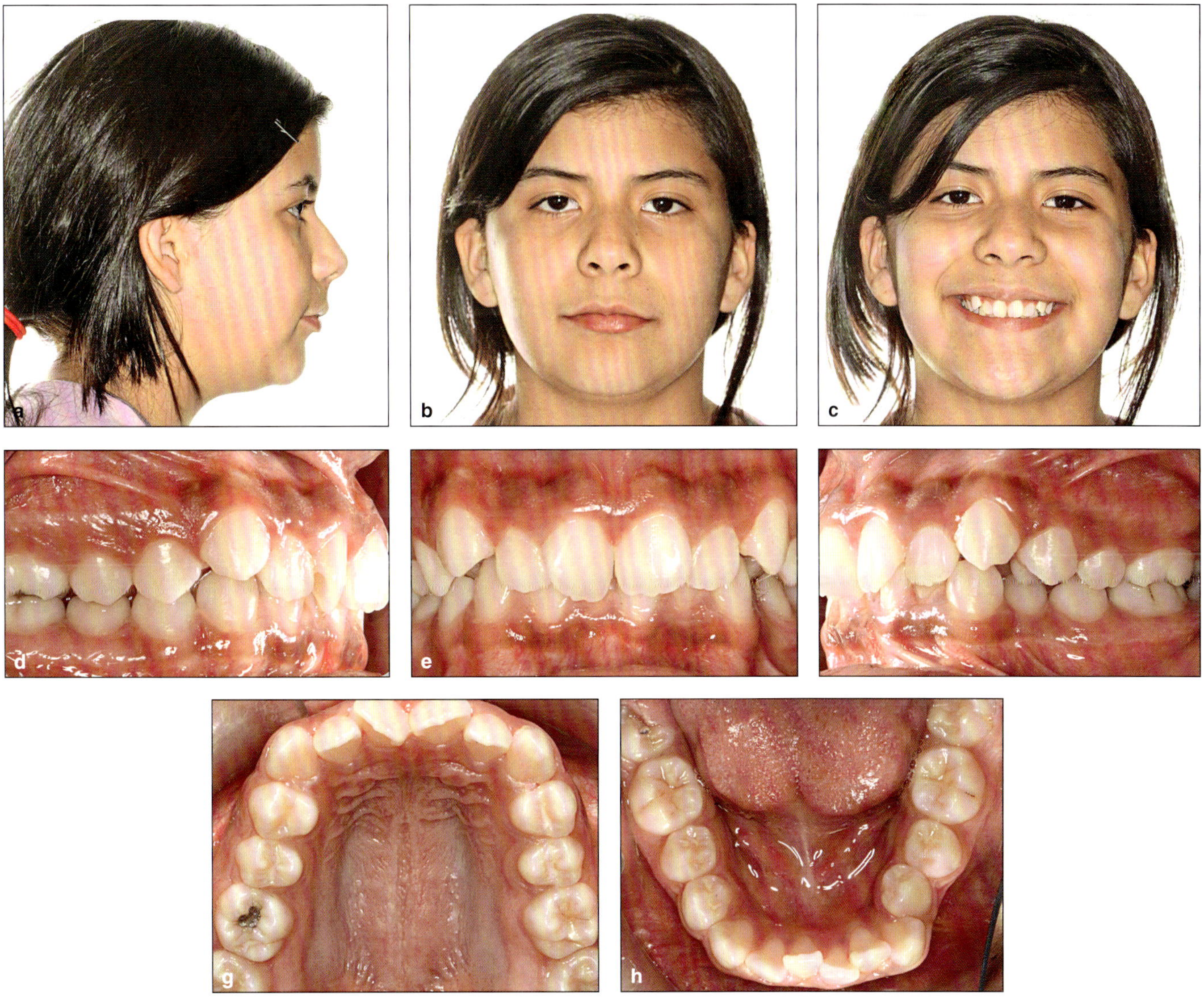

Fig 14-3 *(a to h)* Pretreatment extraoral and intraoral photographs.

Case 3

Initial medical history and chief complaint

A 12-year-old Hispanic girl presented for comprehensive orthodontic treatment with unremarkable medical and dental histories. Her chief compliant was that her teeth were not straight.

Photographic evaluation

Her facial profile was convex (Fig 14-3a), and the lips were competent (Fig 14-3b). She had a nonconsonant smile arc with buccal corridors (Fig 14-3c) and an obtuse nasolabial angle with a deep mentolabial fold. Her upper lip looked thin from the frontal view.

The patient presented in the permanent dentition with a Class II, division 2 malocclusion. She had a deep bite with palatal impingement and a 4-mm overjet as well as severe crowding in the maxillary and mandibular arches with moderately retroclined incisors (Figs 14-3d to 14-3h). The maxillary left first premolar was in crossbite, and there was an excessive curve of Spee in the mandibular arch.

Cephalometric evaluation

The cephalometric evaluation showed a Class II skeletal pattern due to a prognathic maxilla (Table 14-5). The lateral cephalogram confirmed the skeletal relationship with an increased ANB angle and Wits appraisal (Fig 14-3i). The vertical skeletal proportions were within normal limits. The patient appeared to be past the peak of her mandibular growth (CVM stage 5).

Table 14-5 Case 3 pretreatment cephalometric values

Group/measurement	Value	Norm	SD	Dev norm
Maxilla to cranial base				
SNA (degrees)	89.0	82.0	3.5	2.0**
SN-PP (degrees)	5.1	8.0	3.0	–1.0*
SN-OP (degrees)	17.2	14.4	2.5	1.1*
A-N perp (mm)	7.0	0.0	2.0	3.5***
Mandible to cranial base				
SNB (degrees)	80.4	80.9	3.4	–0.1
SNPg (degrees)	80.0	80.0	3.5	0.0
FMA (MP-FH) (degrees)	24.7	24.9	4.5	0.0
SN-MP (degrees)	30.4	32.9	5.2	–0.5
MP-OP (degrees)	13.3	16.2	5.0	–0.6
B-N perp (mm)	–1.6	–6.0	8.0	0.6
Pg-N perp (mm)	–2.5	–5.0	3.0	0.8
y-axis (SGnSN) (degrees)	67.4	67.0	5.5	0.1
Maxilla to mandible				
ANB (degrees)	8.6	1.6	1.5	4.7****
PP-MP (degrees)	25.4	25.0	6.0	0.1
Wits appraisal (mm)	3.3	–1.0	1.0	4.3****
Maxillary length (ANS-PNS) (mm)	43.5	51.6	4.3	–1.9*
Mandibular length (CoGn) (mm)	102.5	116.3	4.0	–3.4***
Cranial base				
BaSN (degrees)	129.3	130.0	5.0	–0.1
Upper incisors to maxilla				
U1-SN (degrees)	101.9	102.5	5.5	–0.1
U1-NA (degrees)	12.9	22.8	5.7	–1.7*
U1-NA (mm)	0.1	4.3	2.7	–1.6*
U1-PP (degrees)	107.1	110.0	5.0	–0.6
Lower incisors to mandible				
L1-MP (degrees)	90.7	95.0	7.0	–0.6
L1-NB (degrees)	24.3	25.3	6.0	–0.2
L1-NB (mm)	5.2	4.0	1.8	0.7
L1 protrusion (L1-APg) (mm)	0.2	1.0	2.3	–0.4
Incisors to each other				
Interincisal angle (U1-L1) (degrees)	134.2	130.0	6.0	0.7
Overjet (Mx1-Md1) (mm)	5.0	3.2	0.4	4.5****
Overbite (Mx1-Md1) (mm)	6.7	3.2	0.7	5.0*****
Soft tissue				
Upper lip to E-plane (mm)	–0.5	–3.0	2.0	1.3*
Lower lip to E-plane (mm)	0.1	–2.5	2.5	1.0*
ILG (HP) (mm)	0.6	2.0	2.0	–0.7
Nasolabial angle (CoLSnUL) (degrees)	123.8	102.0	8.0	2.7**

(cont)

Table 14-5 (cont) **Case 3 pretreatment cephalometric values**

Group/measurement	Value	Norm	SD	Dev norm
H-angle (Pg′UL-Pg′N′) (degrees)	19.4	10.0	4.0	2.3**
Face height (N′Me′) (mm)	107.9	125.0	4.7	–3.6***
UFH (G′Sn′) (mm)	59.0	63.0	3.0	–1.3*
LFH (Sn′Me′) (mm)	68.2	63.0	3.0	1.7*
Facial proportions (hard tissue)				
UFH (N-ANS) (mm)	45.7	50.0	2.5	–1.7*
LFH (ANS-Me) (mm)	61.8	65.0	4.5	–0.7
UFH (N-ANS/[N-ANS+ANS-Me]) (%)	42.6	45.0	5.0	–0.5
LFH (ANS-Me/[N-ANS+ANS-Me]) (%)	57.4	57.0	5.0	0.1
Posterior face height (ArGo) (mm)	47.9	44.0	4.5	0.9
PFH:AFH (CoGo:NMe) (%)	55.9	60.0	1.0	–4.1 ****
Profile				
Convexity (NA-APg) (degrees)	19.5	7.3	3.0	4.1 ****
Facial angle (FH-NPg) (degrees)	88.5	87.6	3.0	0.3

Dev norm, deviation from the norm; PP, palatal plane; OP, occlusal plane; MP, mandibular plane; U1, maxillary incisor; L1, mandibular incisor; ILG (HP), interlabial gap (horizontal plane); CoL, condylion lateral; UL, upper lip; UFH, upper face height; LFH, lower face height; PFH:AFH, posterior face height to anterior face height.
*Each asterisk represents a standard deviation (SD).

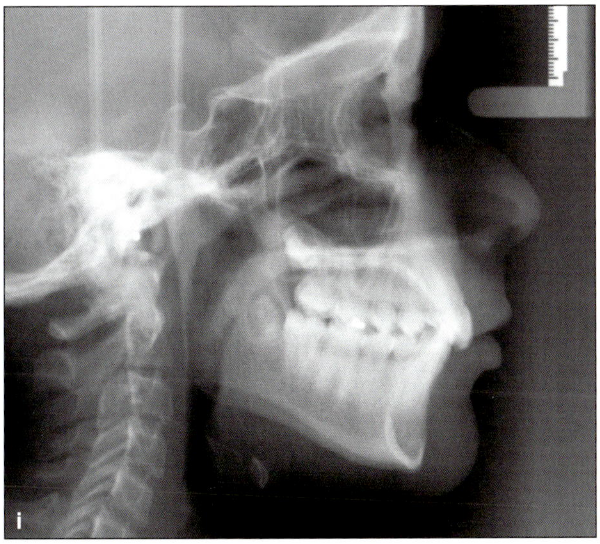

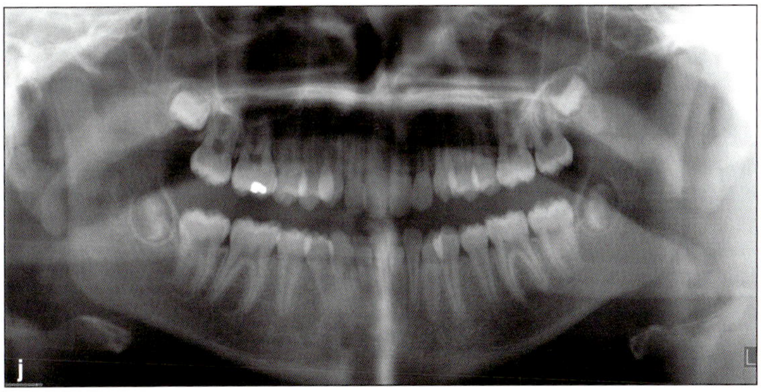

Fig 14-3 *(cont)* *(i)* Pretreatment cephalogram. *(j)* Pretreatment panoramic radiograph.

Panoramic evaluation

The panoramic radiograph showed the presence of all permanent teeth with the third molars in their various stages of development (Fig 14-3j).

Treatment plan

The treatment plan included extraction of all maxillary first premolars and mandibular second premolars and fixed orthodontic appliances with a cervical traction headgear and a Nance appliance to correct the malocclusion and finish in Class I molar and canine occlusion. Anchorage was maximized by placing a Nance appliance.

The maxillary and mandibular teeth were bonded with 0.018-inch American Orthodontics (AO) brackets. AO bands with a headgear tube were used. A Nance appliance was initially delivered before referring the patient for premolar extraction; then a cervical-pull headgear was delivered, and the patient was asked to wear it for 10 to 12 hours per day. The maxil-

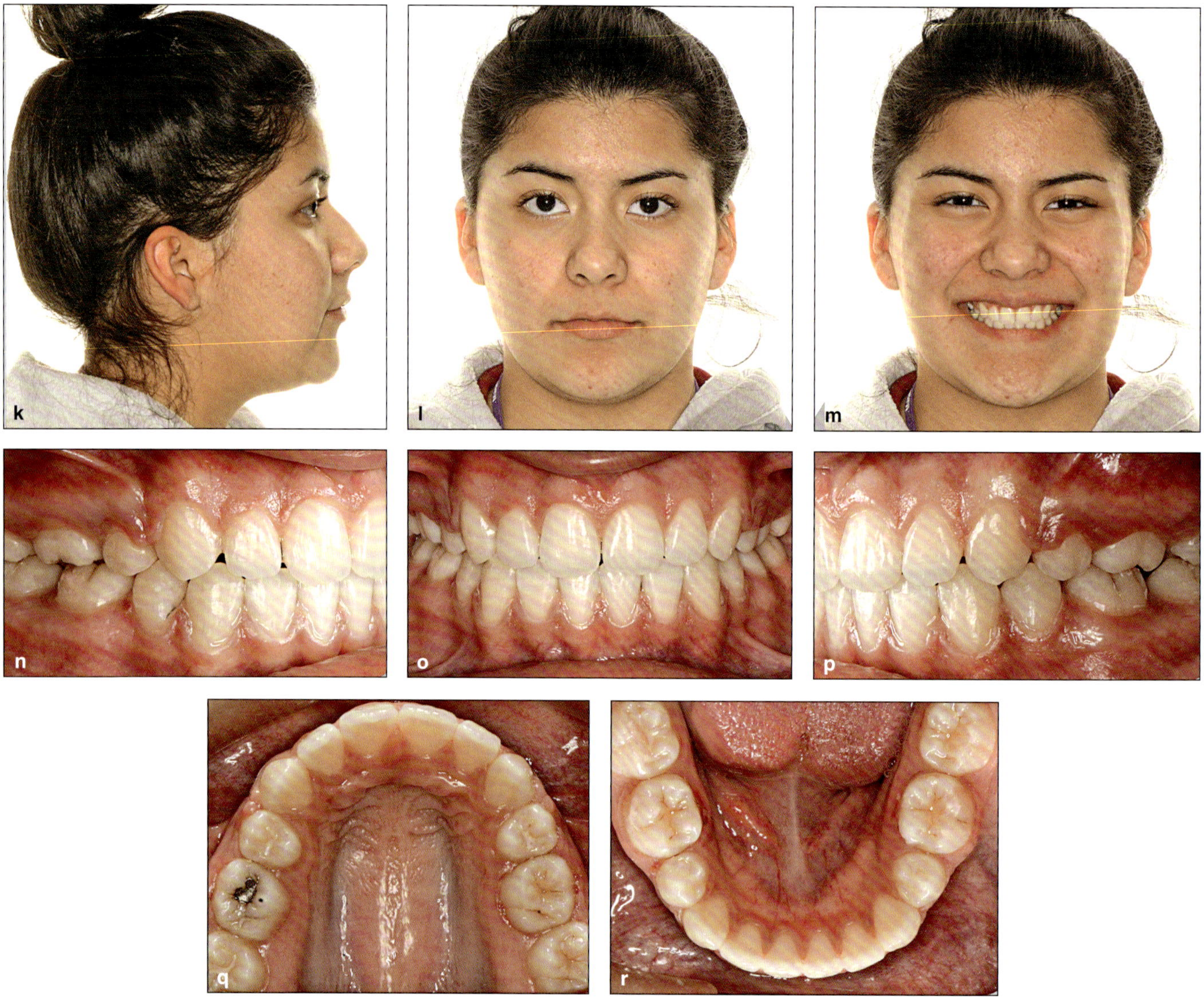

Fig 14-3 *(cont)* *(k to r)* Posttreatment extraoral and intraoral photographs.

lary and mandibular arches were leveled and aligned using 0.016-inch Nitinol wires. The excessive curve of Spee was leveled using a 0.016 × 0.022–inch reverse-curve nickel-titanium wire. Rotations were corrected with progressive archwires. The remaining spaces were consolidated with a 0.016 × 0.022–inch stainless steel (SS) archwire. Then 0.017 × 0.025–inch SS and titanium molybdenum alloy (TMA) archwires were used for the maxillary and mandibular dental arches. Vertical seating elastics were used to improve the interdigitation.

Final evaluation

The posttreatment extraoral photographs show a convex soft tissue profile with a relatively well-balanced face (Figs 14-3k to 14-3m). The midlines are coincident, the molars and maxillary canines are in Class I relationships, and the arches are well coordinated (Figs 14-3n to 14-3r). Figure 14-3s shows the posttreatment panoramic radiograph.

Cephalometric analysis

The anteroposterior skeletal relation maintained in Class II (Fig 14-3t). The ANB angle slightly decreased because of the normal growth. Vertically, the MPA and the face ratio were maintained. The inclination of the maxillary incisors decreased with a value of 99.4 degrees, while the inclination of the mandibular incisors in relation to the mandibular plane decreased with a value of 88.6 degrees (Fig 14-3u and Table 14-6). The lower lip is 2.0 mm behind E-plane, and the nose and chin grew slightly during treatment.

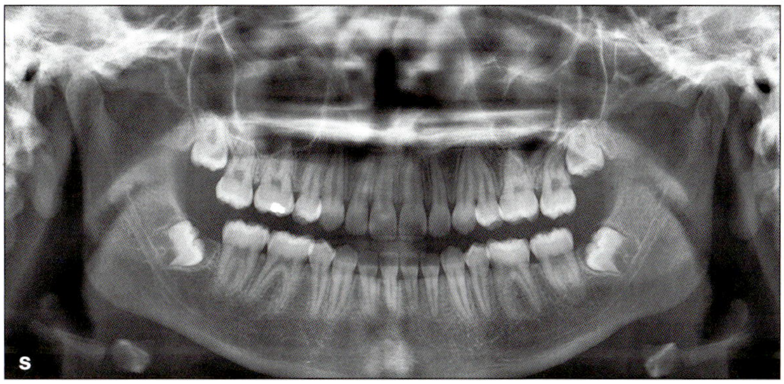

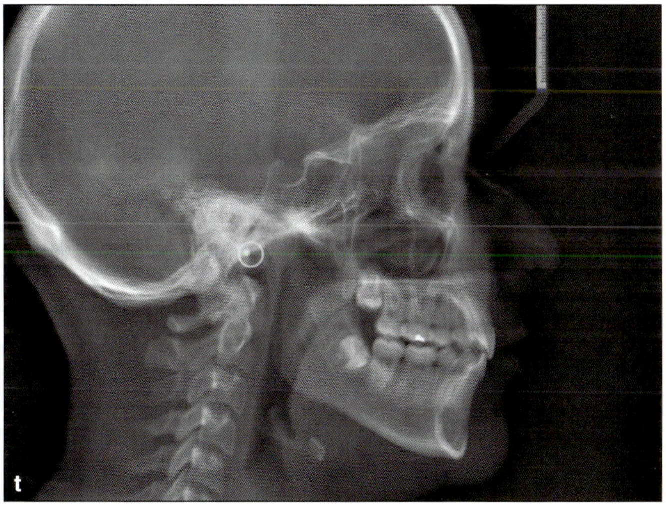

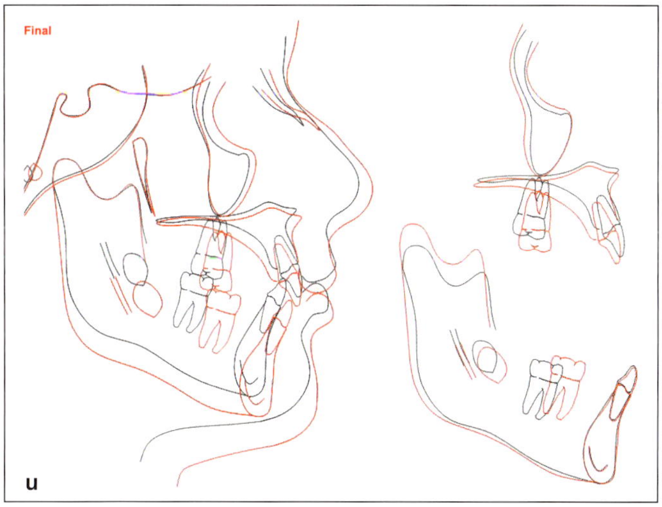

Fig 14-3 *(cont)* *(s)* Posttreatment panoramic radiograph. *(t)* Posttreatment cephalogram. *(u)* Superimposition of pretreatment and posttreatment cephalometric tracings.

Table 14-6 **Case 3 posttreatment cephalometric values**

Group/measurement	Value	Norm	SD	Dev norm
Maxilla to cranial base				
SNA (degrees)	87.9	82.0	3.5	1.7*
SN-PP (degrees)	7.1	8.0	3.0	–0.3
SN-OP (degrees)	19.0	14.4	2.5	1.8*
A-N perp (mm)	4.9	0.0	2.0	2.4**
Mandible to cranial base				
SNB (degrees)	81.1	80.9	3.4	0.1
SNPg (degrees)	80.3	80.0	3.5	0.1
FMA (MP-FH) (degrees)	28.1	23.9	4.5	0.9
SN-MP (degrees)	33.3	32.9	5.2	0.1
MP-OP (degrees)	12.8	17.4	5.0	–0.9
B-N perp (mm)	–2.7	–6.0	8.0	0.4
Pg-N perp (mm)	–4.5	–1.0	3.0	–1.2*
y-axis (SGnSN) (degrees)	67.5	67.0	5.5	0.1

(cont)

Table 14-6 (cont) **Case 3 posttreatment cephalometric values**

Group/measurement	Value	Norm	SD	Dev norm
Maxilla to mandible				
ANB (degrees)	6.8	1.6	1.5	3.5***
PP-MP (degrees)	24.7	25.0	6.0	–0.1
Wits appraisal (mm)	–0.1	–1.0	1.0	0.9
Maxillary length (ANS-PNS) (mm)	47.7	51.6	4.3	–0.9
Mandibular length (CoGn) (mm)	107.2	122.3	4.0	–3.8***
Cranial base				
BaSN (degrees)	125.6	130.0	5.0	–0.9
Upper incisors to maxilla				
U1-SN (degrees)	99.4	102.8	5.5	–0.6
U1-NA (degrees)	11.5	22.8	5.7	–2.0**
U1-NA (mm)	–1.3	4.3	2.7	–2.1**
U1-PP (degrees)	106.5	110.0	5.0	–0.7
Lower incisors to mandible				
L1-MP (degrees)	88.6	95.0	7.0	–0.9
L1-NB (degrees)	25.0	25.3	6.0	–0.1
L1-NB (mm)	5.4	4.0	1.8	0.8
L1 protrusion (L1-APg) (mm)	2.0	1.0	2.3	0.4
Incisors to each other				
Interincisal angle (U1-L1) (degrees)	136.7	130.0	6.0	1.1*
Overjet (Mx1-Md1) (mm)	2.2	3.2	0.4	–2.5**
Overbite (Mx1-Md1) (mm)	2.0	3.2	0.7	–1.7*
Soft tissue				
Upper lip to E-plane (mm)	–4.4	–3.0	2.0	–0.7
Lower lip to E-plane (mm)	–2.0	–2.5	2.5	0.2
ILG (HP) (mm)	0.5	2.0	2.0	–0.8
Nasolabial angle (CoLSnUL) (degrees)	127.2	102.0	8.0	3.2***
H-angle (Pg′UL-Pg′N′) (degrees)	14.5	10.0	4.0	1.1*
Face height (N′Me′) (mm)	115.7	125.0	4.7	–2.0**
UFH (G′Sn′) (mm)	67.5	63.0	3.0	1.5*
LFH (Sn′Me′) (mm)	71.4	63.0	3.0	2.8**
Facial proportions (hard tissue)				
UFH (N-ANS) (mm)	47.6	50.0	2.5	–0.9
LFH (ANS-Me) (mm)	65.5	65.0	4.5	0.1
UFH (N-ANS/[N-ANS+ANS-Me]) (%)	42.1	45.0	5.0	–0.6
LFH (ANS-Me/[N-ANS+ANS-Me]) (%)	57.9	57.0	5.0	0.2
Posterior face height (ArGo) (mm)	50.9	48.5	4.5	0.5
PFH:AFH (CoGo:NMe) (%)	54.4	60.0	1.0	–5.6 *****
Profile				
Convexity (NA-APg) (degrees)	15.8	4.9	3.0	3.6 ***
Facial angle (FH-NPg) (degrees)	87.5	88.6	3.0	–0.4

Dev norm, deviation from the norm; PP, palatal plane; OP, occlusal plane; MP, mandibular plane; U1, maxillary incisor; L1, mandibular incisor; ILG (HP), interlabial gap (horizontal plane); CoL, condylion lateral; UL, upper lip; UFH, upper face height; LFH, lower face height; PFH:AFH, posterior face height to anterior face height.
*Each asterisk represents a standard deviation (SD).

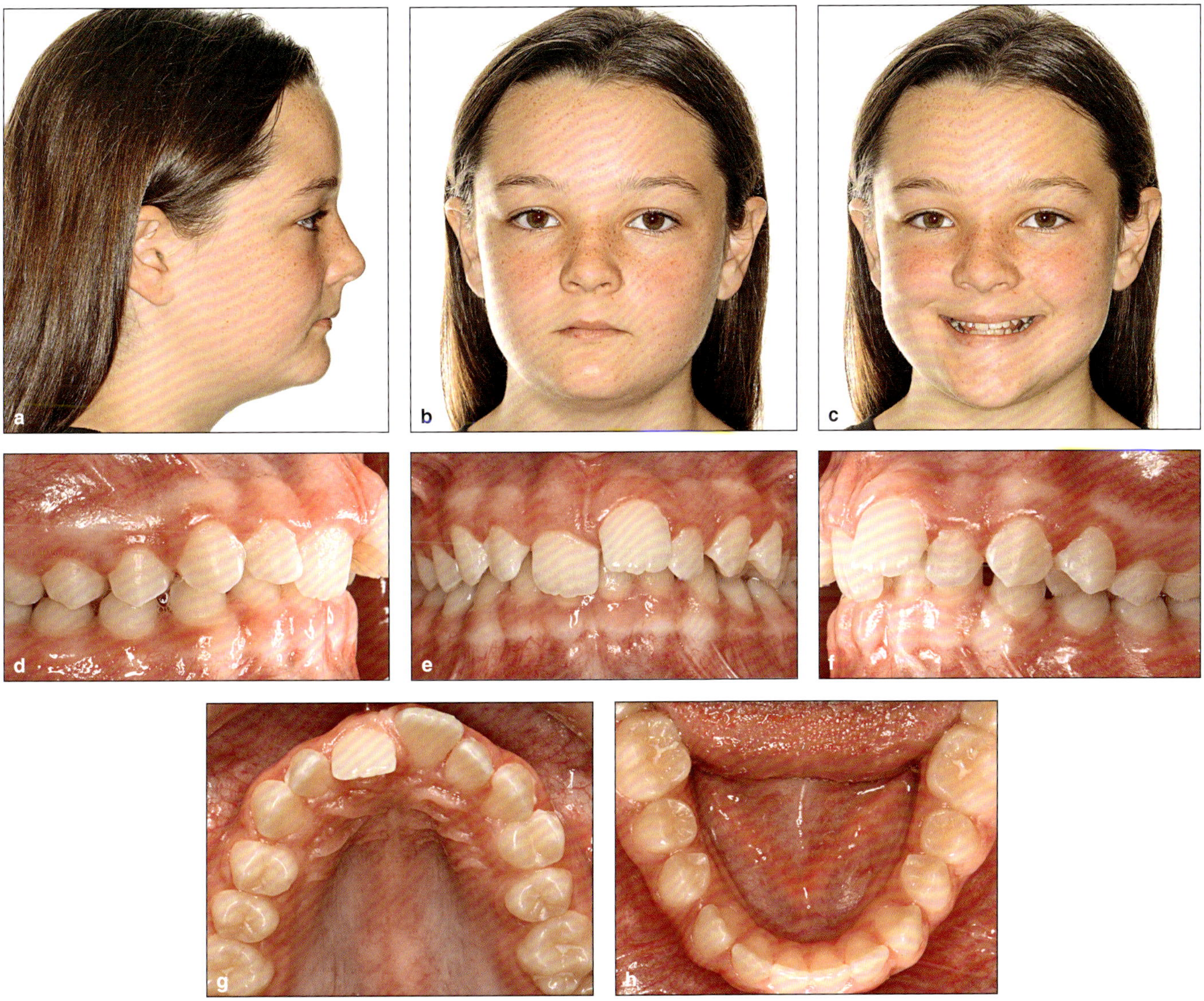

Fig 14-4 *(a to h)* Pretreatment extraoral and intraoral photographs.

Case 4

Initial medical history and chief complaint

An 11-year-old Caucasian girl presented for comprehensive orthodontic treatment with unremarkable medical and dental histories. Her chief complaint was the protruding maxillary left central incisor.

Photographic evaluation

The patient had a convex facial profile (Fig 14-4a). The lips were competent and retrusive based on the esthetic plane, and she had an obtuse nasolabial angle with a deep mentolabial fold. From the frontal view, her upper lip looked thin, with minimal vermilion display (Figs 14-4b and 14-4c). The maxillary midline appeared to be deviated to the left of the facial midline.

The patient presented with a Class II, division 1 malocclusion with more than 9 mm of overjet and palatal impingement (Figs 14-4d to 14-4h). No crowding was present in the maxillary arch or mandibular arch. The maxillary right central incisor was retroclined, and the maxillary left first premolar was in crossbite. The mandibular midline was deviated to the left about 3 mm, and there was an excessive curve of Spee in the mandibular arch.

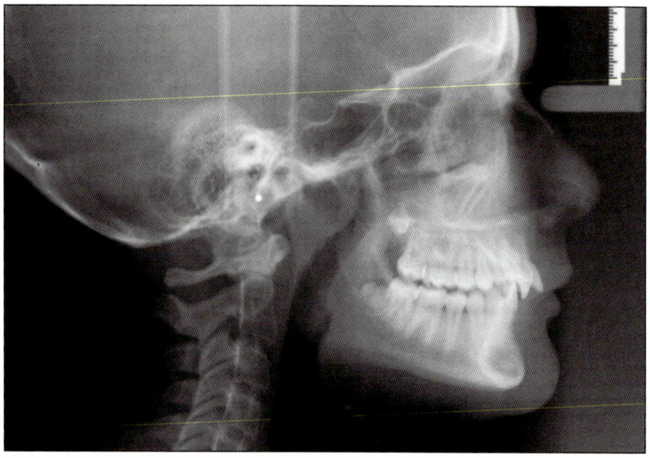

Fig 14-4i Pretreatment cephalogram.

Table 14-7 Case 4 pretreatment cephalometric values

Group/measurement	Value	Norm	SD	Dev norm
Maxilla to cranial base				
SNA (degrees)	83.3	82.0	3.5	0.4
SN-PP (degrees)	9.2	8.0	3.0	0.4
SN-OP (degrees)	6.5	14.4	2.5	–3.2***
A-N perp (mm)	3.3	0.0	2.0	1.7*
Mandible to cranial base				
SNB (degrees)	78.6	80.9	3.4	–0.7
SNPg (degrees)	80.9	80.0	3.5	0.3
FMA (MP-FH) (degrees)	13.7	25.2	4.5	–2.6**
SN-MP (degrees)	20.9	32.9	5.2	–2.3**
MP-OP (degrees)	12.8	15.8	5.0	–0.6
B-N perp (mm)	–1.5	–6.0	8.0	0.6
Pg-N perp (mm)	2.1	–5.0	3.0	2.4**
y-axis (SGnSN) (degrees)	63.9	67.0	5.5	–0.6
Maxilla to mandible				
ANB (degrees)	4.7	1.6	1.5	2.1**
PP-MP (degrees)	10.0	25.0	6.0	–2.5**
Wits appraisal (mm)	6.8	–1.0	1.0	7.8*******
Maxillary length (ANS-PNS) (mm)	46.7	51.6	4.3	–1.1*
Mandibular length (CoGn) (mm)	105.6	114.3	4.0	–2.2**

(cont)

Cephalometric evaluation

The lateral cephalogram confirmed the Class II skeletal relationship with hypodivergent mandible (Fig 14-4i). The mandible was short in length and slightly retrusive to the cranial base. According to the CVM method, the patient appeared to be at CVM stage 4, indicating that the peak in mandibular growth had already occurred. Table 14-7 shows the pretreatment cephalometric values.

Table 14-7 (cont) Case 4 pretreatment cephalometric values

Group/measurement	Value	Norm	SD	Dev norm
Cranial base				
BaSN (degrees)	129.8	130.0	5.0	0.0
Upper incisors to maxilla				
U1-SN (degrees)	116.0	102.4	5.5	2.5**
U1-NA (degrees)	32.7	22.8	5.7	1.7*
U1-NA (mm)	4.0	4.3	2.7	–0.1
U1-PP (degrees)	125.3	110.0	5.0	3.1***
Lower incisors to mandible				
L1-MP (degrees)	87.5	95.0	7.0	–1.1*
L1-NB (degrees)	10.1	25.3	6.0	–2.5**
L1-NB (mm)	–0.2	4.0	1.8	–2.3**
L1 protrusion (L1-APg) (mm)	–4.3	1.0	2.3	–2.3**
Incisors to each other				
Interincisal angle (U1-L1) (degrees)	132.4	130.0	6.0	0.4
Overjet (Mx1-Md1) (mm)	9.8	3.2	0.4	16.5*******
Overbite (Mx1-Md1) (mm)	5.3	3.2	0.7	3.0***
Soft tissue				
Upper lip to E-plane (mm)	–2.5	–3.0	2.0	0.2
Lower lip to E-plane (mm)	–3.7	–2.5	2.5	–0.5
ILG (HP) (mm)	0.9	2.0	2.0	–0.6
Nasolabial angle (CoLSnUL) (degrees)	115.2	102.0	8.0	1.6*
H-angle (Pg′UL-Pg′N′) (degrees)	12.7	10.0	4.0	0.7
Face height (N′Me′) (mm)	106.5	125.0	4.7	–3.9***
UFH (G′Sn′) (mm)	57.7	63.0	3.0	–1.8*
LFH (Sn′Me′) (mm)	62.4	63.0	3.0	–0.2
Facial proportions (hard tissue)				
UFH (N-ANS) (mm)	46.4	50.0	2.5	–1.4*
LFH (ANS-Me) (mm)	54.9	65.0	4.5	–2.2**
UFH (N-ANS/[N-ANS+ANS-Me]) (%)	45.8	45.0	5.0	0.2
LFH (ANS-Me/[N-ANS+ANS-Me]) (%)	54.2	57.0	5.0	–0.6
Posterior face height (ArGo) (mm)	50.2	42.5	4.5	1.7*
PFH:AFH (CoGo:NMe) (%)	62.7	60.0	1.0	2.7**
Profile				
Convexity (NA-APg) (degrees)	5.4	8.1	3.0	–0.9
Facial angle (FH-NPg) (degrees)	91.3	87.3	3.0	1.3*

Dev norm, deviation from the norm; PP, palatal plane; OP, occlusal plane; MP, mandibular plane; U1, maxillary incisor; L1, mandibular incisor; ILG (HP), interlabial gap (horizontal plane); CoL, condylion lateral; UL, upper lip; UFH, upper face height; LFH, lower face height; PFH:AFH, posterior face height to anterior face height.
*Each asterisk represents a standard deviation (SD).

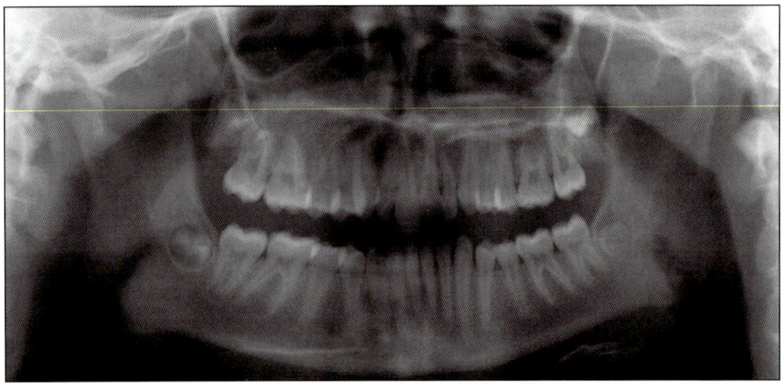

Fig 14-4j Pretreatment panoramic radiograph.

Panoramic evaluation

The panoramic radiograph showed the presence of all permanent teeth with the third molars in their various stages of development (Fig 14-4j).

Treatment plan

The treatment plan objectives were to correct the anteroposterior discrepancy of the jaws using a Forsus appliance to finish in Class I molar and canine occlusion. The maxillary and mandibular teeth were bonded with 0.018-inch AO brackets. AO bands with a headgear tube were used. Maxillary and mandibular arches were leveled and aligned using 0.016-inch Nitinol wires. Rotations were corrected with progressive archwires. The remaining spaces were consolidated with a 0.016 × 0.022–inch SS archwire. Then a Forsus appliance was delivered on 0.017 × 0.025–inch SS archwires for the maxillary and mandibular dental arches. Vertical seating elastics were used to improve the interdigitation.

Final evaluation

The results showed a slightly convex soft tissue profile (Fig 14-4k) based on the angle of convexity (NA-APg) with a relatively well-balanced face (Figs 14-4l and 14-4m). The midlines are coincident, the molars and canines are in Class I relationships, and the arches are well coordinated (Figs 14-4n to 14-4r). Figure 14-4s shows the posttreatment panoramic radiograph.

Cephalometric analysis

SNA decreased by 2 degrees, most likely due to changes in the inclinations of the maxillary incisors, which may affect the position of A-point in the anteroposterior plane. On the other hand, SNB increased by 1 degree (Table 14-8). The skeletal pattern became Class I as ANB changed from 4.7 to 1.4 degrees (Fig 14-4t). In the vertical plane, FMA changed from 13.7 to 18.6 degrees, likely due to the downward and forward movement of the mandible. The inclination of the maxillary incisors decreased by 7.6 degrees, while the inclination of the mandibular incisors increased by 6.6 degrees, reaching the average of the normal range (Fig 14-4u).

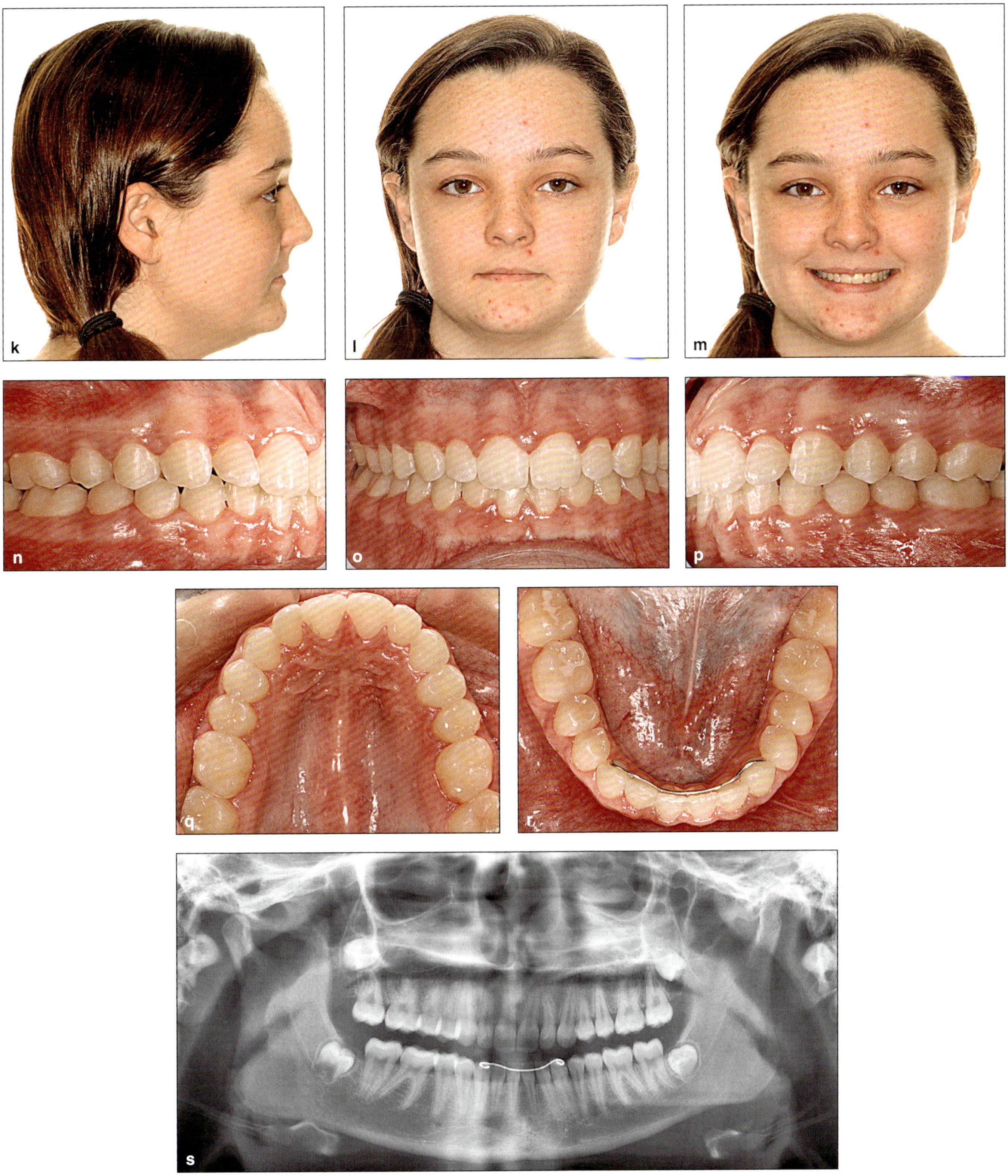

Fig 14-4 *(cont)* *(k to r)* Posttreatment extraoral and intraoral photographs. *(s)* Posttreatment panoramic radiograph.

Table 14-8 Case 4 posttreatment cephalometric values

Group/measurement	Value	Norm	SD	Dev norm
Maxilla to cranial base				
SNA (degrees)	81.0	82.0	3.5	–0.6
SN-PP (degrees)	8.1	8.0	3.0	0.0
SN-OP (degrees)	14.8	14.4	2.5	0.2
A-N perp (mm)	–2.3	0.0	2.0	–1.2*
Mandible to cranial base				
SNB (degrees)	79.6	80.9	3.4	–0.7
SNPg (degrees)	82.0	80.0	3.5	0.6
FMA (MP-FH) (degrees)	18.6	23.9	4.5	–1.2*
SN-MP (degrees)	24.5	32.9	5.2	–1.6*
MP-OP (degrees)	6.5	17.3	5.0	–2.2**
B-N perp (mm)	–5.6	–6.0	8.0	0.0
Pg-N perp (mm)	–0.5	–1.0	3.0	0.2
y-axis (SGnSN) (degrees)	63.3	67.0	5.5	–0.7
Maxilla to mandible				
ANB (degrees)	1.4	1.6	1.5	–0.1
PP-MP (degrees)	13.2	25.0	6.0	–2.0**
Wits appraisal (mm)	–0.3	–1.0	1.0	0.7
Maxillary length (ANS-PNS) (mm)	45.5	51.6	4.3	–1.4*
Mandibular length (CoGn) (mm)	109.9	121.8	4.0	–3.0***
Cranial base				
BaSN (degrees)	131.4	130.0	5.0	0.3
Upper incisors to maxilla				
U1-SN (degrees)	108.4	102.8	5.5	1.0*
U1-NA (degrees)	28.4	22.8	5.7	1.0*
U1-NA (mm)	3.8	4.3	2.7	–0.2
U1-PP (degrees)	116.5	110.0	5.0	1.3*
Lower incisors to mandible				
L1-MP (degrees)	94.1	95.0	7.0	–0.1
L1-NB (degrees)	19.0	25.3	6.0	–1.1
L1-NB (mm)	1.8	4.0	1.8	–1.2*
L1 protrusion (L1-APg) (mm)	–1.3	1.0	2.3	–1.0*
Incisors to each other				
Interincisal angle (U1-L1) (degrees)	131.2	130.0	6.0	0.2
Overjet (Mx1-Md1) (mm)	3.8	3.2	0.4	1.4*
Overbite (Mx1-Md1) (mm)	1.7	3.2	0.7	–2.2**

(cont)

Table 14-8 (cont) **Case 4 posttreatment cephalometric values**

Group/measurement	Value	Norm	SD	Dev norm
Soft tissue				
Upper lip to E-plane (mm)	–7.4	–3.0	2.0	–2.2**
Lower lip to E-plane (mm)	–5.8	–2.5	2.5	–1.3*
ILG (HP) (mm)	0.6	2.0	2.0	–0.7
Nasolabial angle (CoLSnUL) (degrees)	115.8	102.0	8.0	1.7*
H-angle (Pg′UL-Pg′N′) (degrees)	5.7	10.0	4.0	–1.1*
Face height (N′Me′) (mm)	108.1	125.0	4.7	–3.6***
UFH (G′Sn′) (mm)	61.0	63.0	3.0	–0.7
LFH (Sn′Me′) (mm)	61.9	63.0	3.0	–0.4
Facial proportions (hard tissue)				
UFH (N-ANS) (mm)	47.5	50.0	2.5	–1.0*
LFH (ANS-Me) (mm)	57.0	65.0	4.5	–1.8*
UFH (N-ANS/[N-ANS+ANS-Me]) (%)	45.4	45.0	5.0	0.1
LFH (ANS-Me/[N-ANS+ANS-Me]) (%)	54.6	57.0	5.0	–0.5
Posterior face height (ArGo) (mm)	50.2	48.1	4.5	0.5
PFH:AFH (CoGo:NMe) (%)	59.7	60.0	1.0	–0.3
Profile				
Convexity (NA-APg) (degrees)	3.0	5.1	3.0	–3.4***
Facial angle (FH-NPg) (degrees)	89.7	88.6	3.0	0.4

Dev norm, deviation from the norm; PP, palatal plane; OP, occlusal plane; MP, mandibular plane; U1, maxillary incisor; L1, mandibular incisor; ILG (HP), interlabial gap (horizontal plane); CoL, condylion lateral; UL, upper lip; UFH, upper face height; LFH, lower face height; PFH:AFH, posterior face height to anterior face height.
*Each asterisk represents a standard deviation (SD).

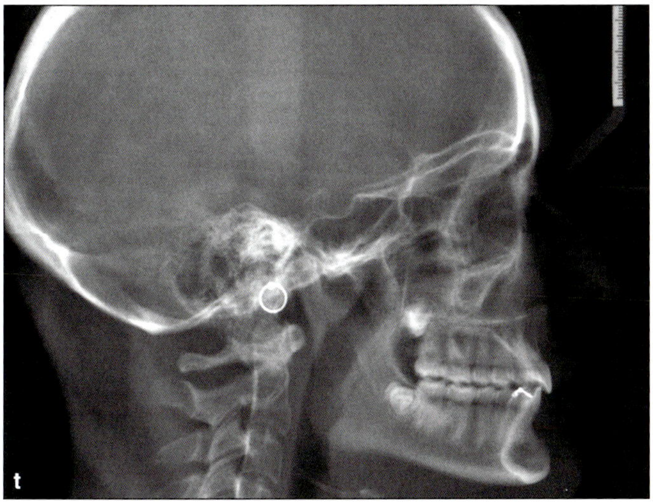
t

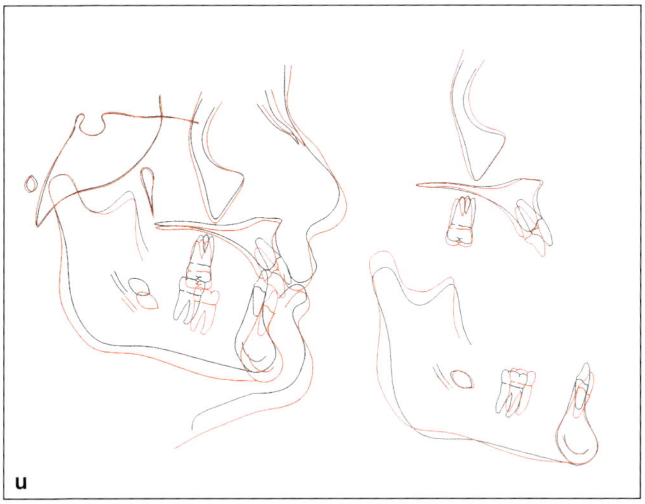
u

Fig 14-4 *(cont)* *(t)* Posttreatment cephalogram. *(u)* Superimposition of pretreatment and posttreatment cephalometric tracings.

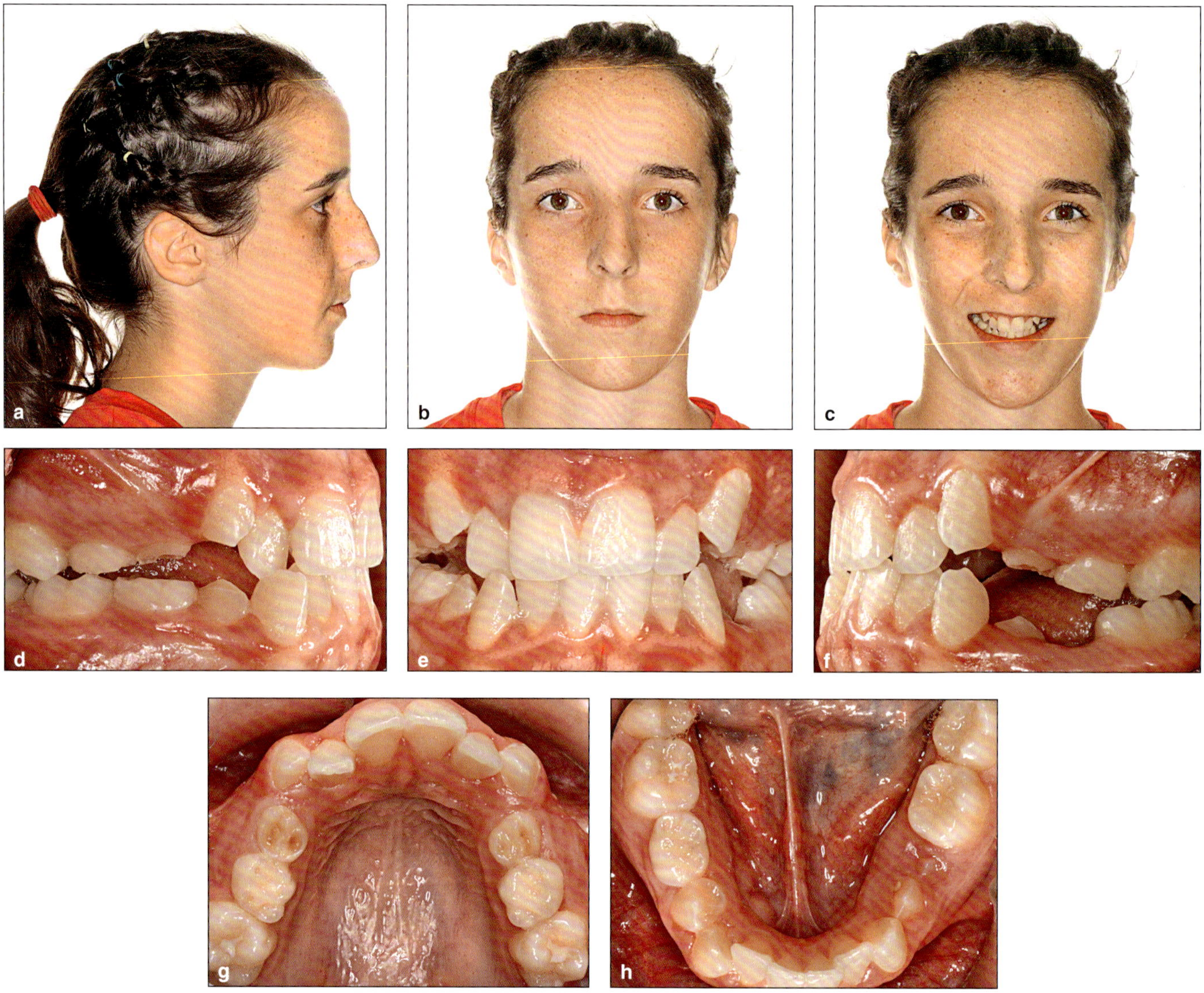

Fig 14-5 *(a to h)* Pretreatment extraoral and intraoral photographs.

Case 5

Initial medical history and chief complaint

A 12-year-old Caucasian girl presented for comprehensive orthodontic treatment with unremarkable medical and dental histories. Her chief complaint was that her teeth were not straight. The etiology of her malocclusion was most likely due to genetic factors.

Photographic evaluation

The patient had a straight facial profile with normal chin development (Fig 14-5a). The lips were competent with a slightly retrusive upper lip, slightly deviated nose, increased lower anterior face height, and a nonconsonant smile arc (Figs 14-5b and 14-5c).

The patient presented in the mixed dentition with a Class III malocclusion. The mandibular incisors were retroclined, and she had a shallow overbite (1.2 mm) and a 1.1-mm overjet (Figs 14-5d to 14-5h). The maxillary right lateral incisor was in anterior crossbite, and the primary first and second molars were in posterior crossbite. She had a short mandible with an excessive curve of spee and a mild curve of Wilson. The maxillary midline was deviated 3 mm to the right, and the mandibular midline was deviated 1 mm to the left in relation to the facial midline.

Cephalometric evaluation

The skeletal base was in Class I relationship with a deficient maxilla and mandible anteroposteriorly. Vertically the patient had a hyperdivergent skeletal pattern (Fig 14-5i and Table 14-9).

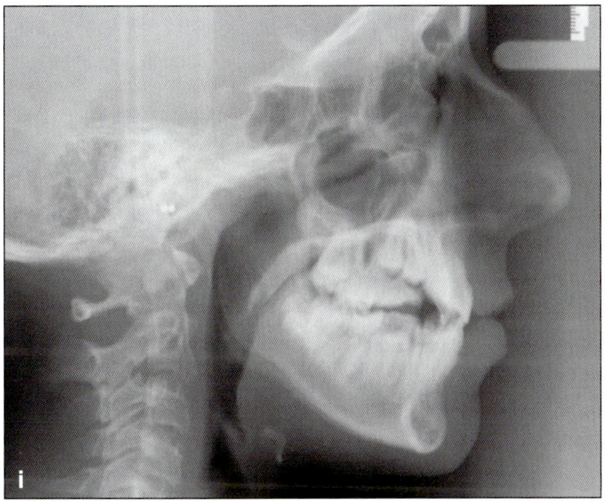

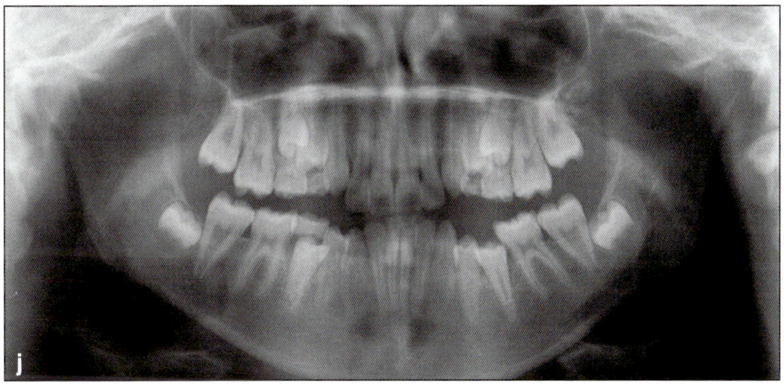

Fig 14-5 *(cont)* *(i)* Pretreatment cephalogram. *(j)* Pretreatment panoramic radiograph.

Table 14-9 **Case 5 pretreatment cephalometric values**

Group/measurement	Value	Norm	SD	Dev norm
Maxilla to cranial base				
SNA (degrees)	72.1	82.0	3.5	–2.8**
SN-PP (degrees)	10.9	8.0	3.0	1.0*
SN-OP (degrees)	22.3	14.4	2.5	3.2***
A-N perp (mm)	–7.6	0.0	2.0	–3.8***
Mandible to cranial base				
SNB (degrees)	69.8	80.9	3.4	–3.3***
SNPg (degrees)	70.7	80.0	3.5	–2.6**
FMA (MP-FH) (degrees)	35.6	24.6	4.5	2.5**
SN-MP (degrees)	41.6	32.9	5.2	1.7*
MP-OP (degrees)	22.9	16.6	5.0	1.3*
B-N perp (mm)	–17.1	–6.0	8.0	–1.4*
Pg-N perp (mm)	–16.7	–5.0	3.0	–3.9***
y-axis (SGnSN) (degrees)	75.7	67.0	5.5	1.6*
Maxilla to mandible				
ANB (degrees)	2.3	1.6	1.5	0.5
PP-MP (degrees)	34.3	25.0	6.0	1.5*
Wits appraisal (mm)	0.8	–1.0	1.0	1.8*
Maxillary length (ANS-PNS) (mm)	49.8	51.6	4.3	–0.4
Mandibular length (CoGn) (mm)	108.5	118.1	4.0	–2.4**

(cont)

Panoramic evaluation

The panoramic radiograph confirmed the late mixed dentition stage and showed the presence of all permanent teeth except the maxillary right third molar (Fig 14-5j).

Treatment plan

The treatment plan involved comprehensive orthodontics. The patient was given and accepted a nonextraction treatment plan with fixed orthodontic appliances to correct the malocclusion and finish in Class I molar and canine occlusion. An

Table 14-9 (cont) Case 5 pretreatment cephalometric values

Group/measurement	Value	Norm	SD	Dev norm
Cranial base				
BaSN (degrees)	136.0	130.0	5.0	1.2*
Upper incisors to maxilla				
U1-SN (degrees)	90.1	102.6	5.5	–2.3**
U1-NA (degrees)	18.0	22.8	5.7	–0.8
U1-NA (mm)	2.1	4.3	2.7	–0.8
U1-PP (degrees)	101.0	110.0	5.0	–1.8*
Lower incisors to mandible				
L1-MP (degrees)	83.8	95.0	7.0	–1.6*
L1-NB (degrees)	19.8	25.3	6.0	–0.9
L1-NB (mm)	4.0	4.0	1.8	0.0
L1 protrusion (L1-APg) (mm)	1.9	1.0	2.3	0.4
Incisors to each other				
Interincisal angle (U1-L1) (degrees)	139.9	130.0	6.0	1.7*
Overjet (Mx1-Md1) (mm)	1.1	3.2	0.4	–4.8****
Overbite (Mx1-Md1) (mm)	1.2	3.2	0.7	–4.1****
Soft tissue				
Upper lip to E-plane (mm)	–4.9	–3.0	2.0	–0.9
Lower lip to E-plane (mm)	–0.8	–2.5	2.5	0.7
ILG (HP) (mm)	0.5	2.0	2.0	–0.8
Nasolabial angle (CoLSnUL) (degrees)	114.7	102.0	8.0	1.6*
H-angle (Pg′UL-Pg′N′) (degrees)	13.0	10.0	4.0	0.8
Face height (N′Me′) (mm)	123.2	125.0	4.7	–0.4
UFH (G′Sn′) (mm)	64.3	63.0	3.0	0.4
LFH (Sn′Me′) (mm)	69.1	63.0	3.0	2.0**
Facial proportions (hard tissue)				
UFH (N-ANS) (mm)	53.1	50.0	2.5	1.2*
LFH (ANS-Me) (mm)	66.8	65.0	4.5	0.4
UFH (N-ANS/[N-ANS+ANS-Me]) (%)	44.3	45.0	5.0	–0.1
LFH (ANS-Me/[N-ANS+ANS-Me]) (%)	55.7	57.0	5.0	–0.3
Posterior face height (ArGo) (mm)	40.0	45.4	4.5	–1.2*
PFH:AFH (CoGo:NMe) (%)	43.7	60.0	1.0	–16.3 *******
Profile				
Convexity (NA-APg) (degrees)	2.9	6.6	3.0	–1.2 *
Facial angle (FH-NPg) (degrees)	81.3	87.9	3.0	–2.2 **

Dev norm, deviation from the norm; PP, palatal plane; OP, occlusal plane; MP, mandibular plane; U1, maxillary incisor; L1, mandibular incisor; ILG (HP), interlabial gap (horizontal plane); CoL, condylion lateral; UL, upper lip; UFH, upper face height; LFH, lower face height; PFH:AFH, posterior face height to anterior face height.
*Each asterisk represents a standard deviation (SD).

appliance with 0.022-inch 3M brackets with MBT prescription was used with bands on the maxillary and mandibular molars and brackets bonded to all maxillary and mandibular teeth. The teeth were leveled and aligned and then detailed with finishing archwires.

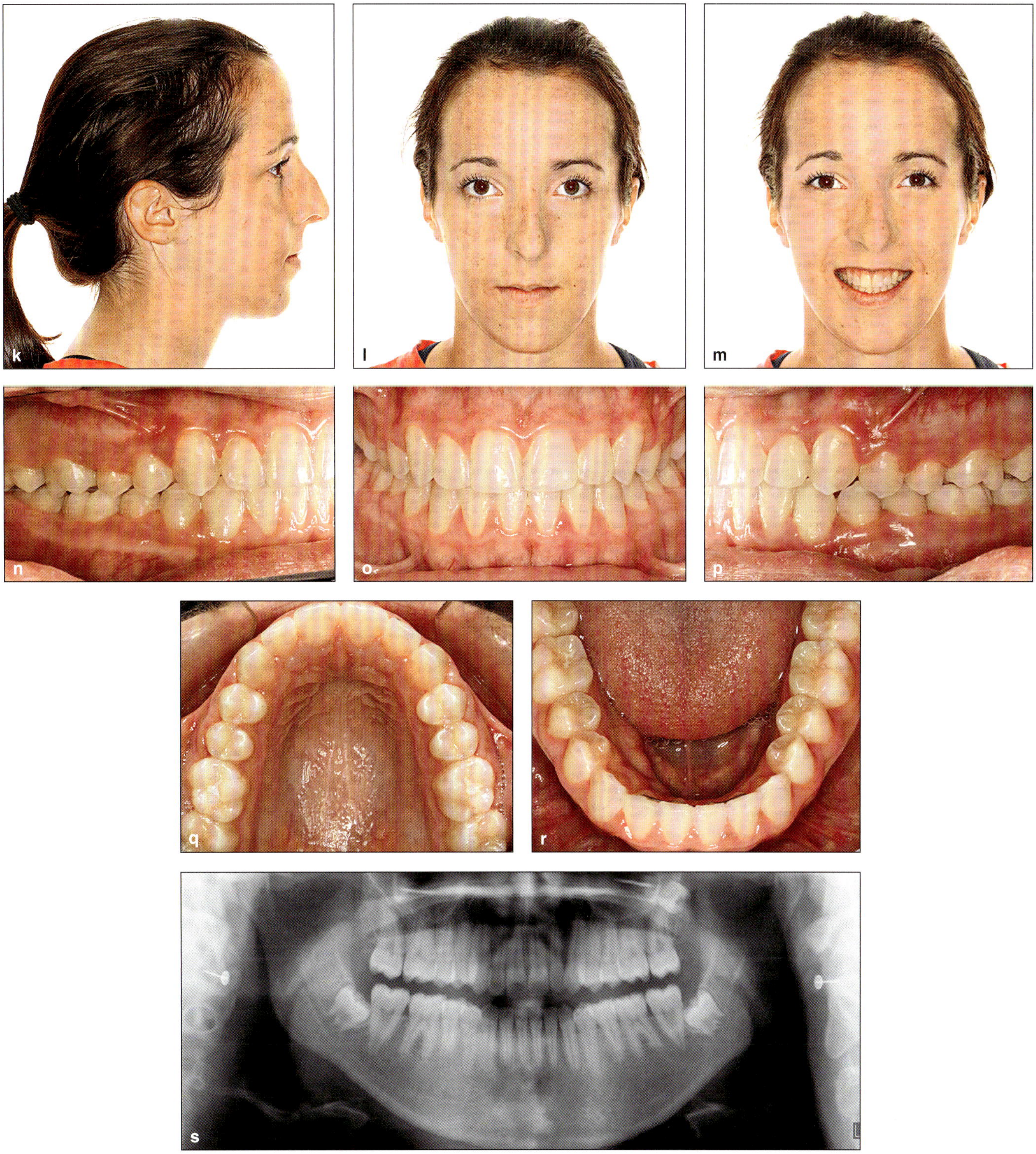

Fig 14-5 *(cont) (k to r)* Posttreatment extraoral and intraoral photographs. *(s)* Posttreatment panoramic radiograph.

Final evaluation

No significant changes were observed in the esthetics of the facial profile (Fig 14-5k). The maxillary midline is coincident with the facial midline, and there is an improvement in the alignment of the teeth with minimal buccal corridors and a consonant smile arc (Figs 14-5l to 14-5r). Figure 14-5s shows the posttreatment panoramic radiograph.

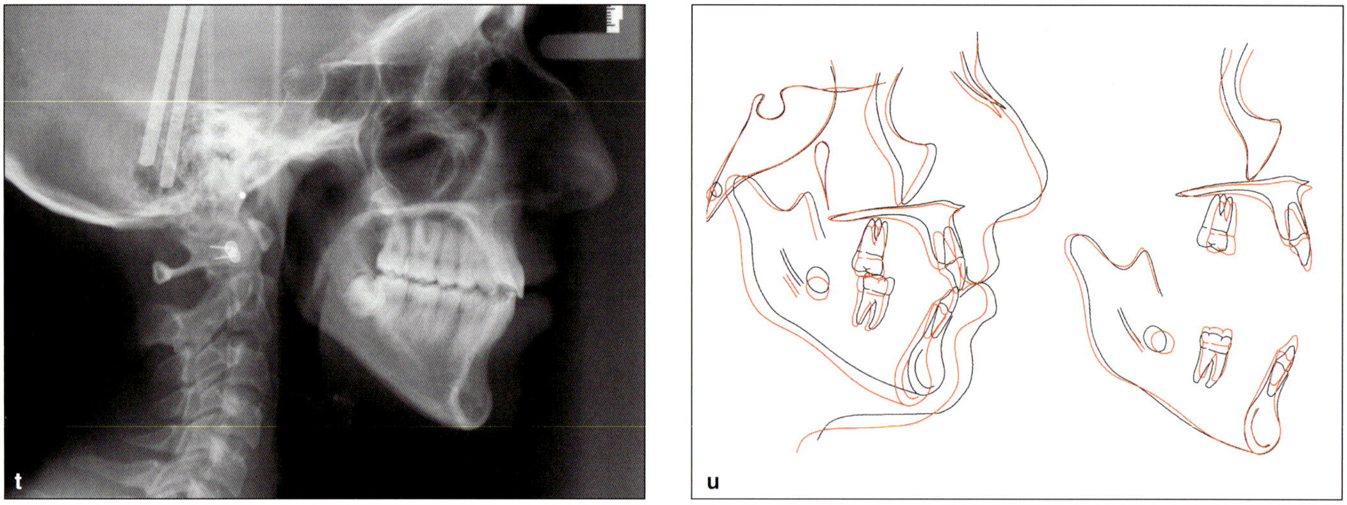

Fig 14-5 *(cont)* *(t)* Posttreatment cephalogram. *(u)* Superimposition of pretreatment and posttreatment cephalometric tracings.

Table 14-10 **Case 5 posttreatment cephalometric values**

Group/measurement	Value	Norm	SD	Dev norm
Maxilla to cranial base				
SNA (degrees)	72.1	82.0	3.5	–2.8**
SN-PP (degrees)	10.6	8.0	3.0	0.9
SN-OP (degrees)	23.4	14.4	2.5	3.6***
A-N perp (mm)	–6.8	0.0	2.0	–3.4***
Mandible to cranial base				
SNB (degrees)	68.9	80.9	3.4	–3.5***
SNPg (degrees)	70.1	80.0	3.5	–2.8**
FMA (MP-FH) (degrees)	39.4	23.9	4.5	3.5***
SN-MP (degrees)	46.3	32.9	5.2	2.6**
MP-OP (degrees)	26.1	17.4	5.0	1.7*
B-N perp (mm)	–17.0	–6.0	8.0	–1.4*
Pg-N perp (mm)	–16.3	–1.0	3.0	–5.1*****
y-axis (SGnSN) (degrees)	77.4	67.0	5.5	1.9*

(cont)

Cephalometric analysis

SNA remained the same, and SNB decreased by about 1 degree. Consequently, ANB changed from 2.3 to 3.2 degrees to correct the skeletal discrepancy between the jaws (Fig 14-5t and Table 14-10). The hyperdivergency of the mandible increased significantly as SN-MP changed from 41.6 to 46.3 degrees. Proclination of the maxillary incisors increased from 90.1 to 94.4 degrees, while the inclination of the mandibular incisors remained the same (Fig 14-5u).

Table 14-10 (cont) **Case 5 posttreatment cephalometric values**

Group/measurement	Value	Norm	SD	Dev norm
Maxilla to mandible				
ANB (degrees)	3.2	1.6	1.5	1.0*
PP-MP (degrees)	38.9	25.0	6.0	2.3**
Wits appraisal (mm)	1.6	–1.0	1.0	2.6**
Maxillary length (ANS-PNS) (mm)	43.2	51.6	4.3	–2.0**
Mandibular length (CoGn) (mm)	108.3	122.3	4.0	–3.5***
Cranial base				
BaSN (degrees)	134.3	130.0	5.0	0.9
Upper incisors to maxilla				
U1-SN (degrees)	94.4	102.8	5.5	–1.5*
U1-NA (degrees)	22.3	22.8	5.7	–0.1
U1-NA (mm)	3.6	4.3	2.7	–0.3
U1-PP (degrees)	104.9	110.0	5.0	–1.0*
Lower incisors to mandible				
L1-MP (degrees)	83.8	95.0	7.0	–1.6*
L1-NB (degrees)	23.6	25.3	6.0	–0.3
L1-NB (mm)	5.5	4.0	1.8	0.8
L1 protrusion (L1-APg) (mm)	2.6	1.0	2.3	0.7
Incisors to each other				
Interincisal angle (U1-L1) (degrees)	131.0	130.0	6.0	0.2
Overjet (Mx1-Md1) (mm)	2.4	3.2	0.4	–2.0**
Overbite (Mx1-Md1) (mm)	1.5	3.2	0.7	–2.4**
Soft tissue				
Upper lip to E-plane (mm)	–6.8	–3.0	2.0	–1.9*
Lower lip to E-plane (mm)	–1.5	–2.5	2.5	0.4
ILG (HP) (mm)	1.9	2.0	2.0	0.0
Nasolabial angle (CoLSnUL) (degrees)	112.2	102.0	8.0	1.3*
H-angle (Pg'UL-Pg'N') (degrees)	11.6	10.0	4.0	0.4
Face height (N'Me') (mm)	121.0	125.0	4.7	–0.8
UFH (G'Sn') (mm)	62.3	63.0	3.0	–0.2
LFH (Sn'Me') (mm)	77.8	63.0	3.0	4.9****
Facial proportions (hard tissue)				
UFH (N-ANS) (mm)	52.5	50.0	2.5	1.0*
LFH (ANS-Me) (mm)	69.7	65.0	4.5	1.0*
UFH (N-ANS/[N-ANS+ANS-Me]) (%)	43.0	45.0	5.0	–0.4
LFH (ANS-Me/[N-ANS+ANS-Me]) (%)	57.0	57.0	5.0	0.0
Posterior face height (ArGo) (mm)	39.8	48.5	4.5	–1.9*
PFH:AFH (CoGo:NMe) (%)	40.4	60.0	1.0	–19.6 *******
Profile				
Convexity (NA-APg) (degrees)	4.3	4.9	3.0	–0.2
Facial angle (FH-NPg) (degrees)	81.6	88.6	3.0	–2.3 **

Dev norm, deviation from the norm; PP, palatal plane; OP, occlusal plane; MP, mandibular plane; U1, maxillary incisor; L1, mandibular incisor; ILG (HP), interlabial gap (horizontal plane); CoL, condylion lateral; UL, upper lip; UFH, upper face height; LFH, lower face height; PFH:AFH, posterior face height to anterior face height.
*Each asterisk represents a standard deviation (SD).

Index

Page references followed by "f" denote figures, and those followed by "t" denote tables.

N

O

P

Q

R

S

T